Penguin Books
The Book of Grass

D1355199

Edited by George Andrews
and SimonVinkenoog

The Book of Grass

An Anthology of Indian Hemp

Penguin Books

Penguin Books Ltd, Harmondsworth,
Middlesex, England
Penguin Books Australia Ltd, Ringwood,
Victoria, Australia

First published by Peter Owen 1967
Published in Penguin Books (with revisions) 1972

Made and Printed in Great Britain by
C. Nicholls & Company Ltd
Set in Linotype Times

Contents

Part Four

POTENTIALITIES FOR INCREASING
CONSCIOUSNESS

Introduction

This book presents a wide variety of personal accounts of experiences induced by Indian hemp. Writers of different cultural traditions and historical periods have left descriptions of this herb. The many points of view which find expression in these pages should help to bring the subject into its proper perspective.

Indian hemp has many names, which causes some confusion. The two most common ones are 'marihuana' (from the Spanish 'Maria Juana') and the Arabic 'hashish'. Marihuana is simply the dried flowers of the female plants. Hashish is the resin with which the flowers are coated, coming off in the form of a golden powder when the plants are shaken. It is then heated and pressed into blocks, which darkens the colour. In both modern American slang and classical Arabic, the term for hemp is 'grass'. This common denominator between different periods of history was a decisive factor in my choice of the title for this anthology.

Although the use of marihuana is widespread, the subject is enshrouded by ignorance. I hope that this book will dispel at least some of the misconceptions about this plant. No practical solution to the problem is possible until the real facts are recognized. In presenting the facts concerning Indian hemp as objectively as I can, I hope to break the taboo which surrounds this subject in our civilization at the present time.

Marihuana has been used freely by a large proportion of the world's population since prehistoric times. It was not prohibited by international agreement until the 1930s. Part One of this book shows it to have been a significant feature of religious rites among the ancient Hindus, Scythians, Iranians, and American Indians. Homer and Solomon sang of it. *The Thousand*

and One Nights are saturated with the odour of hashish. The story of the Assassins shows what can happen when it is used in a destructive way. Among the most well-known users of it in a creative way are a group of nineteenth-century French writers: Baudelaire, Rimbaud, Nerval, and Gautier, for whom the drug revealed completely new dimensions of consciousness, which are reflected in their dazzling poetry. R. Blondel, who was Baudelaire's doctor, once said: 'Each one who takes hashish has the dream that he deserves.' During recent years, painters like Diego Rivera have found that marihuana stimulated their artistic activity, and writers such as Aldous Huxley and Henri Michaux have carried out important experiments in this field.

There is a wide range of variation in the effects of different types of hemp. One of the strangest things about marihuana is the difference in the 'high' depending on where the plant was grown. It has a chameleon-like quality of reproducing the characteristics of its environments. There is a definite relationship between the altitude at which the plant is grown and the kind of 'high' it gives. It grows best on mountain slopes under cedar trees, and the higher up the mountain it grows, the better it is. It may be linked to the legends of the special food of the 'Immortals' who lived on mountain tops in ancient Greece, India, and China.

In Morocco hemp from certain regions is especially valued because it gives the psychic lift without the physical paralysis, so a man can stay 'high' and still do his daily work. From other regions, a pipe in the morning and you stay in bed all day. This wide range of variation in effect makes accurate medical dosage difficult, but upon further investigation it might turn out to be a useful factor in the treatment of disease. Specimens of the different types of hemp now existing in the world should be collected and classified by vintage like wine or tea. Quality is all-important in the use of hemp, as the lower grades stultify rather than activate the brain. Possibilities of mutations in the species should be studied. The legends seem to agree that the plant available today is something different from what the ancients had, giving only a dim echo of that original Soma from the slopes of Mount Meru. The legends mention the plant changing colour after migrations from one region to another. The different types of hemp not only have a wide range of variation in effect, they are also frequently of different colours. Among the marihuana smokers of today, there are a few special names for the extra best: Acapulco gold, Panama or Rangoon red, Yucatan blue, Ketama green, Congo brown, Angola black.

For many centuries and in many different countries its medicinal qualities were readily acknowledged. Just one example, the Indian Pharmacopoeia of 1868, lists it as a remedy for tetanus, hydrophobia, delirium tremens, infantile convulsions, asthma, hay fever and protracted labour. A very complete investigation of great value was carried out by the British Army in India, some extracts from which are to be found in Part Three. The herb was dropped from the American Pharmacopoeia about thirty years ago because no dependable preparation of it was known. This is hardly surprising in the absence of any classification of the different sub-species according to date and place of harvest. The dried flowers are a dependable enough preparation for millions of people all over the world. British doctors cannot prescribe the herb itself, but they can prescribe tinctures and ointments containing an extract of it. The ointment is particularly useful in the treatment of certain types of ulcers.

Another point of interest is the similarity in effect between marihuana and LSD. There is a wide gap between normal four-dimensional consciousness and the multi-dimensional consciousness experienced with LSD. Most people find it extremely difficult to bring the two states into coherent relation with each other. Marihuana provides a point of transition between them, making it possible to open up multi-dimensional consciousness without losing contact with four-dimensional consciousness. This point of transition may well be of major importance in bridging the gap. However, legal restrictions have hindered research during the whole period of the development of modern psychiatry. Recently an American professor of psychology, Dr Timothy Leary, was sentenced to thirty years of prison plus a thirty thousand dollar fine for being in possession of a small personal supply of marihuana. His article on 'The Politics of Consciousness Expansion' appears in Part Four.

As Alan Watts points out in the same section, marihuana can 'bring about certain alterations of sense perception, of emotional level and tone, of identity feeling, of the interpretation of sense data, and of the sensations of time and space'. In many cultures other than our own, marihuana has been traditionally linked with phenomena of extrasensory perception. Tribal medicine men all over the world have used it since the immemorial past, yet the doctors of today have difficulty in carrying out research with the herb on human subjects because of legal restrictions. Tinctures and ointments contain only a fraction of the active principle of the plant, and to experience the complete effect one must use the plant itself.

In spite of the fact that it is illegal, throughout the Middle East hashish smoking and eating is widespread, though considered a lower-class habit. In India too, those who practise it are regarded as old-fashioned by the rest of the population. The reverse is true in the United States and recently in Great Britain, where smokers tend to consider themselves an exclusive and advanced 'in-group'. Penalties for possession of marihuana vary considerably, but are heaviest in the United States. In spite of these heavy penalties, the black market in marihuana continues to grow. Its use is increasingly prevalent among young people, especially students, both in the United States and Great Britain.

If society persistently treats a group of young people as criminals, it is difficult for them not to become criminals. If one thinks of marihuana smoking as a vice, it slants the experience in a negative direction, tending to make the activity anti-social. A vicious circle is started, driving society and the smoker to a more and more extreme antagonism. If one considers the herb as a stimulant like any other, beneficial if used with moderation under the proper circumstances, something to be kept in the cupboard to celebrate special occasions, the experience is channelled in a positive direction. However, this attitude is difficult for a smoker to maintain in a society where possesson of a small personal supply is treated as a crime.

Scientific evidence supports the view that the present drug laws in the United States are unwise, and, apparently, based on misconceptions. Judge Murtagh of New York stated publicly in 1959: 'Our drug laws are immoral in principle and ineffectual in action'. It is a well-known fact that a powerful lobby exists which has every interest in perpetuating the obscurity of the present situation. The drug laws now in effect in the United States and in certain other countries are a greater gold mine for gangsters than the Prohibition Act ever was. In view of this, would it not be preferable to allow smokers to obtain a small personal supply, by legal means, from their local pharmacies?

*

I would like to thank some of the people who made this book possible. Simon Vinkenoog worked just as hard as I did during the early stages of it. He selected many of the texts, translated material from Dutch and German, and did everything in his power to keep the project going. Elfreda Powell was a great help during the later stages. I am responsible for the French translations. It was Ira Cohen who originally gave me the idea for the book; Piero Heliczer suggested the title. I would also like to thank *Ciba Symposia* for their kind help in supplying some of the illustrations; and Pamela Badyk, Asa Benveniste, Daniel Bittlestone, Robert Browne, Yoran Cazac, John Hopkins, Michael Corner, Philippe d'Arschot, Dr O. M. de Vaal, John Esam, Chris Gaiger, Olivia de Haulleville, Professor Heim, Laura Huxley, Bill Jahrmarkt, Fred and Laura Klein, Anton Kothuys, Tuli Kupferberg of Birth Press, Dr R. D. Laing, Gretl Learned, Jean-Jacques Lebel, Gene Mahon,

Nazli Nour, Daniel Richter, Barbara Rubin, Jasper Newsome, Lex de Bruijn, D. H. Sniderman, and Shinkichi Tajiri, Judy Ahern, Christopher Case, Peter Roberts and Nigel Lesmoir Gordon.

GEORGE ANDREWS

Part One
Traces in the Course of History

Indian hemp has been in use for thousands of years. Records from the Ancient Egyptians and Assyrians mention it, and so do some of the earliest Chinese medical books. However, the first substantial literature on the subject comes from India where it appears as 'soma' in the Rig-Veda.

Soma

A. L. Basham

The Rig-Veda is the chief of the four Yedas of ancient India, which consist of hymns and prayers used in the worship of the gods. Research suggests that these hymns were being sung well before 800 B.C.

Like wild winds the draughts have raised me up.
Have I been drinking soma?

The draughts have borne me up, as swift steeds a chariot.
Have I been drinking soma?

Frenzy has come upon me, as a cow to her dear calf.
Have I been drinking soma?

As a carpenter bends the seat of a chariot, I bend this frenzy round
  my heart.
Have I been drinking soma?

Not even as a mote in my eye do the five tribes count with me.
Have I been drinking soma?

The heavens above do not equal one half of me.
Have I been drinking soma?

In my glory I have passed beyond the sky and the great earth.
Have I been drinking soma?

I will pick up the earth, and put it here or put it there.
Have I been drinking soma?

(Rig-Veda x, 119. 2-9)

Soma was a divinity of special character. Soma was originally a plant, not certainly identified, from which a potent drink
was produced, which was drunk only at sacrifices, and which
caused the most invigorating effects. The Zoroastrians of Persia
had a similar drink, which they called 'haoma', the same word
as soma in its Iranian form; the plant identified with 'haoma'
by the modern Parsis is a bitter herb, which has no specially
inebriating qualities, and which cannot have been the soma of
the Veda. The drink prepared from the plant can scarcely have
been alcoholic, for it was made with great ceremony in the
course of the sacrifice, when the herb was pressed between
stones, mixed with milk, strained, and drunk on the same day.
Sugar and honey, which produce fermentation, were not usually mixed with it, and the brief period between its brewing
and consumption cannot have been long enough for the generation of alcohol in any appreciable quantity. The effects of
soma, with vivid hallucinations, and the sense of expanding to
enormous proportions, are rather like those attributed to such
drugs as hashish. Soma may well have been hemp, which grows
wild in many parts of India, Central Asia and South Russia,
and from which modern Indians produce a narcotic drink
called 'bhang'.

Like many ancient peoples, the Indians connected the
growth of plants with the moon, with which soma, the king of
plants, was later identified. So important was the god Soma
considered by the ancient editors of the Rig-Veda that they
extracted all the hymns in his honour and placed them in a
separate book (mandala), the ninth of the ten which constitute the whole.

Most of the gods were good-natured. Guilt-offerings and
thank-offerings, of the kind offered by the ancient Hebrews,
are almost unheard of in the Veda.

Nevertheless the ceremony must have had its element of
awe and wonder. The worshippers, inebriated with soma, saw
wondrous visions of the gods; they experienced strange sensations of power; they could reach up and touch the heavens;
they became immortal; they were gods themselves. The priests,

who alone knew the rituals whereby the gods were brought to the sacrifice, were masters of a great mystery. With these ideas, which are explicitly stated in the hymns, went others less obvious. Often in the Rig-Veda we read of a mysterious entity called 'brahman'; in some contexts brahman is the magical power in the sacred utterance (mantra), but often it has a wider connotation, and implies a sort of supernatural electricity, known to students of primitive religion as 'mana'.

The following translation describes Indra's fight with the cloud-dragon Vrtra. The hymn evidently refers to a well-known legend, which has since been forgotten, but which was probably a variant of the creation myth of Mesopotamia, in which the god Marduk slays the demon of chaos, Tiamat, and creates the universe.

> Let me proclaim the valiant deeds of Indra,
> the first he did, the wielder of the thunder,
> when he slew the dragon and let loose the waters,
> and pierced the bellies of the mountains.

> He slew the dragon lying on the mountain,
> for Tvastr made him a heavenly thunderbolt.
> The waters suddenly, like bellowing cattle,
> descended and flowed on, down to the ocean.

> In his strength he chose the soma –
> from three cups he drank the essence.
> The Generous seized his thunderbolt,
> and smote the first-born of the dragons.

> When, Indra, you slew the first-born of dragons,
> and frustrated the arts of the sorcerers,
> creating sun and heaven and dawn,
> you found no enemy to withstand you.

The Vedic Hymns

Traditional

The following extracts, also from the Vedas, give an idea of the part that the soma plant played in the religion of the ancient Hindus.

> O Poet, O all-knowing Soma, you are the ocean.
> Yours is the space of the five regions of the sky!
> You have risen above the sky and the earth.
> You are the stars, the sun, O clear Soma!

(Rig-Veda ix, 86. 29)

1

The wave of honey has risen from the breast of the ocean,
together with the stalk of Soma she has attained the land of the
    immortals,
she has mastered the secret name of the ritual Ghee:
'tongue of the gods', navel of immortality.

2

We are going to proclaim the name of the ritual Ghee,
we are going to sustain it by our praise in this sacrifice.
As soon as it is spoken, may the priest take heed!
It comes from the Buffalo with four horns.

3

The Buffalo has four horns, three feet,
he has two heads and seven hands.
Held by three chains, the Bull roars powerfully:
the mighty god has entered the land of the mortals.

4

The gods discovered the ritual Ghee in the primordial Cow,
although it had been concealed by the demons in three forms.

Indra created one, the Sun another,
the last was extracted from the Poet's own flesh.

5
This flowing Ghee spreads from the ocean of spirits;
a hundred barriers prevent the enemy from seeing it.
I ardently contemplate this flowing Ghee,
which surrounds Soma's golden phallus.

6
Words flow like rivers,
clarifying through thought what is in the heart.
These waves of Ghee spread
like gazelles who flee before a hunter.

7
Like whirlpools in the current of a river,
they leap forth and catch the wind,
these young waves of Ghee, like nuts growing wild
which break their shells, swelling with the waves.

8
They sprinkle the Fire smiling
like beautiful women on their way to a feast.
The waves of Ghee caress the logs,
and the Fire, happy to play their game, courts them.

9
I ardently contemplate them, they are like girls
who are painting their faces before being married.
There where the Soma is pressed, where the sacrifice is made,
the flowing Ghee pours to be clarified.

10
Let glorious praise flow forth,
celebrate a tournament with abundant cattle,
bring us good fortune and wealth! Lead this our sacrifice to the
    gods!
The flowing Ghee is clarified like honey.

11

The entire universe is fixed on your essence,
on the internal ocean, on the heart, on the number of life-breaths.
May we master your wave made of honey
which was brought to the place where Soma is mixed with water
in the presence of the gods!

(Rig-Veda iv, 58)

1

May Indra conqueror of the demon drink
Soma from Saryanavat
if he wishes to put strength in his soul
to accomplish a heroic deed!
Flow, O liquor, for Indra all around!

2

Purify yourself, master of the dawns,
Soma from Mount Arjika, O benefactor!
You who are pressed with incantations,
with truth, with belief and enthusiasm!
Flow, O liquor, for Indra all around!

3

The daughter of the Sun brought along with her
the Buffalo who was raised by the God of Rain.
Celestial musicians greeted him,
they put into the Soma this fragrance.
Flow, O liquor, for Indra all around!

4

You speak like a holy man, you whose aura is holy,
you speak in truth, you whose act is true,
you speak according to the belief, O King Soma,
O Soma which the priest carefully prepares.
Flow, O liquor, for Indra all around!

5

High, with power that is real,
its flowing blends together,

together blend the fragrances of the fragrant,
purifying you by the formula, O wild god.
Flow, O liquor, for Indra all around!

6

There where the priest, O purified Soma,
speaking the language of poets,
is exalted by Soma, holding in his hand the stone,
creating ecstasy for himself through Soma.
Flow, O liquor, for Indra all around!

7

There where the light that cannot be extinguished is,
the world where the sun was placed,
in this immortal world, O clear Soma,
in this inexhaustible world place me!
Flow, O liquor, for Indra all around!

8

There where the King of Death lives,
at the frontier of the sky,
where the fountain of youth is,
in that place make me immortal!
Flow, O liquor, for Indra all around!

9

There where beings move at will
in the third firmament, the third sky of the sky,
there where the worlds made of light are,
in that place make me immortal!
Flow, O liquor, for Indra all around!

10

There where desires and inclinations are,
there where the sun is at its peak,
where the funeral ceremony is and the reward of the dead,
in that place make me immortal!
Flow, O liquor, for Indra all around!

11

There where happiness and joy are
where pleasure and delight live,
where the desires of desires are fulfilled,
in that place make me immortal!
Flow, O liquor, for Indra all around!

(Rig-Veda ix, 113)

It is thanks to Soma that the gods are vigorous,
thanks to Soma that the world is wide.
And even in the lap of the constellations
Soma has been placed.

People think they are drinking Soma
when they crush the juice from the plant.
But the Soma that the Brahmins know,
nobody consumes it.

Guarded by those whose task it is to watch,
protected by inhabitants of the sky, O Soma,
you keep listening to the stones.
No terrestrial being consumes you.

(Rig-Veda x, 85. 2,3,4)

Eight wheels, nine doors
has the impregnable castle of the gods.
In it resides the golden disc,
celestial and brilliant.

The golden castle, colour of Soma,
which shines from far away, all covered
with glory – the Brahmin enters there,
into this impregnable castle.

(*Atharva'Veda* x, 2, 31, 33)

Sanskrit Sources

Uday Chand Dutt and George King

Cannabis sativa has been used from a very remote period both in medicine and as an intoxicating agent. A mythological origin has been invented for it. It is said to have been produced in the shape of nectar while the gods were churning the ocean with the mountain called Mandara. It is the favourite drink of Indra the king of gods, and is called 'vijaya', because it gives success to its votaries. The gods through compassion on the human race sent it to this earth so that mankind by using it habitually may attain delight, lose all fear, and have their sexual desires excited. On the last day of the Durga pooja, after the idols are thrown into water, it is customary for the Hindus to see their friends and relatives and embrace them. After this ceremony is over it is incumbent on the owner of the house to offer to his visitors a cup of 'bhang' and sweet-meats for tiffin.

An intoxicating agent with such recommendations cannot but be popular and so we find it in general use amongst all classes especially in the north-west provinces and Beham ... Sir William O'Shaughnessy has so well described the preparations of Indian hemp that I cannot do better than quote his account of them.

Siddhi, subjee, and *bhang* (synonymous) are used with water as a drink which is thus prepared: About three tola's weight (540 troy grains) are well washed with cold water, then rubbed to powder, mixed with black pepper, cucumber and melon seeds, sugar, half-a-pint of milk and an equal quantity of water. This is considered sufficient to intoxicate an habituated person. Half the quantity is enough for a novice ... intoxication will ensue in half an hour. Almost invariably the inebriation is of the most cheerful kind, causing the person to sing and dance, to eat food with great relish, and to seek aphrodisiac enjoyments. In persons of a quarrelsome nature it occasions, as might be expected, an exasperation of their natural tendency. The intoxication lasts about three hours, when sleep supervenes. No nausea or sickness of the stomach succeeds, nor are the bowels at all affected; next day there is slight giddiness and vascularity of the eyes, but no other symptom worth recording.

The *Majoon* or hemp confection, is a compound of sugar, butter, flour, milk, and *siddhi* or *bhang*. The process has been repeatedly performed before us by Ameer, the proprietor of a celebrated place of resort for hemp devotees in Calcutta and who is considered the best artist in his profession. Four ounces of *siddhi* and an equal quantity of *ghee* are placed in an earthen vessel, a pint of water added, and the whole warmed over a charcoal fire. The mixture is constantly stirred until the water all boils away, which is known by the crackling noise of the melted butter on the sides of the vessel. The mixture is then removed from the fire, squeezed through cloth while hot, by which an oleaginous solution of the active principles and colouring matter of the hemp is obtained; and the leaves, fibres, etc., remaining on the cloth are thrown away. The green oily solution soon concretes into a buttery mass and is then well washed by the hand in soft water, so long as the water becomes coloured. The colouring matter and an extractive substance are thus removed and a very pale green mass, of the consistence of simple ointment, remains. The washings are thrown away. Ameer says that these are intoxicating, and produce constriction of the throat, great pain and very disagreeable and dangerous symptoms.

The operator then takes two pounds of sugar, and adding a little water, places it in a pipkin over the fire. When the sugar dissolves and froths, two ounces of milk are added; a thick scum rises and is removed; more milk and a little water are added from time to time, and the boiling continued about an hour, the solution being carefully stirred until it becomes an adhesive clear syrup, ready to solidify on a cold surface; four ounces of tyre (new milk dried before the sun) in fine powder are now stirred in, and lastly the prepared butter of hemp is introduced, brisk stirring being continued for a few minutes. A few drops of attar of roses are then quickly sprinkled in, and the mixture poured from the pipkin on a flat cold dish or slab. The mass concretes immediately into a thick cake, which is divided into small lozenge-shaped pieces ... The taste is sweet and the odour very agreeable. Ameer states that sometimes by special order of customers he introduces stramonium seeds, but never nux vomica; that all classes of persons including the lower Portuguese and especially their females consume the drug; that it is most fascinating in its effects, producing extatic [sic] happiness, a persuasion of high rank, a sensation of flying, voracious appetite and intense aphrodisiac desire.

The leaves of Cannabis sativa are purified by being boiled in milk before use. They are regarded as heating, digestive, astringent and narcotic. The intoxication produced by 'bhang' is said to be of a pleasant description and to promote talkativeness.

In sleeplessness, the powder of the dried leaves is given in suitable doses for inducing sleep and removing pain.

The Ancient Greeks

Pascal Brotteaux

It is estimated that roughly at the same time the Vedic Hymns were known to be in use in India, in 800 B.C., Homer's Odyssey was being composed.

A controversial question is the one of Homer's 'nepenthe'. Is this drug hashish? Virey, Guyon, and Hahn seem to think so. They rest their case on the testimony of Diodorus of Sicily, who stated that the women of Thebes chased away anxiety with a drug whose active principle was hemp. It is well known that 'nepenthe' is derived from 'ne' negative and 'penthos' anxiety. What is one to think of this interpretation?

Telemachus, the son of Ulysses, has just left Ithaca to go and search for his father. Peisistratos, the son of Nestor, takes him from Pylos to Sparta, where Menelaus receives them hospitably. Telemachus describes the siege of Troy to them and insists on the painful losses of the Achaeans:

Menelaus' words brought them all to the brink of tears. Helen of Argos, child of Zeus, broke down and wept. Telemachus and

Menelaus did the same. Nor could Nestor's son keep his eyes dry when he thought of his brother . . .

At this moment, slaves are preparing the banquet. Thus, before the meal:

Helen, the child of Zeus, had a happy thought. Into the bowl in which their wine was mixed, she slipped a drug that had the power of robbing grief and anger of their sting and banishing all painful memories. No one that swallowed this dissolved in wine could shed a single tear that day, even for the death of his mother and father, or if they put his brother or his own son to the sword and he were there to see it done. This powerful anodyne was one of many useful drugs which had been given to the daughter of Zeus by an Egyptian lady, Polydamna, the wife of Thon. For the fertile soil of Egypt is most rich in herbs, many of which are wholesome in solution, though many are poisonous. And in medical knowledge the Egyptian leaves the rest of the world behind. He is a true son of Paeëon the Healer.

When Helen had thrown the drug into the wine and seen that their cups were filled, she turned to the company once more . . .

It seems difficult to attribute this effect on the memory to hashish. As we will see further on, the intoxication produced by Indian hemp does not suppress the memory; however, it does produce a state of euphoria. In our opinion, the brew in question could have contained hemp, but probably associated in the proper proportions with some venomous herb of the 'solanum' family, such as henbane, datura, or belladonna, which do act upon the memory. What confirms us in this opinion that 'nepenthe' was a complex preparation is that in another passage of the *Odyssey* Homer substituted the term 'pharmakos' (drug) for the term 'nepenthe'. In any case, the use of hashish seems to have been widespread at the period when the author (or the authors) of the *Odyssey* were writing.

This may well have been true also of the potion that the Old Man of the Mountain gave his followers. Hemp was too widely known in the Middle East at that time to explain by itself the unprecedented success his mixture had, although it was obviously one of the important ingredients.

Humphrey Osmond, D.P.M. states in A Review of the Clinical Effects of Psychotomimetic Agents *that: 'The effect of datura on hashish has been known for many years in India, and it is said to have been used by professional robbers in that country to produce temporary madness in their victims.'*

Ancient Scythia and Iran

Mircea Eliade

The Getae were described by Herodotus as the most valiant and law-abiding of the Thracian tribes. What chiefly impressed the Greeks was their belief in the immortality of the soul. They were expert in the use of the bow and arrow while on horseback. Their name first appears in connection with the expedition of Darius Hystaspes against the Scythians (515 B.C.) They were conquered briefly by the Romans, but regained their independence.

Only one document appears to indicate the existence of a Getic shamanism: it is Strabo's account of the Mysian Kapnobatai, a name that has been translated, by analogy with Aristophanes' Aerobates, as 'those who walk in clouds', but which should be translated as 'those who walk in smoke'. Presumably the smoke is hemp smoke, a rudimentary means of ecstasy known to both the Thracians and the Scythians. The Kapnobatai would seem to be Getic dancers and sorcerers who used hemp smoke for their ecstatic trances.

Herodotus has left us a good description of the funerary customs of the Scythians. The funeral was followed by purifications. Hemp was thrown on heated stones and all inhaled the smoke; 'the Scythians howl in joy for the vapour-bath'.

Karl Meuli has well brought out the shamanic nature of the funerary purification; the cult of the dead, the use of hemp, the vapour bath, and the 'howls' compose a specific religious ensemble, the purpose of which could only be ecstasy. In this connection Meuli cites the Altaic seance described by Radlov, in which the shaman guided to the underworld the soul of a woman who had been dead forty days. The shaman-psychopomp is not found in Herodotus' description; he speaks only of purifications following a funeral. But among a number of Turko-Tatar peoples such purifications coincide with the shaman's escorting the deceased to his new home, in the nether regions ...

One fact, at least, is certain: shamanism and ecstatic intoxication produced by hemp smoke were known to the Scythians. As we shall see, the use of hemp for ecstatic purposes is also attested among the Iranians, and it is the Iranian word for hemp that is employed to designate mystical intoxication in central and north Asia ...

The Cinvat bridge plays an essential role in Iranian funerary mythology; crossing it largely determines the destiny of the soul; and the crossing is a difficult ordeal, equivalent, in structure, to initiatory ordeals ...

The Gathas make three references to this crossing of the Cinvat bridge. In the first two passages Zarathustra, according to H. S. Nyberg's interpretation, refers to himself as a psychopomp. Those who have been united to him in ecstasy will cross the bridge with ease; the impious, his enemies, will be 'for all time ... dwellers in ... the House of the Lie'. The bridge, then, is not only the way for the dead; in addition – and we have frequently encountered it as such – it is the road of ecstatics. It is likewise in ecstasy that Artay Viraf crosses the Cinvat bridge in the course of his mystical journey. According to Nyberg's interpretation, Zarathustra would seem to have been an ecstatic very close to a 'shaman' in his religious experiences. The Swedish scholar considers that the Gathic term *Maga* is proof that Zarathustra and his disciples induced an ecstatic experience by ritual songs intoned in chorus in a closed, consecrated space. In this sacred space (*Maga*) communication between heaven and earth became possible – that is, in accordance with a universally disseminated dialectic, the sacred space became a 'centre'. Nyberg stresses the fact that the communion was ecstatic, and he compares the mystical experience of the 'singers' with Shamanism proper. This interpretation has been attacked by the majority of Iranists ... Thus, though the question of the possible 'shamanic' experience of Zarathustra himself must remain open, there is no doubt that the most elementary technique of ecstasy, intoxication by hemp, was known to the ancient Iranians ... The importance of the intoxication sought from hemp is further confirmed by the extremely wide dissemination of the Iranian term through central Asia. In a number of Ugrian languages the Iranian word for hemp, *Bangha,* has come to designate both the pre-eminently shamanic mushroom ... and intoxication ... These facts prove that the magico-religious value of intoxication for achieving ecstasy is of Iranian origin. Added to the other Iranian influences on central Asia ... *Bangha* illustrates the high degree of religious prestige attained by Iran ...

There is every reason to believe that the use of narcotics was encouraged by the quest for 'magical heat'. The smoke from certain herbs, the 'combustion' of certain plants had the virtue of increasing 'power' ... We must also take into consideration the symbolic value of narcotic intoxication. It was equivalent to a 'death', the intoxicated person left his body, acquired the condition of ghosts and spirits. Mystical ecstasy being assimilated to a temporary 'death' or leaving the body, all intoxications that produced the same result were given a place among the techniques of ecstasy.

Other authors have frequently stated that the Scythians threw hemp seeds on to burning coals and inhaled the smoke. As any smoker knows, the seeds are the least interesting part of the plant to smoke. The Scythians were obviously throwing dried hemp flowers on the burning coals: the seeds being far less

combustible than the dried flowers would be the last to burn,
and would tend to drop down among the ashes, leaving the
remains discovered by archaeologists and described by his-
torians of antiquity who observed the rite without participat-
ing in it.

Remnants from Prehistoric Times

W. Reininger

Remnants of hemp dating from prehistoric times were discovered in 1896 in northern Europe when the German archaeolo-
gist, Hermann Busse, opened a tomb containing a funerary
urn at Wilmersdorf (Brandenburg). The vessel in question contained sand in which were mixed remnants of plants. It dated
from the fifth century B.C. The botanist, Ludwig Wittmaack
(1839–1929), was able to find among this plant debris fragments
of the seed and pericarp of *Cannabis sativa L.* At the session of
the Berlin Society for Anthropology, Ethnology and Prehis-
tory on 15 May 1897, Busse presented a report on his discovery
and drew the conclusion that hemp had already been known
in northern Europe in prehistoric times. But Rudolf Virchow
(1821–1902) threw doubt on this interpretation that hemp had
already been known in northern Europe at such an early time.
He expressed the hypothesis that the hemp in question might
have been introduced into the vase much later. The close examination of the place where the urn was found, and of its
position, which Busse undertook at the time of discovery
showed that this conjecture could be discarded. Furthermore,
one must agree with C. Hartwich that hemp was already employed in northern Europe at the same time that it was by the
Chinese and the Scythians for food and pleasure. All that remains is to determine whether hemp was imported from the
Orient or whether it was already cultivated in the country.

The use of hemp in the manufacture of ropes and fabrics seems to have been introduced rather late. Not a single passage is to be found in the writings and mural inscriptions of the ancient Egyptians and Hebrews which makes any allusion to such usage. Herodotus, on the other hand, reports that the inhabitants of Thrace made clothes from hemp fibres. It is related that Hiero (third century B.C.), tyrant of Syracuse, had hemp brought from Rhodanus (the country of the Rhône?) in order to equip a ship. Pausanius (second century B.C.) mentions that hemp and other textile plants were cultivated in Elide; and Pliny the Elder (A.D. 23–79), relates that the sails and cordage of the Roman galleys were made of hemp.

In the second century, Galen wrote that it was customary to give hemp to guests at banquets to promote hilarity and happiness. At the beginning of the third century, the Chinese physician Hoa-Thoa used hemp as an anaesthetic in surgical operations.

In the thirteenth century garments of hemp were in common use throughout southern Europe.

Tracing One Word through Different Languages

Sara Benetowa

As evidence now shows, in antiquity hemp was used in widely differing cultures. In the following article, Sara Benetowa of the Institute of Anthropological Sciences in Warsaw attempts to find out through a comparative study of languages in what cultural environment hemp was first used as a narcotic.

After having compared the words meaning hemp in Indo-European, Finnish, Turkish and Tartar, and Semitic language groups, the conclusion was reached that, leaving aside all the obviously borrowed words, either Finnish, Turkish, Celtic, or

Roman, there remained four groups to investigate: 1. Sanskrit – cana; 2. Slav – konopla; 3. Semitic, for example in Assyro-Babylonia – kannab; 4. Greek: cannabis.

In all these languages the words meaning hemp have a common root: kan. This root with the double meaning of 'hemp' and 'cane' is common to almost all the languages of antiquity.

It is easy to show that 'canna' means both 'hemp' and 'cane'. But what is the meaning of the ending, 'bis'? The answer is not difficult to find if one notices an interesting detail encountered in several Semitic texts from Oriental antiquity. For example, let us look at the original text of the Old Testament and its Aramaic translation, the 'Targum Onculos'. The word 'kane' or 'kene' sometimes appears alone and sometimes linked to the adjective 'bosm' (in Hebrew) or 'busma' (in Aramaic) which means: odorous, smelling good, aromatic. As I demonstrate in detailed fashion in this study, the Biblical 'kane bosm' and the Aramaic 'kene busma' both mean 'hemp'. The linguistic evolution of the terms in question leads to the formation of the unique term 'kanabos' or 'kanbos'. This is encountered in the Mischna, the collection of traditional Hebrew law which contains many Aramaic elements. The astonishing resemblance between the Semitic 'kanbos' and the Scythian 'cannabis' lead me to suppose that the Scythian word was of Semitic origin. These etymological discussions run parallel to arguments drawn from history. The Iranian Scythians were probably related to the Medes, who were neighbours of the Semites and could easily have assimilated the word for hemp. The Semites could also have spread the word during their migrations through Asia Minor.

Taking into account the matriarchal element of Semitic culture, one is led to believe that Asia Minor was the original point of expansion for both the society based on the matriarchal circle and the mass use of hashish.

Let us look for factors which could have contributed to the start of mass use of hashish in the matriarchal circle. One important factor is that in preparing fibre from the plant and during the harvest the strong odour intoxicates the workers.

According to ancient customs still surviving in modern times, all work involving hemp is done in mass. Since antiquity the hemp harvest has been considered as a holiday, especially for the young people. In many countries the harvest is a sort of reunion to which guests come with or without masks and give all sorts of presents to the workers. Here we see an obvious link with the masculine secret societies in the matriarchal circle in which there is mass use of hashish. Another factor is the making of sacrifices to the ancestors, which is a common practice in the masculine secret societies.

Here is another obvious link between the character of this plant used in the cult of the dead and the masculine secret societies founded on this cult. Many particularities of the ancestor cult can be brought forth as evidence of this.

In Poland on the night before Christmas a ritual dish is served made of hemp seeds, called 'hemp soup', because according to popular superstition at that time the souls of the dead visit their friends and family to feast together. Another trace is the Polish habit of throwing a few hemp seeds in the fire 'as a sacrifice' during the harvest.

An obvious link between sacrifices in honour of the dead and the mass use of hashish is to be found in the Scythian funeral ceremony.

After the burial, the Scythians purified themselves in the following manner: they washed and anointed their heads and, after having planted posts in the ground and wrapped cloth around them, they threw hemp into receptacles filled with red-hot stones.

By comparing the old Slavic word 'kepati' and the Russian 'kupati' with the Scythian 'cannabis' Schrader developed and justified Meringer's supposition that there is a link between the Scythian baths and Russian vapour baths.

In the entire Orient even today to 'go to the bath' means not only to accomplish an act of purification and enjoy a pleasure, but also to fulfil the divine law. Vambrey calls 'bath' any club in which the members play chequers, drink coffee, and smoke hashish or tobacco.

The tobacco imported from America spread so rapidly through Europe because the way had been prepared for it by hemp.

NAMES OF THE PLANT

anascha – Russia	hampr – Finland
banga – Sanskrit	hanf – Germany
bangi – Congo	hanpr – Norway
bhang – India	haschisch – France
boo – USA	hashish – Africa, Asia
cabza – India	hemp – Great Britain
canab – Brittany	hennep – Holland
canaib – Ireland	herbe – France
canappa – Italy	hierba – Mexico
canna – Persia	hsien ma tze – China
cannapis – Rumania	Indian hay – USA
chanvre – France	intsangu – South Africa
charas – India	jive – USA
charge – USA	joint – USA
dagga – South Africa	joy – USA
dawamesk – Algeria	juana – Mexico
diamba – Brazil	juanita – Mexico
djamba – South Africa	kanapes – Lithuania
esrar – Turkey, Persia	kanas – Brittany
ganjah – India	kanbun – Chaldean
ganjika – Sanskrit	kanebosm – Hebrew
gauge – USA	kanebusma – Aramaic
goni – Sanskrit	kanep – Albania
goo – USA	kannab – Arabia
grass – USA	kanopia – Czechoslovakia
grifa – Spain, Mexico	kendir – Tartar
haenep – Old English	kendiros – Tartar
hamp – Denmark	khanchha – Cambodia
hampa – Sweden	kif – North Africa

kinder – Tartar
konop – Bulgaria
konopie – Poland
konoplja – Russia
liamba – Brazil
loco weed (confused with
    datura) – USA
maconha – Brazil
majoun – North Africa,
    Middle East
marihuana – Mexico, USA,
    Europe
marijuana – Mexico, USA,
    Europe
mary jane – USA
matakwane – Sotho (South
    Africa)
mbangi – Tanzania
momea – Tibet
mora – Mexico
morisqueta – Mexico
mota – Mexico
muggles – USA
muta – USA

nena – Mexico
nsangu – Zulu
pajuela – Mexico
pot – USA
qunubu – Assyrian
rap – India
reefer – USA
rosamaria – Mexico
rup – India
sana – Sanskrit
shanapu – Sanskrit
shora – Mexico
so-la-ra-dsa – Tibet
sonadora – Mexico
stick – USA
suruma – Ronga (Africa)
takrouri – Tunisia
tea – USA
tiamba – Brazil
tirsa – Mexico
umya – Xhosa (Africa)
weed – USA
wheat – Europe

Fragments from a Search

Melvin Clay

The recipe from the wilderness. The Suama plant. The area around Tell Abu Matar. The recipe found on urns and cups, workmanship of high quality, used at religious feasts, the roots boiled and drunk or the leaves smoked.

'To report none of their secrets even though tortured to death.'

A holy hermit named Zin, also called Aqrabbim, first author of recipe, clothed only with what grew on trees, ate only wild food, took cold water baths, renounced pleasure other than his brew, devoted to peaceful acts, members of his family lived for over a hundred years, artisan and craftsman, would not make weapons, could read ancient symbols, wrote a new language of his own symbols, studied herbs and roots, always fasted the longest, would not offer animal sacrifice, excluded from the Temple of Jerusalem, made brews for foretelling the future.

'Studies have shown that the roots of the Suama plant were boiled to make a drink producing states of bliss and overt joy.'

The recipe: Suama plant found in region of Kadesh-barnea, north-eastern Sinai, the site of the Ascent of Aqrabbim.

Dr W. F. Cartwell of Oriental Institute has no recollection of recipe, but speaks of leaves smoked and inhaled at a Palestine synagogue during the writing of the Hasteric Scrolls (Books of Joy). He adds that 'The Suama plant is known to us from the time of the Pentateuch. Some very early discoveries have been made concerning the Suama plant. We find it coming up again and again under different names. Smoking its leaves or using its roots as a herbal drink always produces states of flashing colours and euphoric bliss. Here is a specimen of a type of recipe credited to a hermit named Zin . . .'

28 December 1963 . . . heartiest congratulations . . . discovery . . . no possible doubt . . . the Light of Zin . . . hermit called Zin . . . smoking the Suama plant . . . brewing the roots . . . recipes do exist . . . third century B.C. . . . incredible . . . perhaps older . . . not the slightest doubt . . . preserved in caves . . . visions and cures . . . genuine . . . incredible . . .

The Song of Solomon

It is possible that the word translated as 'calamus' in the following passage really refers to hemp.

Thy lips, O my spouse, drop as the honeycomb: honey and milk are under thy tongue; and the smell of thy garments is like the smell of Lebanon.

A garden inclosed is my sister, my spouse; a spring shut up, a fountain sealed.

Thy plants are an orchard of pomegranates, with pleasant fruits; camphire, with spikenard,

Spikenard and saffron; calamus and cinnamon, with all trees of frankincense; myrrh and aloes, with all the chief spices:

A fountain of gardens, a well of living waters, and streams from Lebanon.

Awake, O north wind; and come, thou south; blow upon my garden, that the spices thereof may flow out. Let my beloved come into his garden, and eat his pleasant fruits.

(Ch. 4, vv. 11-16)

The Tale of Two Hashish-Eaters

Traditional

There was once, my lord and crown upon my head, a man in a certain city, who was a fisherman by trade and a hashish-eater by occupation. When he had earned his daily wage, he would spend a little of it on food and the rest on a sufficiency of that hilarious herb. He took his hashish three times a day: once in the morning on an empty stomach, once at noon, and once at sundown. Thus he was never lacking in extravagant gaiety. Yet he worked hard enough at his fishing, though sometimes in a very extraordinary fashion. On a certain evening, for instance, when he had taken a larger dose of his favourite drug than usual, he lit a tallow candle and sat in front of it, asking himself eager questions and answering with obliging wit. After some hours of this delight, he became aware of the cool silence of the night about him and the clear light of a full moon above his head, and exclaimed affably to himself: 'Dear friend, the silent streets and the cool of the moon invite us to a walk. Let us go forth, while all the world is in bed and none may mar our solitary exaltation.' Speaking in this way to himself, the fisherman left his house and began to walk towards the river; but, as he went, he saw the light of the full moon lying in the roadway and took it to be the water of the river. 'My dear old friend the fisherman,' he said, 'get your line and take the best of the fishing, while your rivals are indoors.' So he ran back and fetched his hook and line, and cast into the glittering patch of moonlight on the road.

Soon an enormous dog, tempted by the smell of the bait, swallowed the hook greedily and then, feeling the barb, made desperate efforts to get loose. The fisherman struggled for some time against this enormous fish, but at last he was pulled over and rolled into the moonlight. Even then he would not let go his line, but held on grimly, uttering frightened cries. 'Help, help, good Mussulmans!' he shouted. 'Help me to secure this mighty fish, for he is dragging me into the deeps! Help, help, good friends, for I am drowning!' The guards of that quarter ran up at the noise and began laughing at the fisherman's antics; but when he yelled: 'Allah curse you, O sons of bitches! Is it a time to laugh when I am drowning?' they grew angry and, after giving him a sound beating, dragged him into the presence of the kadi.

At this point Shahrazad saw the approach of morning and discreetly fell silent.

BUT WHEN
THE SEVEN-HUNDRED-AND-NINETY-EIGHTH NIGHT
HAD COME

SHE said:

Allah had willed that the kadi should also be addicted to the use of hashish; recognizing that the prisoner was under that jocund influence, he rated the guards soundly and dismissed them. Then he handed over the fisherman to his slaves that they might give him a bed for calm sleep.

After a pleasant night and a day given up to the consumption of excellent food, the fisherman was called to the kadi in the evening and received by him like a brother. His host supped with him; and then the two sat opposite the lighted candles and each swallowed enough hashish to destroy a hundred-year-old elephant. When the drug exalted their natural dispositions, they undressed completely and began to dance about, singing and committing a thousand extravagances.

Now it happened that the Sultan and his wazir were walking through the city, disguised as merchants, and heard a strange noise rising from the kadi's house. They entered through the unlatched door and found two naked men, who stopped dancing at their entrance and welcomed them without the least embarrassment. The Sultan sat down to watch his venerable kadi dance again; but when he saw that the other man had a dark and lively zabb, so long that the eye might not carry to the end of it, he whispered in his wazir's startled ear: 'As Allah lives, our kadi is not as well hung as his guest!' 'What are you whispering about?' cried the fisherman. 'I am the Sultan of this city and I order you to watch my dance respectfully, otherwise I will have your head cut off. I am the Sultan, this is my wazir; I hold the whole world like a fish in the palm of my right hand.' The Sultan and his wazir realized that they were in the presence of two hashish-eaters, and the wazir, to amuse his master, addressed the fisherman, saying: 'How long have you been Sultan, dear master, and can you tell me what has happened to your predecessor?' 'I deposed the fellow,' answered the fisherman. 'I said: "Go away!" and he went away.' 'Did he not protest?' asked the wazir. 'Not at all,' replied the fisherman. 'He was delighted to be released from the burden of kingship. He abdicated with such good grace that I keep him by me as a servant. He is an excellent dancer. When he pines for his throne, I tell him stories. Now I want to piss.' So saying, he lifted up his interminable tool and, walking over to the Sultan, seemed to be about to discharge upon him. 'I also want to piss,' exclaimed the kadi, and took up the same threatening position in front of the wazir. The two victims shouted with laughter and fled from that house, crying over their shoulders: 'God's curse on all hashish-eaters!'

Next morning, that the jest might be complete, the Sultan called the kadi and his guest before him. 'O discreet pillar of our law,' he said, 'I have called you to me because I wish to learn the most convenient manner of pissing. Should one squat and carefully lift the robe, as religion prescribes? Should one stand up, as is the unclean habit of unbelievers? Or should one undress completely and piss against one's friends, as is the custom of two hashish-eaters of my acquaintance?'

Knowing that the Sultan used to walk about the city in disguise, the kadi realized in a flash the identity of his last night's visitors, and fell on his knees, crying: 'My lord, my lord, the hashish spake in these indelicacies, not I!' But the fisherman, who by his careful daily taking of the drug was always under its effect, called somewhat sharply: 'And what of it? You are in your palace this morning, we were in our palace last night.' 'O sweetest noise in all our kingdom,' answered the delighted King, 'as we are both Sultans of this city, I think you had better henceforth stay with me in my palace. If you can tell stories, I trust that you will at once sweeten our hearing with a chosen one.' 'I will do so gladly, as soon as you have pardoned my wazir,' replied the fisherman; so the Sultan bade the kadi rise and sent him back forgiven to his duties.

The Assassins

Philip K. Hitti

The Assassin movement, called the 'new propaganda' by its members, was inaugurated by al-Hasan ibn-al-Sabbah (died in 1124), probably a Persian from Tus, who claimed descent from the Himyarite kings of South Arabia. The motives were evidently personal ambition and desire for vengeance on the part of the heresiarch. As a young man in al-Rayy, al-Hasan received instruction in the Batinite system, and after spending a year and a half in Egypt returned to his native land as a Fatimid missionary. Here in 1090 he gained possession of the strong mountain fortress Alamut, north-west of Qazwin. Strategically situated on an extension of the Alburz chain, 10,200 feet above sea level, and on the difficult but shortest road between the shores of the Caspian and the Persian highlands, this 'eagle's nest', as the name probably means, gave ibn-al-Sabbah and his successors a central stronghold of primary importance. Its possession was the first historical fact in the life of the new order.

From Alamut the grand master with his disciples made surprise raids in various directions which netted other fortresses. In pursuit of their ends they made free and treacherous use of the dagger, reducing assassination to an art. Their secret organization, based on Ismailite antecedents, developed an agnosticism which aimed to emancipate the initiate from the trammels of doctrine, enlightened him as to the superfluity of prophets and encouraged him to believe nothing and dare all. Below the grand master stood the grand priors, each in charge of a particular district. After these came the ordinary propagandists. The lowest degree of the order comprised the 'fida'is', who stood ready to execute whatever orders the grand master issued. A graphic, though late and secondhand, description of the method by which the master of Alamut is said to have hypnotized his 'self-sacrificing ones' with the use of hashish has come down to us from Marco Polo, who passed in that neighbourhood in 1271 or 1272. After describing in glowing terms the magnificent garden surrounding the elegant pavilions and palaces built by the grand master at Alamut, Polo proceeds:

Now no man was allowed to enter the Garden save those whom he intended to be his Ashishin. There was a fortress at the entrance to the Garden, strong enough to resist all the world, and there was no other way to get in. He kept at his Court a number of the youths of the country, from twelve to twenty years of age, such as had a taste for soldiering.... Then he would introduce them into his Garden, some four, or six, or ten at a time, having first made them drink a certain potion which cast them into a deep sleep, and then causing them to be lifted and carried in. So when they awoke they found themselves in the Garden.

When therefore they awoke, and found themselves in a place so charming, they deemed that it was Paradise in very truth. And the ladies and damsels dallied with them to their hearts' content...

So when the Old Man would have any prince slain, he would say to such a youth: 'Go thou and slay So and So; and when thou returnest my Angels shall bear thee into Paradise. And shouldst thou die, natheless even so will I send my Angels to carry thee back into Paradise.'

(from *The Book of Ser Marco Polo, the Venetian*, translated by Henry Yule, London, 1875)

The assassination in 1092 of the illustrious vizir of the Saljuq sultanate, Nizam-al-Mulk, by a fida'i disguised as a Sufi, was the first of a series of mysterious murders which plunged the Muslim world into terror. When in the same year the Saljuq Sultan Malikshah bestirred himself and sent a disciplinary force against the fortress, its garrison made a night sortie and repelled the besieging army. Other attempts by caliphs and sultans proved equally futile until finally the Mongolian Hula-gu, who destroyed the caliphate, seized the fortress in 1256 together with its subsidiary castles in Persia. Since the Assassin books and records were then destroyed, our information about this strange and spectacular order is derived mainly from hostile sources.

As early as the last years of the eleventh century the Assassins had succeeded in setting firm foot in Syria and winning as convert the Saljuq prince of Aleppo, Ridwan ibn-Tutush (died in 1113). By 1140 they had captured the hill fortress of Masyad and many others in northern Syria, including al-Kahf, al-Qadmus and al-'Ullayqah. Even Shayzar (modern Sayjar) on the Orontes was temporarily occupied by the Assassins, whom Usamah calls Isma'ilites. One of their most famous masters in Syria was Rachid-al-Din Sinan (died in 1192), who resided at Masyad and bore the title *shakh al-jabal'*, translated by the Crusades' chroniclers as 'the old man of the mountain'. It was Rashid's henchmen who struck awe and terror into the hearts of the Crusaders. After the capture of Masyad in 1260 by the Mongols, the Mamluk Sultan Baybars in 1272 dealt the Syrian Assassins the final blow. Since then the Assassins have been sparsely scattered through northern Syria, Persia, 'Uman, Zanzibar and especially India, where they number about a hundred and fifty thousand and go by the name of Thojas or Mowlas. They all acknowledge as titular head the Aga Khan of Bombay, who claims descent through the last grand master of Alamut from Isma'il, the seventh imam, receives over a tenth of the revenues of his followers, even in Syria, and spends most of his time as a sportsman between Paris and London.

The Hodja

Traditional

Nasreddin Hodja is believed to have lived in the fourteenth century, though opinions vary. Stories concerning his feats have passed into the folklore of many Middle Eastern countries. The following is retold by Taner Baybars.

The Hodja was very curious to know how he would react to hashish. One day he plucked up the courage and bought himself a handful from the apothecary's, smoked it and then went to a Turkish bath. Some time passed, but he felt no change in himself. 'They must have given me the wrong thing,' he kept on saying. 'I must go and find out. I'm not going to be cheated like this.'

So he rushed out naked.

'Hodja, what is the matter?' people asked him. 'Where are you going like this, with nothing on?'

'Don't ask me,' he said. 'I thought smoking hashish would do something to me. But as you can see, I'm still what I was. I'm going to get the real stuff from the apothecary's. I have a feeling he's cheated me.'

A Moroccan Folk Tale

Traditional

One day the Sultan woke up in a bad mood. He walked over to a group of his counsellors and ordered them to make a chain of sand. They were silent. To say 'no' to a request from the Sultan meant instant death. To say 'yes' and then to be unable to carry it out meant instant death. To give no answer also meant instant death. The silence grew longer and heavier. But fortunately there was a man among them who smoked a lot of kif, and he said: 'If your majesty will show us how to start the chain, then we will be glad to finish it.' So they were spared from the wrath of the king.

The Herb Pantagruelion

François Rabelais

Pantagruel took leave of the good Gargantua, who offered up fervent prayers for the success of his son's voyage, and a few days later he arrived at the port of Thalassa, near Saint Malo, accompanied by Panurge, Epistemon, Friar John of the Hashes, Abbot of Thélème, and others of the royal house, notably by Xenomanes, the great traveller and journeyer by perilous ways, who had come at Panurge's command, since he had some small holding in the domain of Salmigundia. When they got there, Pantagruel equipped a fleet of vessels, equal in number to those which Ajax of Salamis once gathered to escort the Greeks to Troy. He collected sailors, pilots, boatswains, interpreters, craftsmen, and soldiers, also provisions, artillery, munitions, clothes, money, and other such goods as were needed for a long and perilous voyage. These he took on board, and amongst the cargo I noticed a great store of his herb Pantagruelion,* both in its raw green state and also prepared and manufactured.

The herb Pantagruelion has a small, hardish, roundish root, ending in a blunt point, and does not strike more than a foot and a half into the ground. From the root grows a single round, umbelliferous stem, green on the outside, white within and hollow like the stems of Smyrnium, Olus atrum, beans, and gentian. It is woody, straight, friable, and slightly denticulated after the fashion of a lightly fluted column; and it is full of fibres, in which lie all the virtue of the herb, particularly in the part called *Mesa*, or middle, and in that called *Mylasea*. Its height is commonly from five to six feet. But sometimes it is taller than a lance; that is to say when it grows in a sweet, spongy, light soil, moist but not cold, like that of Olonne, and

*This will prove to be hemp.

that of Rosea, near Praeneste in Sabine territory, and provided that it does not lack rain around the fisherman's festivals and the summer solstice. Then it grows higher than some trees, and so, on Theophrastus's authority, is called *dendromalache*, although the herb dies each year, and has not the root, trunk, peduncles, or permanent branches of a tree.

Great, strong branches issue from the stem. Its leaves are three times longer than they are wide. They are always green, slightly rough like alkanet; toughish, with sickle-shaped indentations all round, like betony; and terminating in points like a Macedonian pike or a surgeon's lancet. Their shape is not very different from that of ash or agrimony leaves; and it is so like hemp-agrimony that many herbalists have called it cultivated hemp-agrimony, and have called hemp-agrimony wild pantagruelion. The leaves sprout out all round the stalk at equal distances, to the number of five or seven at each level; and it is by a special favour of Nature that they are grouped in these two odd numbers, which are both divine and mysterious. Their scent is strong, and unpleasant to delicate nostrils.

The seeds form near the top of the stalk, and a little below. They are as numerous as those of any herb in existence, spherical, oblong, or rhomboid in shape, black, bright, or brown in colour, hardish, enclosed in a light husk, and much loved by all such singing birds as linnets, goldfinches, larks, canaries, yellowhammers, and others. But in man they destroy the generative seed if eaten often and in quantity; and although the Greeks of old used sometimes to make certain kinds of cakes, tarts, and fritters of them, which they ate after supper as a dainty and to enhance the taste of their wine, still they are difficult to digest, lie heavy on the stomach, make bad blood, and, by their excessive heat, harm the brain, filling the head with noxious and painful vapours. Just as in many plants there are two sexes, male and female – as we see in laurels, palms, oaks, yews, asphodels, mandragora, ferns, agarics, birthwort, cypress, turpentine, pennyroyal, peonies, and others – so in this herb there is a male, which has no flower but plenty of seeds, and a female, which is thick and has little whitish useless flowers, but no seed to speak of; and as in other plants of this kind, the female leaf is larger but less tough than the male, and does not grow as high.

This Pantagruelion is sown at the first coming of the swallows, and pulled out of the ground when the cicadas begin to get hoarse.

Pantagruelion is prepared at the autumn equinox in different ways according to the fancies of the people and to national preferences. Pantagruel's first instructions were to strip the stalk of its leaves and seeds; to soak it in still – not in running – water for five days, if the weather is fine and the water warm, and for nine to twelve if the weather is cloudy and the water cold; then to dry it in the sun, and afterwards in the shade, remove the outside, separate the fibres – in which, as has been said, lies all its use and value – from the woody part, which is useless except to make a fire blaze, as kindling, or for blowing up pigs' bladders to amuse children. Sometimes also gluttons will find a sly use for them, as syphons to suck up new wine through the bung-hole.

Some modern Pantagruelists, to avoid the manual labour entailed in making this separation, use certain pounding instruments, formed in the shape in which the angry Juno held the fingers of her hands together, to prevent the delivery of Alcmena, the mother of Hercules. With the aid of these they bruise and break up the woody part, making it useless, in order to recover the fibres. The only people who practise this process are those who defy the world's opinion, and in a manner considered paradoxical by philosophers earn their livings by walking backwards.* Those who want to make better and more valuable use of the fibre imitate the fabled pastime of the three sister Fates, the nocturnal recreation of the noble Circe, and the lengthy stratagem practised by Penelope to ward off her amorous suitors during the absence of her husband Ulysses.

*These are the ropemakers, who draw the fibre from a bag, and walk backwards as they plait the rope.

In this way it can be put to all its inestimable uses, of which I will tell you some only – for it would be impossible for me to reveal them all – if first I may explain to you the plant's name.

I find the plants are named in different ways. Some have taken their name from the man who first discovered them, recognized them, demonstrated them, cultivated them, domesticated them, and applied them to their uses; as dog's mercury from Mercury; panacea (all-heal) from Panace, the daughter of Aesculapius; artemisia from Artemis, who is Diana; eupatoria from king Eupator; telephium from Telephus; euphorbium from Euphorbus, king Juba's physician; clymenos (honeysuckle) from Clymenus; alcibiadion from Alcibiades; gentian from Gentius, King of Slavonia. And so highly valued of old was this prerogative of giving one's name to a newly discovered plant that, just as there was a controversy between Neptune and Pallas as to which should name the country discovered by them both jointly, which was afterwards called Athens from Athena, that is to say Minerva – even so did Lyncus, King of Scythia attempt treacherously to murder the young Triptolemus, who was sent by Ceres to show mankind wheat, which was till then unknown. For by the youth's death Lyncus hoped to give the grain his own name and, to his honour and immortal glory, to be called the discoverer of a food both useful and necessary to the life of man. But, for his treachery, he was transformed by Ceres into an ounce or lynx. Similarly, great and long wars were waged of old between certain kings in and around Cappadocia, their only difference being which of them should give his name to a certain herb. Owing to their quarrel, the name it eventually received was *Polemonia*, since it was the cause of war.

Others have kept the names of the regions from which they were once brought; Median apples – or lemons – for instance from Media where they were first found; Punic apples – that is pomegranates – which were brought from the Punic country, which is Carthage; ligusticum – that is lovage – which came from Liguria, the coast of Genoa; rhubarb, from the barbarian river called Rha, as Ammianus testifies; also sontonica, fenu-greek, chestnuts, peaches, Sabine juniper, and stoechas, which owe their name to my own islands of Hyères, called in ancient days the Stoechades, also *spica celtica*, et cetera.

Others take their names by antiphrasis or irony; absinthe for instance, because it is the contrary of *pynthe* – the Greek for beverage – being unpleasant to drink; holosteon, which means all bone, because there is no herb in all Nature more fragile and tender.

Others derive their names from their properties and uses, as aristolochia, which helps women in childbirth; lichen, which heals the skin eruptions so called; mallow, which mollifies; callithricum, which beautifies the hair, alyssum, ephemerum, bechium, nasturtium – or nose-twister, which is a breath-catching cress – pig-nut, henbane, and others.

Others derive their names from the admirable qualities dis-covered in them, as heliotrope, or *solsequium*, follower of the sun, which opens as the sun rises, climbs as it ascends, declines as the sun sinks, and closes as it disappears; adiantum, or waterless, since it never retains any moisture, although it grows near the water, and even though it be plunged in water for a considerable time; also hieracia, eryngion, et cetera.

Others get their names from men or women who have been transformed into them, as daphne, the laurel, from Daphne; the myrtle from Myrsine; pitys, the stonepipe, from Pitys; cynara, which is the artichoke; narcissus; crocus, the saffron; smilax, et cetera.

Others from physical resemblance, as hippuris, or horse-tail, since it is like a horse's tail; alopecuros, which is like a fox's tail; psyllion, which is like a flea; delphinium, like a dol-phin; bugloss, like an ox's tongue; iris, whose flowers are like a rainbow; myosotis, like a mouse's ear; coronopus, like a crow's foot, et cetera.

Reciprocally, some men have taken their names from plants; the Fabii from beans, the Pisones from peas, the Lentuli from lentils, and the Ciceros from chick-peas. And again from more exalted similarities come Venus' navel, venushair, Venus' basin, Jupiter's beard, Jupiter's eye. Mars's blood, Mercury's fingers, hermodactyls, et cetera.

Others again, are named from their form, as trefoil, which has three leaves; pentaphyllon, which has five leaves; serpillum, which creeps along the ground; helxine or pellitory from its clinging properties; petasites or sunshades, and myrobolan plums, which the Arabs call *been*, for they are acorn-shaped and oleaginous.

The plant Pantagruelion got its name in all these ways – always excepting the mythological one. For Heaven forbid that we should in any way resort to myth in this most truthful history. Pantagruel was its discoverer; I do not mean the discoverer of the plant, but of a certain application of it. Thus applied, it is more loathed and abhorred by robbers, and is their more unremitting enemy than are dodder and choke-weed to flax, than reed to ferns, than horse-tail to mowers, than broom-rape to chick-peas, than darnel to barley, than hatchet-weed to lentils, than antranium to beans, than tares to wheat, than ivy to walls; than the water-lily *Nymphaea heraclea* to lecherous monks; than the strap and the birch to the scholars of the College of Navarre; than the cabbage to the vine, garlic to magnetic iron, onion to the eyes, fern-seed to pregnant women, the seed of willow to immoral nuns, and the yew-tree's shade to those who sleep beneath it; than wolf's bane to panthers and wolves; than the smell of a fig tree to mad bulls, than hemlock to goslings, than purslane to the teeth, than oil to trees. For we have seen many robbers end their lives high and briefly because of its use, after the manner of Phyllis, Queen of the Thracians; of Bonosus, Emperor of Rome; of Amata, wife of King Latinus; of Iphis, Auctolia, Lycambes, Arachne, Phaedra, Leda, Achaeus, King of Lydia, and others, whose only complaint was that, without their being otherwise sick, the channels through which their witticisms came out and their dainty snacks went in were stopped by the herb Pantagruelion, more scurvily than ever they could have been by the dire spasms or the mortal quinsy.

Others we have heard, at the moment when Atropos was cutting their life-thread, woefully lamenting and complaining that Pantagruel had them by the throat. But, gracious me, it wasn't Pantagruel at all. He never broke anyone on the wheel. It was Pantagruelion, doing duty as a halter, and serving them as a cravat. Besides they were speaking incorrectly and committing a solecism, unless they could be excused on the plea that they were using the figure synecdoche, taking the inventor for the invention, as one uses Ceres for bread, and Bacchus for wine. I swear to you here, by the wit residing in that bottle, cooling there in the tub, that Pantagruel never took anyone by the throat, except such men as neglect to ward off an impending thirst.

Pantagruelion is also so called by similarity. For when he was born into the world Pantagruel was as tall as the herb in question; and it was easy to make this measurement since he was born in a time of drought when they gather the said herb, and when Icarus' dog, by barking at the sun, makes every man a troglodyte, forcing the whole world to live in caves and subterranean places.

Pantagruelion owes its name also to its virtues and peculiarities. For as Pantagruel has been the exemplar and paragon of perfect jollity – I don't suppose that any one of you boozers is in any doubt about that – so in Pantagruelion I recognize so many virtues, so much vigour, so many perfections, so many admirable effects, that if its full worth had been known when, as the Prophet tells us, the trees elected a wooden king to reign over them and govern them, it would no doubt have gained the majority of their votes and suffrages. Shall I go further? If Oxylus, son of Oreius, had begotten it on his sister Hamadryas, he would have taken more delight in its worth alone than in his eight children, so celebrated by our mythologists, who have caused their names to be eternally remembered. The eldest, a daughter, was called the vine; the next, a son, was called the fig; the next, the walnut; the next, the oak; the next, the sorb-apple; the next, the mountain-ash; the next, the poplar: and the last, the elm, which was a great surgeon in its time.

I shall forbear to tell you how the juice of this herb, squeezed and dropped into the ears, kills every kind of vermin that may have bred there by putrefaction, and any other beast that may have got in. If you put some of this juice into a bucket of water, you will immediately see the water coagulate like curds, so great are its virtues; and this coagulated water is a prompt remedy for horses with colic and broken wind. Its root, boiled in water, softens hardened sinews, contracted joints, sclerotic gout, and gouty swellings. If you want quickly to heal a scald or a burn, apply some Pantagruelion raw; that is to say just as it comes out of the earth, without any preparation or treatment; and be sure to change it as soon as you see it drying on the wound.

Without it kitchens would be a disgrace, tables repellent, even though they were covered with every exquisite food, and beds pleasureless, though adorned with gold, silver, amber, ivory, and porphyry in abundance. Without it millers would not carry wheat to the mill, or carry flour away. Without it, how could advocates' pleadings be brought to the sessions hall? How could plaster be carried to the workshop without it? Without it, how could water be drawn from the well? What would scribes, copyists, secretaries, and writers do without it? Would not official documents and rent-rolls disappear? Would not the noble art of printing perish? What would window screens be made of? How would church bells be rung? It provides the adornment of the priests of Isis, the robes of the pastophores, and the coverings of all human beings in their first recumbent position. All the woolly trees of Northern India, all the cotton plants of Tylos on the Persian Gulf, of Arabia, and of Malta have not dressed so many people as this plant alone. It protects armies against cold and rain, much more effectively than did the skin tents of old. It protects theatres and amphitheatres against the heat; it is hung round woods and coppices for the pleasure of hunters; it is dropped into sweet water and sea-water for the profit of fishermen. It shapes and makes serviceable boots, high-boots, heavy boots, leggings, shoes, pumps, slippers, and nailed shoes. By it bows are strung, arbalests bent, and slings made. And as though it were a sacred plant, like verbena, and reverenced by the Manes and Lemurs, the bodies of men are never buried without it.

I will go further. By means of this herb, invisible substances are visibly stopped, caught, detained and, as it were, imprisoned; and by their capture and arrest great, heavy mill-wheels are lightly turned to the signal profit of humankind. It astounds me that the practicability of such a process was hidden for so many centuries from the ancient philosophers, considering the inestimable benefit it provides and the intolerable labours they had to perform in their mills through lack of it. By its powers of catching the waves of the air, vast merchant ships, huge cabined barges, mighty galleons, ships with a crew of a thousand or ten thousand men are launched from their moorings and driven forward at their pilots' will. By its help nations which Nature seemed to keep hidden, inaccessible, and unknown, have come to us, and we to them: something beyond the power of birds, however light of wing, and whatever freedom to swim down the air Nature may have given them. Ceylon has seen Lapland, Java has seen the Riphaean Mountains, Phebol shall see Thélème; the Icelanders and Greenlanders shall see the Euphrates. By its help Boreas has seen the mansion of Auster, Eurus has visited Zephyrus; and as a result, those celestial intelligences, the gods of the sea and land, have all taken fright. For they have seen the Arctic peoples, in full sight of the Antarctic peoples, by the aid of this blessed Pantagruelion, cross the Atlantic sea, pass the twin Tropics, go down beneath the torrid zone, measure the entire Zodiac, disport themselves below the Equinoctial Line, and hold both Poles in view on the level of their horizon. In a similar fright the gods of Olympus cried: 'By the power and uses of this herb of his, Pantagruel has given us something new to think about, which is costing us a worse headache than ever the Aloides did. He will shortly be married. His wife will bear him children. This is fated and we cannot prevent it. It has passed through the hands and over the spindles of the fatal sisters, the daughters of necessity. Perhaps his children will discover a plant of equal power, by whose aid mortals will be able to visit the sources of the hail, the flood-gates of the rain, and the smithy of the thunder; will be able to invade the regions of the moon, enter the territory of the celestial signs, and there take lodging, some at the Golden Eagle, others at the Ram, others at the Crown, others at the Harp, others at the Silver Lion; and sit down with us at table there, and marry our goddesses; which is their one means of rising to the gods.'

In the end they decided to deliberate on a means of preventing this, and called a council.

American Indians in 1626

Jean Leander

The following extract is taken from Traité du Tabac du Panacée Universelle *which was published in Lyons in 1626. Dr Leander is describing American Indian priests, whom he calls 'Bubites', obviously referring to the traditional tribal medicine men.*

When they want to know the outcome of something, they perfume themselves with tobacco to ravish themselves into ecstasy, and when in this state question the devil as to the subject about which they want to know. The priest, having been questioned, burns dry tobacco leaves and, with a hollow stalk or a pipe such as is in common use among us, draws in the smoke and is transported to the point of losing all contact with his surroundings as if in ecstasy, letting himself fall to the ground, where he lies for the rest of the day or the night, completely relaxed and motionless. Then he pretends that he has talked with the devil and gives oracles, thus doing wrong to these unfortunate Indians. The doctors of these poor barbarians also used it in order to communicate with the gods.

The Garden of Health (1633)

HEMPE

1. The seede expelleth windinesse. 2. If a man taketh a little too much of it, it dryeth up natural seed, and the milke of women. 3. Jaundies and stopping of the liver, stamp the seed, and drink it with wine. 4. Care paine, and hermine [?] therein, put in the juice of the greene leaves. 5. Gout, a shrinking of sinews, seethe the root in water, and apply it. 6. Hens to lay apace, give them the seeds. 7. Gnats to best, lay the moyst branches by thee. 8. Belly bound, stamp the seeds, and seethe them in running water, and streine it and drinke a good draught when thou goest to bed. 9. Oyle to make, stamp the seed, and sprinkle it with a little wine, and heat it in a new earthen panne well glazed, and when thou canst not suffer thy hand any longer in it, presse out the oyle through a square bag, and drink one ounce of it, to make thee merry, fierce, hardy to fight, and comely to see; and in like sort thou mayest drain oyle out of all seeds. 10. Cough dry, seethe the seeds in milk, and use it. Give a horse as much seed to eat as thou mayest take up with both thy hands to cause him presently to pisse and void the chollick and stone, but he must not drink of two hours after. 11. Fever quarten, take the juice of Hempe before the fit. [See Fenigreke.] Sinewes shrunk, seethe the roots in wine, and apply them. 12. Eares noyle [?], purge with pills Hiera picra, and put on oyle of Hemp-seed marine with a little vinegar, but if it come of great heat, then with womans milke, and leap on the foot on the same side often, and provoke sneezing. 13. Breast suppuration and mattering, seethe Hemp-seed in water, and use the milk thereof. 14. Stamp the seed and strain it with water, and put it two rosted Egs, and take it fasting to stop the bloudy flux. 15. Eares worms, put in the cleare juice of the leaves and seeds. 16. Appetite to cause, steep the seeds in ale

one night, then rub them betweene your hands till the husks be off, and wash them clean, and stamp them, and make it like an Almond candell, and use it often. 17. Kankar of fever, burn Hemp-seed and Rye-meal, & mix the powder with the juice of smallage & hony, & dip tents of linnen therein, & put it in. 18. Seethe the seeds in goats milk to ye third part, & drink it 3 daies to avoid all inward poison.

Culpeper's Herbal and English Physician Enlarged (1731 Edition)

HEMP

This is so well known to every good housewife in the country, that I shall not need to write any description of it.

Government and virtues: It is a plant of Saturn, and good for something else, you see, than to make halters only. The seed of Hemp consumes wind, and by too much use thereof disperses it so much that it dries up the natural seed for pro-creation; yet, being boiled in milk and taken, helps such as have a hot dry cough. The Dutch make an emulsion out of the seed, and give it with good success to those that have the jaundice, especially in the beginning of the disease, if there be no ague accompanying it, for it opens obstructions of the gall, and causes digestion of choler. The emulsion or decoction of the seed stays lasks and continual fluxes, eases the cholic, and allays the troublesome humours in the bowels, and stays bleeding at the mouth, nose, or other places, some of the leaves being fried with the blood of them that bleed, and so given them to eat. It is held very good to kill the worms in men or beasts; and

*From the above it is obvious that it was common practice to prepare one's own extract of cannabis in Elizabethan England without bothering to go to a chemist's shop. This means that the plant was growing in abundance and could be found without difficulty. As the recommended dose of the extract is a full ounce, it must have been far less potent than the African and Asian varieties of hemp, but would of course have had a similar effect.

the juice dropped into the ears kills worms in them; and draws forth earwigs, or other living creatures gotten into them. The decoction of the root allays inflammations of the head, or any other parts: the herb itself, or the distilled water thereof doth the like. The decoction of the root eases the pains of the gout, the hard humours of knots in the joints, the pains and shrinking of the sinews, and the pains of the hips. The fresh juice mixed with a little oil and butter, is good for any place that hath been burnt with fire, being thereto applied.

Diary Notes

George Washington

The following entries from George Washington's Diary show that he personally planted and harvested hemp. As it is known that the potency of the female plants decreases after they have been fertilized by the males, the fact that he regrets having separated the male from the female plants too late (after fertilization) clearly indicates that he was cultivating the plant for medicinal purposes as well as for its fibre.

1765
May 12-13—Sowed Hemp at Muddy hole by Swamp.
August 7—began to separate [*sic*] the Male from the Female hemp at Do—rather too late.

Two Celebrated Hashish Eaters

W. Reininger

The investigations on hashish and its effects that the physician J. J. Moreau de Tours carried out around 1840 led to the rise of a hashish fashion (*mode du hachisch*) among the bohemians of Paris to which a number of artists became addicted for some time. Of these, we must mention the poets Théophile Gautier (1811-72) and Charles Baudelaire (1821-67) who published observations gathered in the course of experiments that they carried out by consuming hashish as was done in their circle. Quite apart from their literary value, these notes have some scientific importance since they are concerned with the determination of the effects of hashish. The first article published by Théophile Gautier in the journal *La Presse*, entitled 'Le Club des Hachischins', was even reproduced by Moreau in his monograph on hashish that appeared in 1845 to characterize a kind of intoxication typical of hashish.

The 'Club des Hachischins' founded by Gautier held its meeting at the Hotel Pimodan on the Ile Saint-Louis. Gautier, and much later Baudelaire, occupied attic rooms in it for several years. It was Moreau who provided Gautier with the first samples of hashish. This is how the poet described his first hashish intoxication:

At the end of several minutes, a general numbness spread through me. It seemed to me that my body dissolved and became transparent. In my chest I saw very clearly the hashish that I had eaten, in the form of an emerald that gave off millions of tiny sparkles. My eyelashes grew longer and longer without stopping, and like gold threads rolled up on little ivory spinning wheels that revolved completely alone with dazzling rapidity. Around me streamed and rolled precious stones of all colours. In space, flower patterns branched off ceaselessly in such a way that I know of nothing better with which to compare them than the play of a kaleidoscope. At certain

moments, I saw my comrades again, but they were distorted; they
appeared as half men, half plants, with the thoughtful air of an ibis,
standing on an ostrich foot and beating their wings. So strange was
this sight that I was convulsed with laughter in my corner and in
order to join in the buffoonery of this spectacle I began to throw my
pillows in the air, catching them again, and making them go
around with the rapidity of an Indian juggler. One of these gentle-
men began to converse with me in Italian, but which the hashish by
its omnipotence translated into Spanish for me. The questions and
answers were almost reasonable and dealt with trivial matters, with
theatrical and literary news.

The first bout reached its end. After several minutes, I had recovered completely my composure, without a headache or any of
the symptoms that accompany intoxication produced by wine, and
greatly astonished by what had happened – Hardly had half an
hour passed when I again fell under the sway of hashish. This time
the vision was more complicated and extraordinary. In an atmosphere of confusedly flitting lights there were thousands of swarming butterflies whose wings rustled like fans. Gigantic flowers with
crystal calices, enormous hollyhocks, gold and silver lilies rose and
opened around me with a crackling like a bouquet of fireworks.
My hearing was prodigiously developed: I heard the sound of colours. Green, red, blue, and yellow sounds came to me in perfectly
distinct waves. A glass that was upset, a creaking armchair, a softly
spoken word vibrated and re-echoed in me like the rumbling of
thunder. My own voice seemed to me so powerful and loud that I
dared not speak for fear of causing the walls to collapse or of making myself burst like a bomb. More than five hundred clocks sang
the time with their flute-like, coppery, silvery voices. Each flowered
object emitted a sound of a harmonica or of an aeolian harp. I
swam or rather floated in an ocean of sound in which, like islands
of light, were motifs from *Lucia* or the *Barber* (of Seville). Never
had such waves of bliss filled my being. I was so much a part of the
wave, so far from myself and so devoid of my own being, this odi-
ous witness which accompanies us everywhere, that I understood
for the first time what the existence of elementary spirits, of angels
and souls separated from the body may be like. I was like a sponge
in the middle of the sea; each moment waves of happiness traversed
me, entering and leaving by my pores, for I had become permeable
and, to the tiniest capillary vessel, my entire being was injected with
the colour of the fantastic *milieu* in which I was plunged. Sounds,

perfumes, light came to me through multitudes of tubes as thin as hairs, in which I heard the whistle of magnetic currents – According to my calculation, this state lasted about three hundred years, for the sensations were so numerous and followed each other so closely that any real appreciation of time became impossible – The attack passed, and I saw that it had lasted a quarter of an hour.

What is distinctive of hashish intoxication is that it is not continuous. It seizes one and leaves one; you rise to the sky and come back to earth without transition – As in madness, one has moments of lucidity – A third attack, the last and the most bizarre ended my oriental soirée; in this last one I had double vision – Two images of each object were reflected on my retina and produced a complete symmetry. But soon the magic paste, completely digested, acted with great power on my brain and I became completely mad for an hour. All the pantagruelion dreams passed through my fantasy: ibises, bridled geese, unicorns, griffins, incubus, entire menageries of monstrous dreams trotted, skipped, fluttered about, yelped and squeaked through the room ... The visions became so queer and whimsical that I was seized by a desire to draw them, and to make in less than five minutes a portrait of the doctor ... (probably Dr Moreau de Tourse), as he appeared to me, seated at the piano in a Turkish costume with the sun in the back of his jacket. The notes were represented as escaping from the piano in the form of firework rockets and capriciously corkscrewed spirals. Another sketch bearing this caption – an animal of the future – represented a live locomotive with a swan's neck ending in the face of a serpent from which spurted clouds of smoke and with monstrous paws composed of wheels and pulleys. Each pair of paws was accompanied by a pair of wings, and on the tail of the animal one saw the Mercury of antiquity who acknowledged himself vanquished despite his winged heels. Thanks to the hashish I was able to make a portrait of an elf from nature. Until the present I only heard them groaning and moving about in the night in my old buffet ...

Under the same title, 'Le Club des Hachischins,' Théophile Gautier published another article on hashish in the *Revue des Deux Mondes* of 1 February 1846. This article, however, contains a great deal more literary embellishment than the one quoted above and which it seems is in agreement with scientific observation. Nevertheless, Gautier's second article which is often mentioned in the literature has a certain importance for the history of hashish intoxication because of its exact descriptions of the *milieu* in which the club met.

Charles Baudelaire, who was introduced into the 'Club des Hachischins' in 1844 by the painter Joseph Ferdinant Boissard de Boisdenier (1813–66), devoted to hashish a rather large study which first appeared in September 1858, in the *Revue contemporaine*, under the title, 'De l'idéal artificiel', and which the poet republished two years later under the title 'Le poème du hachisch' in his book, *Les Paradis artificiels*, of which it constituted the first part. Much later, Baudelaire presented a brief extract of this study in an article entitled 'Du vin et du hashish, comparés commes moyens de multiplication de l'individualité'.

As the *Paradis artificiels* of Baudelaire is well known, we will only mention the most characteristic passages that deal with hashish. In his historical exposé of hashish addiction and in his description of hashish intoxication, Baudelaire presents hardly any important new facts. That which gives this study a scientific value is the reflections of the author on the psychological attitude of the hashish eater and on the moral consequences of this passion. Under the heading, 'L'Homme-Dieu', Baudelaire in the fourth paragraph of his essay presents an analysis, which is very interesting from the psychological point of view, of the exaltation of the personality aroused by the drug in the course of hashish intoxication, an exaltation which inspires, often to the point of madness, the feeling that one is about to become a truly all-powerful divinity. In the fifth paragraph, entitled 'Morale', the poet explains this self-deification, which is manifested in hashish intoxication, by the desire of all hashish addicts to escape from the overwhelming reality of daily life, and he arrives at this conclusion:

Every man who does not accept the conditions of life, sells his soul. It is easy to grasp the connection which exists between the satanic creations who are often devoted to stimulants. Man wanted to be God, but before long by virtue of an uncontrollable moral law, he fell even lower than his real nature. It is a soul which sells itself piece-meal.

Although Baudelaire in his writings almost always speaks of the experiences of his friends with hashish, and only rarely mentions his own trials, it can be said that most of the details that he presents rest on observations made on himself. Some of the biographers of Baudelaire have even suggested that one of the causes of his death was his abuse of opium and hashish, but recent researches seem to contradict this assertion. Nevertheless, it is fairly well established that at the end of 1844 the poet repeatedly used these two intoxicants although at very irregular intervals and in varied doses.

Concerning Hashish

Charles Baudelaire

Sometimes strange things happen among the male and female workers during the hemp harvest. It seems as if some dizzy spirit rises from the harvest which circulates around their legs and mounts mischievously to the brain. The head of the harvester is full of whirlpools, at other times loaded with daydreams. The limbs weaken and refuse to be of service. Similar phenomena happened to me as a child when I was playing and rolling around in heaps of lucerne.

There have been attempts to make hashish out of hemp grown in France. So far they have all been unsuccessful, and the obstinate ones who wish to procure themselves enchanted enjoyment at no matter what price continue to use hashish from across the Mediterranean, that is to say made from Indian or Egyptian hemp. Hashish is composed of a decoction of Indian hemp, butter, and a little bit of opium.

Here is a green jam, strangely odorous, so odorous that it provokes a certain repulsion, as any fine odour does when carried to its maximum force and density. Take a piece as big as a walnut, fill a small spoon with it, and you possess happiness; absolute happiness with all its frenzies, its youthful follies, and also its infinite beatitudes. Happiness is there in the form of a little piece of jam; take it without fear, no one dies from it; the physical organs are hardly touched. Perhaps your will-power may be diminished, but that is another matter.

Usually in order to give the hashish all its strength and powers of development, it is mixed with very hot black coffee and drunk on an empty stomach. Supper should be taken late that evening, at about ten o'clock or midnight. A very light soup is the only food permitted. Breaking this simple rule produces either vomiting, as the food quarrels with the drug, or it cancels the effect of the hashish. Many ignorant or stupid people who have broken this rule accuse hashish of being powerless.

No sooner has the little amount of drug been swallowed (an act which requires a certain determination, as the mixture has such a strong odour that it provokes nausea in some people) than you find yourself placed in a state of anxious waiting. You have heard vaguely about the marvellous effects of hashish, your imagination has already formed its particular idea of an ideal intoxication, and you are impatient to find out if the result will in reality live up to your preconception. The amount of time that passes between drinking the drug and feeling the first effects varies according to temperaments and also according to habit. People who know their way around with hashish sometimes feel the first effects after half an hour.

I forgot to say that as hashish causes an exaggeration of the personality at the same time as a very sharp feeling for circumstances and surroundings, it is best to use it only in favourable circumstances and surroundings. All joy and happiness being super-abundant, all sorrow and anguish is immensely profound. Do not experiment with it if you have to accomplish some disagreeable matter of business, if you are feeling melancholy, or if you have a bill to pay. Hashish is not suited for action. It does not console as wine does, all it does is to develop immeasurably the human personality in the actual circumstances where it is placed. As far as possible, one should have a beautiful apartment or landscape, a free clear mind, and some accomplices whose intellectual temperament is akin to your own; and a little music too, if possible.

Novices at their first initiation almost always complain about how slow the effects are, and as it is not going fast enough to suit them, they begin boasting incredulously, which is very amusing to those who know about the way hashish works. It is not one of the least comic things to see the first effects appear and multiply themselves right in the middle of this incredulity. First a certain absurd and irresistible hilarity comes over you. The most ordinary words, the most simple ideas take on a strange new aspect. This gaiety becomes insupportable to you, but it is useless to revolt. The demon has invaded you, all the efforts you make to resist only accelerate his progress. You laugh at your own silliness and folly; your companions make fun of you, and you are not angry, for benevolence has begun to manifest itself.

This languishing gaiety, uneasiness in joy, insecurity, unhealthy indecision usually lasts only a short while. It sometimes happens that people not at all suited to word games improvise interminable series of puns, bringing the most improbable ideas together, made to mislead the strongest masters of this absurd art. After several minutes the relationships become so vague, the threads which connect your conceptions are so tenuous, that only your accomplices, members of the same religion, can understand you. Your folly, your bursts of laughter seem extremely stupid to anyone who is not in the same state as you.

The sobriety of this unfortunate person amuses you boundlessly, his composure pushes you to the last limits of irony; he seems to you the most insane and ridiculous of human beings. As for your comrades, you understand them perfectly. Soon you will only communicate with the eyes. The fact is that it is a very amusing situation: people enjoying a gaiety which is incomprehensible to anyone who is not situated in the same world as they are, regard him with profound pity. From then on the idea of superiority dawns on your mental horizon. Soon it will increase immeasurably.

I was a witness to two rather grotesque scenes during this first phase. A famous musician who knew nothing about the properties of hashish, and who had probably never heard of it, arrived in the middle of a group where almost everyone had taken it. They tried to make him understand its marvellous effects. He laughed it off politely, like a man who is willing to pose for a few minutes in a spirit of propriety because he has been well brought up. There was a lot of laughter; for the person who has taken hashish is endowed with a marvellous awareness of the comic during the first phase. Bursts of laughter, incomprehensible enormities, inextricable word games, baroque gestures continued. The musician declared that this 'charge' was bad for artists, and that besides it must be very tiring for them.

The joy increased. He said 'This charge may be good for you, but not for me.' One of the intoxicated egotistically replied 'It suffices that it be good for us.' Interminable bursts of laughter filled the room. The man got angry and wanted to leave. Someone locked the door and hid the key. Someone else kneeled down before him, and, speaking for the whole group, declared with tears in his eyes that although they were moved by a most profound pity for him and for his inferiority, they would not be any the less animated by an eternal benevolence.

He was begged to play some music, and finally agreed. The violin had hardly begun to be heard when the sounds spreading through the apartment took possession of some of the intoxicated here and there. Nothing but deep sighs, sobs, heartbreaking groans, torrents of tears. The horrified musician stopped, he thought he was in a lunatic asylum. He approached the one whose beatitude was making the most noise, and asked him if he was suffering very much, and what should be done to help him. A down-to-earth person, who also had not taken the beatific drug, suggested lemonade and bitters. The intoxicated one, ecstasy in his eyes, looked at him with unutterable contempt, only pride preventing the most serious insults. Indeed, what could be more exasperating to someone sick with joy than to want to cure him?

Here is a phenomenon that seems extremely curious to me: a servant who was asked to bring tobacco and refreshments to people who had taken hashish, upon seeing herself surrounded by strange heads with enormous eyes, by an unhealthy atmosphere, by a collective insanity, burst into hysterical laughter, dropped the tray which broke with all its cups and glasses, and fled in horror as fast as she could. Everybody laughed. She admitted the next day that she had felt something strange for several hours, to have been 'all queer, I don't know how'. However, she had not taken hashish.

The second phase announces itself by a sensation of coolness at the extremities, a great weakness; you have, as they say, butter-fingers, a heavy head, and general stupefaction in all your being. Your eyes get bigger, they are as if pulled in all directions by an implacable ecstasy. Your face becomes pale, then livid and greenish. The lips withdraw, shrink, and seem to want to enter the interior of your mouth. Raucous and profound sighs escape from your chest, as if your old nature could not support the weight of your new nature. The senses become extraordinarily delicate and sharp. The eyes pierce the infinite. The ear hears the tiniest sounds in the middle of the loudest noises.

The hallucinations begin. External objects take on monstrous appearances. They reveal themselves to you in previously unsuspected forms. Then they deform themselves, transform themselves, and finally they enter into your being, or else you enter into theirs. The most singular ambiguities, the most inexplicable transpositions of ideas take place. Sounds have a colour, colours have a music. Musical notes are numbers, and you solve with frightening rapidity prodigious arithmetical calculations while the music unfolds in your ear. You are seated and you are smoking; you think that you are sitting in your pipe and it is you that your pipe is smoking; it is yourself that you exhale in the form of blue clouds.

You feel well, there is only one thing that bothers and worries you. How will you manage to get out of your pipe? This hallucination lasts for an eternity. An interval of lucidity permits you to make a great effort and look at the clock. The eternity has lasted one minute. Another current of ideas carries you off; it will carry you for a minute in its living whirlpool, and this minute will be another eternity. The proportions of time and of the being are upset by an innumerable multitude of intense sensations and ideas. One lives several human lives in the space of an hour. That is certainly the subject of *Peau de chagrin*. There is no longer an equation between the organs and the joys.

From time to time the personality disappears. The objecivity which some pantheist poets and great actors have becomes so great that you confuse yourself with external beings. Here you are a tree moaning to the wind and recounting vegetable melodies to nature. Now you are flying in the blue of an immensely enlarged sky. All pain has disappeared. You resist no longer, you are carried away, no longer your own master and no longer caring. Soon the idea of time will disappear completely. From time to time still a little awakening takes place. It seems to you that you are leaving a fantastic and marvellous world. It is true that you retain the ability to observe yourself, and the next day you will be able to remember some of your sensations. But you cannot make use of this psychological ability. I defy you to sharpen a pen or a pencil; it will be a labour beyond your strength.

At other times music recites infinite poems to you, placing you in frightening or fantastic dramas. It associates itself with objects that are before your eyes. Paintings on the ceiling come to life in a frightening way even if they are mediocre or bad. Clear enchanting water flows. Nymphs with radiant flesh look at you with large eyes clearer than water and the sky. You take your place and your part in the most mediocre paintings, the crudest pictures hung on the walls of hotel rooms.

I have noticed that water takes on a frightening charm for artistically inclined natures illuminated by hashish. Running water, fountains, harmonious waterfalls, and the blue immensity of the sea roll, sleep, and sing at the bottom of your being. It might not be a good idea to leave a man in this condition on the bank of a clear stream; like the fisherman in the ballad, he might allow himself to be carried away by a water-sprite.

One can eat towards the end of the evening, but this operation is not accomplished without difficulty. You find yourself so much above material facts that you would certainly prefer to remain sprawled out in the depths of your intellectual paradise. Sometimes, however, the appetite develops in an extraordinary way, but it takes a lot of courage to move a bottle, a fork, and a knife.

The third phase, which is separated from the second by a redoubled crisis, a dizzying intoxication followed by a new uneasiness, is something indescribable. It is what Orientals call the 'kief', it is absolute happiness. It is no longer something spinning and tumultuous. It is a calm and motionless beatitude. All philosophical problems are resolved. All the difficult questions about which theologians argue and which make reasonable men despair are clear and transparent. All contradiction has become unity. Man has become god.

There is something in you which says: 'You are superior to all men, no one understands what you think, what you are feeling now. They are even incapable of understanding the immense love you have for them. But you must not hate them for that, you must have pity on them. An immensity of happiness and virtue is opening itself before you. No one will ever know what degree of virtue and intelligence you have reached. Live in the solitude of your thoughts, and avoid harming others.'

One of the grotesque effects of hashish is the fear of hurting anyone at all, which is pushed to the point of the most meticulous folly. If you had the strength, you would even disguise the extra-natural state in which you are in order to avoid upsetting the least important people.

In this supreme state among artistic and tender spirits love-making takes on the most singular forms and abandons itself to the most baroque combinations. Unbridled debauchery can be mixed with an ardent and affectionate fatherly feeling.*

*The hashish jam which Baudelaire ate probably contained cantharides and other drugs.

My final observation will not be the least curious. The next morning, when you see daylight in your room, your first sensation is one of profound astonishment. Time has completely disappeared. A little while ago it was night, now it is day. 'Have I slept, or have I not slept? Did my intoxication last all night, and the notion of time being suppressed the whole night flashed by in a second for me? Or else have I been buried in the veils of a sleep full of visions?' It is impossible to know.

You seem to feel a well-being and a marvellous lightness of spirit, no fatigue. But as soon as you stand up the aftermath of the intoxication manifests itself. Your weak legs carry you timidly, you are afraid of breaking yourself as though you were a fragile object. A great languor, which is not without its charm, takes over your spirit. You are incapable of work and active energy.

It is a merited punishment for the impious prodigality with which you have spent so much of your nervous energy. You have scattered your personality to the four winds, and now you have difficulty in regathering and concentrating it.

I do not say that hashish produces all the effects I have just described on all men. The phenomena I have described usually took place, with a few exceptions, among people of an artistic and philosophic spirit. But there are temperaments upon which the drug only develops a noisy insanity, a violent gaiety that resembles vertigo, dances, leaps, stamping, bursts of laughter. It can be said that their hashish is entirely materialistic. They are intolerable to those of a spiritual nature, who have great pity for them. The ugliness of their personalities becomes obvious. Once I saw a respectable judge, an honourable man, as people of this type call themselves, one of those men whose artificial gravity is always so imposing, at the moment when the hashish invaded him, suddenly begin to leap around doing a most indecent dance. The true internal monster revealed itself. This man who judged the actions of his fellows, this 'Togatus' had in secret learned how to do the can-can.

Thus it can be affirmed that this impersonal quality, this

objectivity which I previously mentioned and which is only the excessive development of the poetic spirit, will never be found in the hashish of those other people.

Supernaturalist

Gérard de Nerval

The following is taken from Gérard de Nerval's dedication of Les Filles de feu *to Alexandre Dumas. Nerval was one of the founding members of the Club des Hachischins, to which Dumas also belonged. It is interesting that Nerval uses the word 'supernaturalist' to describe the state we moderns call 'high'. This passage was quoted by André Breton in the first Surrealist Manifesto.*

And since you have had the imprudence to cite one of the sonnets composed in that state of day-dreaming the Germans would call *supernaturalist,* you must hear them all. You will find them at the end of the volume. They are hardly more obscure than the metaphysics of Hegel or the 'Memorabilia' of Swedenborg, and would lose their charm by being explained, if such a thing were possible . . .

Morning of Drunkenness

Arthur Rimbaud

O *my* Good! O *my* Beautiful! Atrocious fanfare in which I do not falter! Enchanted rack! Hurrah for the undreamed-of work and for the marvellous body, for the first time! It began with the laughter of children, with their laughter it will end. This poison will remain in all our veins even when, by a turn of the fanfare, we shall be returned to the old disharmony. O may we now, so deserving of these tortures! fervently consummate that superhuman promise made to our created body and soul: that promise, that madness! Elegance, science, violence! We have been promised that the tree of good and evil shall be buried in darkness, that tyrannical respectabilities shall be exiled, so that we may bring here our very pure love. It began with a certain amount of disgust and it ends – we being unable to seize at once this eternity – it ends in a riot of perfumes.

Laughter of children, discretion of slaves, austerity of virgins, horror of the faces and objects of this place, be you made holy by the memory of this vigil. It began in all vulgarity, behold it ends with angels of flame and ice.

Little drunken vigil, holy! if only for the mask you granted us. We affirm you, method! We do not forget that yesterday you glorified each one of our ages. We have faith in the poison. We know how to give our whole life every day.

Now is the time of the ASSASSINS.

VOWELS

A black, E white, I red, U green, O blue: vowels,
Some day I shall tell of your potential incarnations:
A, black corset hairy with shining flies
Which buzz around cruel foul odours,

Gulfs of shadow; E, candours of vapours and of tents,
Lances of proud glaciers, white kings, tremors of flower bells;
I, purple, spat blood, laughter from beautiful lips
In anger or drunk with penitence;

U, cycles, divine vibrations of green seas,
Peace of pastures dotted with animals, peace of the furrows
Which alchemy prints on great studious foreheads;

O, supreme Trumpet-call full of strange urgency,
Silences crossed by Worlds and by Angels;
O the Omega, violet ray of Her Eyes!

Nietzsche's Letter to Peter Gast

Friedrich Würzbach

From Nietzsche's letter to Peter Gast, Torino, 2 December 1888: 'I have just returned from a great concert, which made the strongest impression on me of any concert in my life – my face made grimaces constantly to overcome an extreme feeling of well-being, including for ten minutes the grimaces of tears.'

Biographer's note: If one did not know about the end of Nietzsche, no one would have considered the passage 'my face made grimaces constantly' to be of importance. It often occurs that someone makes grimaces in order to avoid strong emotions being noticed. However, in this context it counts as proof that Nietzsche had taken a drug which causes grimaces, laughing cramps, and gradual loss of self-control. This brings to mind the 'suspect' passage in 'Ecce Homo': 'When one wants to get rid of an insupportable pressure, one needs hashish.'

Nietzsche wants to explain his attitude to Wagner's music by this comparison. Had he therefore tried the action of hashish? His sister had said that Nietzsche received a bottle of a Javanese sedative* from a Dutchman, and that once when he took too much of it he was convulsed with laughing cramps on the floor. As we know, hashish has this effect. If we agree that Nietzsche had taken the poisonous exhilaration of narcotics, let us remember the words of Baudelaire, who described so well the effect of hashish, and who says quite rightly that one will not find anything admirable in hashish intoxication except one's own sharpened nature. Thus we get a Nietzsche with all his natural characteristics of genius strengthened and intensified.

*The Javanese sedative referred to was probably a mixture of hemp with other drugs. Nietzsche had his breakdown on 3 January 1889.

Sitting Bull's Vision of Victory

Stanley Vestal

No one seems to know precisely what herbs, besides the bark of the red willow, went into the mixture Sitting Bull smoked before dancing into a prophetic trance, but hemp may well have been among the ingredients, since it is known to have grown wild in the region where Sitting Bull lived.

Sitting Bull did not spend all his time at councils of war. Horses and guns were needed, of course. But he soon went about something far more vital to his success. One day he loosened the braids of his long hair, removed the feathers from his head, washed off the red paint he habitually wore on his face, and filled his long pipe with tobacco. Then he bound silvery sprays of wild aromatic sage – a sacred plant – about his pipestem. When he was all ready to start, he called his nephew White Bull, his adopted brother Jumping Bull, and the son of his close friend and fellow-chief Black Moon. He asked them to go with him to the top of a butte some distance south of the old camp-site, down-river. The four reached the hilltop about noon.

There Sitting Bull renewed his vow before witnesses. He stood facing the Sun, holding the pipestem upward and wailing for mercy. When he had wailed for a while, he made his prayer: 'My God, save me and give me all my wild game animals. Bring them near me, so that my people may have plenty to eat this winter. Let good men on earth have more power, so that all the nations may be strong and successful. Let them be of good heart, so that all Sioux people may get along well and be happy. If you do this for me, I will perform the sun-gazing dance two days, two nights, and give you a whole buffalo.'

Then all four smoked the pipe in communion, and after Sitting Bull had wiped his face with the sage, set out for camp.

Sitting Bull immediately went hunting. He shot three buffalo. Of these he chose the fattest. Then, with the help of his nephew, he rolled the cow upon her belly, and together they stretched out the legs in four directions to prop it so. The head was stretched out also. Then Sitting Bull stood with raised hands and wailed for pity. Afterwards, he prayed: 'Wakan Tanka, this is the one I offered you awhile back. Here it is.' In this manner he offered the buffalo to God, and made his vow good.

Within a few days, the Sun Dance was begun. Black Moon conducted it, holding the office of Intercessor. Sitting Bull, having vowed the dance, was Chief of the Dancers.

That was a big Sun Dance, well remembered by the Sioux and Cheyennes, scores of whom now living were present. Because of the wonderful prophecy that Sitting Bull made there, and because he vowed the ceremony, it has ever since been known as 'Sitting Bull's Sun Dance'.

All the people – both Sioux and Cheyennes – went into camp in one big circle for the ceremony. The camp was on the west bank of the Rosebud, not far from the carved rocks, where the prehistoric pictures are. There the ceremony began. The virgin cut the sacred tree, the chiefs carried it into the camp circle on poles, as if it had been the body of an enemy. It was dedicated and decorated with its symbols and its offerings. A square 'bed' of ground was smoothed for the altar, a buffalo skull placed thereon, and a pipe set up against the little scaffold before the skull. All the elaborate ritual of the Sun Dance was gone through with. It was all familiar to Sitting Bull: he had danced the Sun Dance many times, and his breast and back bore the scars of the torture. At last it came time for him to fulfil his vow made last autumn – to give his flesh to Wakan Tanka. Naked to the waist, he went forward to the sacred pole.

This time he had decided to give one hundred pieces of flesh – that is to say, skin – from his arms. Jumping Bull had agreed to do the cutting.

Jumping Bull came forward, bringing a sharp steel awl, and a knife ground down to a thin, narrow blade, very sharp. He knelt beside Sitting Bull, who sat leaning back against the sacred pole, his legs straight out on the ground in front of him, and his relaxed arms resting on his thighs. Jumping Bull began at the bottom – near the wrist – of the right arm and worked upwards. He stuck the awl into the skin of the arm, lifted the skin clear of the flesh, and then used the knife. Each time he would cut out a small bit of skin, about the size of the head of a match. Then he would let the skin fall again, withdraw the awl, and begin again just above. Sitting Bull's arm was soon covered with blood.

All the time Jumping Bull was slowly and carefully cutting away on him, Sitting Bull remained perfectly still. He was wailing all the time – not because of the pain – but for mercy to Wakan Tanka, the Great Mysterious. When Jumping Bull had worked up to the top of the right arm and cut out fifty pieces of skin, he then got up and went over to the left side. There he cut in the same manner, beginning at the wrist and working towards the shoulder. Sitting Bull sat there, wailing, never wincing, while that endless piercing, endless cutting went on, cruel and sharp, over and over. Jumping Bull was careful, his hand was sure, he worked as rapidly as he could. But it was a painful ordeal for the half-hour it lasted. White Bull stood looking on. One Bull was dancing. Sitting White Buffalo was pierced at this dance, also. Everybody in camp was looking on.

Having paid his ounce of flesh, it now remained for Sitting Bull to dance the sun-gazing dance. He took his place, and, facing the Sun while the blood ran down his fingers and slowly congealed and closed his wounds, began to bob up and down, staring up towards the Sun. All that day he danced, and that night, and the next day about noon, the crowd noticed that he appeared faint and hardly able to stand.

Black Moon and others took Sitting Bull and laid him down. He was almost unconscious. They threw cold water on him to revive him. His eyes cleared, and he spoke in a low voice to Black Moon. He had had a vision: his offering had been accepted, his prayers were heard.

Black Moon walked out into the middle of the Sun Dance enclosure and called out in a loud voice: 'Sitting Bull wishes to announce that he just heard a Voice from above saying, *"I give you these because they have no ears."* He looked up and saw soldiers and some Indians on horseback coming down like grasshoppers, with their heads down and their hats falling off. They were falling right into our camp.'

Then the people rejoiced. They knew what that meant. Those white men, who would not listen, who made war without just cause, were coming to their camp. Since they were coming upside down, the Indians knew the soldiers would be killed there. The people had what they wanted: Wakan Tanka would care for his own. The Sun Dance was swiftly brought to an end. It was 14 June '76.

Afterwards, Sitting Bull warned the people: 'These dead soldiers who are coming are the gifts of God. Kill them, but do not take their guns or horses. Do not touch the spoils. If you set your hearts upon the goods of the white man, it will prove a curse to this nation.' Twelve lesser chiefs heard this warning, but said nothing. All the people heard of this, but some of them had no ears.

The prophecy, so soon to be fulfilled, fired the Sioux and Cheyennes with martial spirit. Ice and Two Moon, Crazy Horse and Gall, all of them had faith in Sitting Bull, believed in him. They had heard him prophesy before, and nearly always his prophecies came true. Others also divined the future at this camp, and when Custer's troops reached it, ten days later, the Ree scouts found traces of ceremonies that made them tell him, 'The Sioux are sure of winning.'

So long as old-time Indians retain their memories, Sitting Bull's Sun Dance on the Rosebud will never be forgotten. For many years the Sacred Pole where he shed his blood and had his vision of Custer's doom stood on the flat no great distance south of the Northern Cheyenne Reservation. Even after the pole fell, the stump remained, for no Indian would go near the site of a Medicine Lodge – that was holy ground. But at last some white men removed it. And now in the midst of the subdued grandeur of that lovely valley, which Sitting Bull worked so hard to hold his own, the site of that pole is lost beneath the modern motor-road.

Black Elk Speaks of His Great Vision

John Neihardt

Black Elk was a friend of Sitting Bull, and fought beside him. He makes no specific reference to hemp itself, but pipes and herbs of power form an important motif in the theme of his vision.

The next morning the camp moved again, and I was riding with some boys. We stopped to get a drink from a creek, and when I got off my horse, my legs crumpled under me and I could not walk. So the boys helped me up and put me on my horse; and when we camped again that evening, I was sick. The next day the camp moved on to where the different bands of our people were coming together, and I rode in a pony drag, for I was very sick. Both my legs and both my arms were swollen badly and my face was all puffed up.

When we had camped again, I was lying in our tepee and my mother and father were sitting beside me. I could see out through the opening, and there two men were coming from the clouds, head-first like arrows slanting down, and I knew they were the same that I had seen before. Each now carried a long spear, and from the points of these a jagged lightning flashed. They came clear down to the ground this time and stood a little way off and looked at me and said: 'Hurry! Come! Your Grandfathers are calling you!'

Then they turned and left the ground like arrows slanting upwards from the bow. When I got up to follow, my legs did not hurt me any more and I was very light. I went outside the tepee, and yonder where the men with flaming spears were going, a little cloud was coming very fast. It came and stooped and took me and turned back to where it came from, flying fast. And when I looked down I could see my mother and my father yonder, and I felt sorry to be leaving them.

Then there was nothing but the air and the swiftness of the little cloud that bore me and those two men still leading up to where white clouds were piled like mountains on a wide blue plain, and in them thunder beings lived and leaped and flashed.

Now suddenly there was nothing but a world of cloud, and we three were there alone in the middle of a great white plain with snowy hills and mountains staring at us; and it was very still; but there were whispers.

Then the two men spoke together and they said: 'Behold him, the being with four legs!'

I looked and saw a bay horse standing there, and he began to speak: 'Behold me!' he said. 'My life-history you shall see.' Then he wheeled about to where the sun goes down, and said: 'Behold them! Their history you shall know.'

I looked, and there were twelve black horses yonder all abreast with necklaces of bison hoofs, and they were beautiful, but I was frightened, because their manes were lightning and there was thunder in their nostrils.

Then the bay horse wheeled to where the great white giant lives (the north) and said: 'Behold!' And yonder there were twelve white horses all abreast. Their manes were flowing like a blizzard wind and from their noses came a roaring, and all about them white geese soared and circled.

Then the bay wheeled round to where the sun shines continually (the east) and bade me look; and there twelve sorrel horses, with necklaces of elk's teeth, stood abreast with eyes that glimmered like the daybreak star and manes of morning light.

Then the bay wheeled once again to look upon the place where you are always facing (the south), and yonder stood twelve buckskins all abreast with horns upon their heads and manes that lived and grew like trees and grasses.

And when I had seen all these, the bay horse said: 'Your Grandfathers are having a council. These shall take you; so have courage.'

Then all the horses went into formation, four abreast – the blacks, the whites, the sorrels, and the buckskins – and stood behind the bay, who turned now to the west and neighed; and yonder suddenly the sky was terrible with a storm of plunging horses in all colours that shook the world with thunder, neighing back.

Now turning to the north the bay horse whinnied, and yonder all the sky roared with a mighty wind of running horses in all colours, neighing back.

And when he whinnied to the east, there too the sky was filled with glowing clouds of manes and tails of horses in all colours singing back. Then to the south he called, and it was crowded with many coloured, happy horses, nickering.

Then the bay horse spoke to me again and said: 'See how your horses all come dancing!' I looked, and there were horses, horses everywhere – a whole skyful of horses dancing round me.

'Make haste!' the bay horse said; and we walked together side by side, while the blacks, the whites, the sorrels, and the buckskins followed, marching four by four.

I looked about me once again, and suddenly the dancing horses without number changed into animals of every kind and into all the fowls that are, and these fled back to the four quarters of the world from whence the horses came, and vanished.

Then as we walked, there was a heaped up cloud ahead that changed into a tepee, and a rainbow was the open door of it; and through the door I saw six old men sitting in a row.

The two men with the spears now stood beside me, one on either hand, and the horses took their places in their quarters, looking inwards, four by four. And the oldest of the Grandfathers spoke with a kind voice and said: 'Come right in and do not fear.' And as he spoke, all the horses of the four quarters neighed to cheer me. So I went in and stood before the six, and they looked older than men can ever be – old like hills, like stars.

The oldest spoke again: 'Your Grandfathers all over the world are having a council, and they have called you here to teach you.' His voice was very kind, but I shook all over with fear now, for I knew that these were not old men, but the Powers of the World. And the first was the Power of the West; the second, of the North; the third, of the East; the fourth, of the South; the fifth of the Sky; the sixth, of the Earth. I knew this, and was afraid, until the first Grandfather spoke again: 'Behold them yonder where the sun goes down, the thunder beings! You shall see, and have from them my power; and they shall take you to the high and lonely centre of the earth that you may see; even to the place where the sun continually shines, they shall take you there to understand.'

And as he spoke of understanding, I looked up and saw the rainbow leap with flames of many colours over me.

Now there was a wooden cup in his hand and it was full of water and in the water was the sky.

'Take this,' he said. 'It is the power to make live, and it is yours.'

Now he had a bow in his hands. 'Take this,' he said. 'It is the power to destroy, and it is yours.'

Then he pointed to himself and said: 'Look close at him who is your spirit now, for you are his body and his name is Eagle Wing Stretches.'

And saying this, he got up very tall and started running towards where the sun goes down; and suddenly he was a black horse that stopped and turned and looked at me, and the horse was very poor and sick; his ribs stood out.

Then the second Grandfather, he of the North, arose with a herb of power in his hand, and said: 'Take this and hurry.' I took and held it towards the black horse yonder. He fattened and was happy and came prancing to his place again and was the first Grandfather sitting there.

The second Grandfather, he of the North, spoke again: 'Take courage, younger brother,' he said; 'on earth a nation you shall make live, for yours shall be the power of the white giant's wing, the cleansing wind.' Then he got up very tall and started running towards the north; and when he turned towards me, it was a white goose wheeling. I looked about me now, and the horses in the west were thunders and the horses of the north were geese. And the second Grandfather sang two songs that were like this:

> They are appearing, may you behold!
> They are appearing, may you behold!
> The thunder nation is appearing, behold!

> They are appearing, may you behold!
> They are appearing, may you behold!
> The white geese nation is appearing, behold!

And now it was the third Grandfather who spoke, he of where the sun shines continually. 'Take courage, younger brother,' he said, 'for across the earth they shall take you!' Then he pointed to where the daybreak star was shining, and beneath the star two men were flying. 'From them you shall have power,' he said, 'from them who have awakened all the beings of the earth with roots and legs and wings.' And as he said this, he held in his hand a peace pipe which had a spotted eagle outstretched upon the stem; and this eagle seemed alive, for it was poised there, fluttering, and its eyes were looking at me. 'With this pipe,' the Grandfather said, 'you shall walk upon the earth, and whatever sickens there you shall make well.' Then he pointed to a man who was bright red all over, the colour of good and of plenty, and as he pointed, the red man lay down and rolled and changed into a bison that got up and galloped towards the sorrel horses of the east, and they too turned to bison, fat and many.

And now the fourth Grandfather spoke, he of the place where you are always facing (the south), whence comes the power to grow. 'Younger brother,' he said, 'with the powers of the four quarters you shall walk, a relative. Behold, the living centre of a nation I shall give you, and with it many you shall save.' And I saw that he was holding in his hand a bright red stick that was alive, and as I looked it sprouted at the top and sent forth branches, and on the branches many leaves came out and murmured and in the leaves the birds began to sing. And then for just a little while I thought I saw beneath it in the shade the circled villages of people and every living thing with roots or legs or wings, and all were happy. 'It shall stand in the centre of the nation's circle,' said the Grandfather, 'a cane to walk with and a people's heart; and by your powers you shall make it blossom.'

Then when he had been still a little while to hear the birds sing, he spoke again: 'Behold the earth!' So I looked down and saw it lying yonder like a hoop of peoples, and in the centre bloomed the holy stick that was a tree, and where it stood there crossed two roads, a red one and a black. 'From where the giant lives (the north) to where you always face (the south) the red road goes, the road of good,' the Grandfather said, 'and on it shall your nation walk. The black road goes from where the thunder beings live (the west) to where the sun continually shines (the east), a fearful road, a road of troubles and of war. On this also you shall walk, and from it you shall have the power to destroy a people's foes. In four ascents you shall walk the earth with power.'

I think he meant that I should see four generations, counting me, and now I am seeing the third.

Then he rose very tall and started running towards the south, and was an elk; and as he stood among the buckskins yonder, they too were elks.

Now the fifth Grandfather spoke, the oldest of them all, the Spirit of the Sky. 'My boy,' he said, 'I have sent for you and you have come. My power you shall see!' He stretched his arms and turned into a spotted eagle hovering. 'Behold,' he said, 'all the wings of the air shall come to you, and they and the winds and the stars shall be like relatives. You shall go across the earth with my power.' Then the eagle soared above my head and fluttered there; and suddenly the sky was full of friendly wings all coming towards me.

Now I knew the sixth Grandfather was about to speak, he

who was the Spirit of the Earth, and I saw that he was very old, but more as men are old. His hair was long and white, his face was all in wrinkles and his eyes were deep and dim. I stared at him, for it seemed I knew him somehow; and as I stared, he slowly changed, for he was growing backward into youth, and when he had become a boy, I knew that he was myself with all the years that would be mine at last. When he was old again, he said: 'My boy, have courage, for my power shall be yours, and you shall need it, for your nation on the earth will have great troubles. Come.'

He rose and tottered out through the rainbow door, and as I followed I was riding on the bay horse who had talked to me at first and led me to that place.

Then the bay horse stopped and faced the black horses of the west, and a voice said: 'They have given you the cup of water to make live the greening day, and also the bow and arrow to destroy.' The bay neighed, and the twelve black horses came and stood behind me, four abreast.

The bay faced the sorrels of the east, and I saw that they had morning stars upon their foreheads and they were very bright. And the voice said: 'They have given you the sacred pipe and the power that is peace, and the good red day.' The bay neighed, and the twelve sorrels stood behind me, four abreast.

My horse now faced the buckskins of the south, and a voice said: 'They have given you the sacred stick and your nation's hoop, and the yellow day; and in the centre of the hoop you shall set the stick and make it grow into a shielding tree, and bloom.' The bay neighed, and the twelve buckskins came and stood behind me, four abreast.

Then I knew that there were riders on all the horses there behind me, and a voice said: 'Now you shall walk the black road with these; and as you walk, all the nations that have roots or legs or wings shall fear you.'

So I started, riding towards the east down the fearful road, and behind me came the horsebacks four abreast – the blacks, the whites, the sorrels, and the buckskins – and far away above the fearful road the daybreak star was rising very dim.

I looked below me where the earth was silent in a sick green light, and saw the hills look up afraid and the grasses on the hills and all the animals; and everywhere about me were the cries of frightened birds and sounds of fleeing wings. I was the chief of all the heavens riding there, and when I looked behind me, all the twelve black horses reared and plunged and thundered and their manes and tails were whirling hail and their nostrils snorted lightning. And when I looked below again, I saw the slant hail falling and the long, sharp rain, and where we passed, the trees bowed low and all the hills were dim.

Now the earth was bright again as we rode. I could see the hills and valleys and the creeks and rivers passing under. We came above a place where three streams made a big one – a source of mighty waters – and something terrible was there. Flames were rising from the waters and in the flames a blue man lived. The dust was floating all about him in the air, the grass was short and withered, the trees were wilting, two-legged and four-legged beings lay there thin and panting, and wings too weak to fly.

Then the black horse riders shouted 'Hoka hey!' and charged down upon the blue man, but were driven back. And the white troop shouted, charging, and was beaten; then the red troop and the yellow.

And when each had failed, they all cried together: 'Eagle Wing Stretches, hurry!' And all the world was filled with voices of all kinds that cheered me, so I charged. I had the cup of water in one hand and in the other was the bow that turned into a spear as the bay and I swooped down, and the spear's head was sharp lightning. It stabbed the blue man's heart, and as it struck I could hear the thunder rolling and many voices that cried 'Un-hee!', meaning I had killed. The flames died. The trees and grasses were not withered any more and murmured happily together, and every living being cried in gladness with whatever voice it had. Then the four troops of horsemen charged down and struck the dead body of the blue man, counting coup; and suddenly it was only a harmless turtle.

You see, I had been riding with the storm clouds, and had

come to earth as rain, and it was drouth that I had killed with the power that the Six Grandfathers gave me. So we were riding on the earth now down along the river flowing full from the source of waters, and soon I saw ahead the circled village of a people in the valley. And a Voice said: 'Behold a nation; it is yours. Make haste, Eagle Wing Stretches!'

I entered the village, riding, with the four horse troops behind me – the blacks, the whites, the sorrels, and the buckskins; and the place was filled with moaning and with mourning for the dead. The wind was blowing from the south like fever, and when I looked around I saw that in nearly every tepee the women and the children and the men lay dying with the dead.

So I rode around the circle of the village, looking in upon the sick and dead, and I felt like crying as I rode. But when I looked behind me, all the women and the children and the men were getting up and coming forth with happy faces.

And a Voice said: 'Behold, they have given you the centre of the nation's hoop to make it live.'

So I rode to the centre of the village, with the horse troops in their quarters round about me, and there the people gathered. And the Voice said: 'Give them now the flowering stick that they may flourish, and the sacred pipe that they may know the power that is peace, and the wing of the white giant that they may have endurance and face all winds with courage.'

So I took the bright red stick and at the centre of the nation's hoop I thrust it in the earth. As it touched the earth it leaped mightily in my hand and was a rustling tree, very tall and full of leafy branches and of all birds singing. And beneath it all the animals were mingling with the people like relatives and making happy cries. The women raised their tremolo of joy, and the men shouted all together: 'Here we shall raise our children and be as little chickens under the mother prairie hen's wing.'

Then I heard the white wind blowing gently through the tree and singing there, and from the east the sacred pipe came flying on its eagle wings, and stopped before me there beneath the tree, spreading deep peace around it.

Then the daybreak star was rising, and a Voice said: 'It shall be a relative to them; and who shall see it, shall see much more, for thence comes wisdom; and those who do not see it shall be dark.' And all the people raised their faces to the east, and the star's light fell upon them, and all the dogs barked loudly and the horses whinnied.

Then when the many little voices ceased, the great Voice said: 'Behold the circle of the nation's hoop, for it is holy, being endless, and thus all powers shall be one power in the people without end. Now they shall break camp and go forth upon the red road, and your Grandfathers shall walk with them.' So the people broke camp and took the good road with the white wing on their faces, and the order of their going was like this:

First, the black horse riders with the cup of water; and the white horse riders with the white wing and the sacred herb; and the sorrel riders with the holy pipe; and the buckskins with the flowering stick. And after these the little children and the youths and maidens followed in a band.

Second, came the tribe's four chieftains, and their band was all young men and women.

Third, the nation's four advisers leading men and women neither young nor old.

Fourth, the old men hobbling with their canes and looking to the earth.

Fifth, old women hobbling with their canes and looking to the earth.

Sixth, myself all alone upon the bay with the bow and arrows that the First Grandfather gave me. But I was not the last; for when I looked behind me there were ghosts of people like a trailing fog as far as I could see – grandfathers of grandfathers and grandmothers of grandmothers without number. And over these a great Voice – the Voice that was the South – lived, and I could feel it silent.

And as we went the Voice behind me said: 'Behold a good nation walking in a sacred manner in a good land!'

Then I looked up and saw that there were four ascents

ahead, and these were generations I should know. Now we were on the first ascent, and all the land was green. And as the long line climbed, all the old men and women raised their hands, palms forward, to the far sky yonder and began to croon a song together, and the sky ahead was filled with clouds of baby faces.

When we came to the end of the first ascent we camped in the sacred circle as before, and in the centre stood the holy tree, and still the land about us was all green.

Then we started on the second ascent, marching as before, and still the land was green, but it was getting steeper. And as I looked ahead, the people changed into elks and bison and all four-footed beings and even into fowls, all walking in a sacred manner on the good red road together. And I myself was a spotted eagle soaring over them. But just before we stopped to camp at the end of that ascent, all the marching animals grew restless and afraid that they were not what they had been, and began sending forth voices of trouble, calling to their chiefs. And when they camped at the end of that ascent, I looked down and saw that leaves were falling from the holy tree.

And the Voice said: 'Behold your nation, and remember what your Six Grandfathers gave you, for thenceforth your people walk in difficulties.'

Then the people broke camp again, and saw the black road before them towards where the sun goes down, and black clouds coming yonder; and they did not want to go but could not stay. And as they walked the third ascent, all the animals and fowls that were the people ran here and there, for each one seemed to have his own little vision that he followed and his own rules; and all over the universe I could hear the winds at war like wild beasts fighting. (At this point Black Elk remarked: 'I think we are near that place now, and I am afraid something very bad is going to happen all over the world.' He cannot read and knows nothing of world affairs.)

And when we reached the summit of the third ascent and camped, the nation's hoop was broken like a ring of smoke that spreads and scatters and the holy tree seemed dying and all its birds were gone. And when I looked ahead I saw that the fourth ascent would be terrible.

Then when the people were getting ready to begin the fourth ascent, the Voice spoke like some one weeping, and it said: 'Look there upon your nation.' And when I looked down, the people were all changed back to human, and they were thin, their faces sharp, for they were starving. Their ponies were only hide and bones, and the holy tree was gone.

And as I looked and wept, I saw that there stood on the north side of the starving camp a sacred man who was painted red all over his body, and he held a spear as he walked into the centre of the people, and there he lay down and rolled. And when he got up, it was a fat bison standing there, and where the bison stood a sacred herb sprang up right where the tree had been in the centre of the nation's hoop. The herb grew and bore four blossoms on a single stem while I was looking – a blue, a white, a scarlet, and a yellow – and the bright rays of these flashed to the heavens.

I know now what this meant, that the bison were the gift of a good spirit, and were our strength, but we should lose them, and from the same good spirit we must find another strength. For the people all seemed better when the herb had grown and bloomed, and the horses raised their tails and neighed and pranced around, and I could see a light breeze going from the north among the people like a ghost; and suddenly the flowering tree was there again at the centre of the nation's hoop where the four-rayed herb had blossomed.

I was still the spotted eagle floating, and I could see that I was already in the fourth ascent and the people were camping yonder at the top of the third long rise. It was dark and terrible about me, for all the winds of the world were fighting. It was like rapid gunfire and like whirling smoke, and like women and children wailing and like horses screaming all over the world.

I could see my people yonder running about, setting the smoke-flap poles and fastening down their tepees against the wind, for the storm cloud was coming on them very fast and black, and there were frightened swallows without number fleeing before the cloud.

Then a song of power came to me and I sang it there in the midst of that terrible place where I was. It went like this:

> A good nation I will make live.
> This the nation above has said.
> They have given me the power to make over.

And when I had sung this, a Voice said: 'To the four quarters you shall run for help, and nothing shall be strong before you. Behold him!'

Now I was on my bay horse again, because the horse is of the earth, and it was there my power would be used. And as I obeyed the Voice and looked, there was a horse all skin and bones yonder in the west, a faded brownish black. And a Voice there said: 'Take this and make him over'; and it was the four-rayed herb that I was holding in my hand. So I rode above the poor horse in a circle, and as I did this I could hear the people yonder calling for spirit power, 'A-hey! a-hey! a-hey! a-hey!' Then the poor horse neighed and rolled and got up, and he was a big, shiny, black stallion with dapples all over him and his mane about him like a cloud. He was the chief of all the horses; and when he snorted, it was a flash of lightning and his eyes were like the sunset star. He dashed to the west and neighed, and the west was filled with a dust of hoofs, and horses without number, shiny black, came plunging from the dust. Then he dashed towards the north and neighed, and to the east and to the south, and the dust clouds answered, giving forth their plunging horses without number – whites and sorrels and buckskins, fat, shiny, rejoicing in their fleetness and their strength. It was beautiful, but it was also terrible.

Then they all stopped short, rearing, and were standing in a great hoop about their black chief at the centre, and were still. And as they stood, four virgins, more beautiful than women of the earth can be, came through the circle, dressed in scarlet, one from each of the four quarters, and stood about the great black stallion in their places; and one held the wooden cup of water, and one the white wing, and one the pipe, and one the nation's hoop. All the universe was silent, listening; and then the great black stallion raised his voice and sang. The song he sang was this:

> My horses, prancing they are coming.
> My horses, neighing they are coming;
> Prancing, they are coming.
> All over the universe they come.
> They will dance; may you behold them.
> (4 times)
> A horse nation, they will dance. May you behold them.
> (4 times)

His voice was not loud, but it went all over the universe and filled it. There was nothing that did not hear, and it was more beautiful than anything can be. It was so beautiful that nothing anywhere could keep from dancing. The virgins danced, and all the circled horses. The leaves on the trees, the grasses on the hills and in the valleys, the waters in the creeks and in the rivers and the lakes, the four-legged and the two-legged and the wings of the air – all danced together to the music of the stallion's song.

And when I looked down upon my people yonder, the cloud passed over, blessing them with friendly rain, and stood in the east with a flaming rainbow over it.

Then all the horses went singing back to their places beyond the summit of the fourth ascent, and all things sang along with them as they walked.

And a Voice said: 'All over the universe they have finished a day of happiness.' And looking down I saw that the whole wide circle of the day was beautiful and green, with all fruits growing and all things kind and happy.

Then a Voice said: 'Behold this day, for it is yours to make. Now you shall stand upon the centre of the earth to see, for there they are taking you.'

I was still on my bay horse, and once more I felt the riders of the west, the north, the east, the south, behind me in formation, as before, and we were going east. I looked ahead and saw the mountains there with rocks and forests on them, and from the mountains flashed all colours upwards to the heavens. Then I was standing on the highest mountain of them all, and round about beneath me was the whole hoop of the world. (Black Elk said the mountain he stood upon in his vision was Harney Peak in the Black Hills. 'But anywhere is the centre of the world,' he added.) And while I stood there I saw more than I can tell and I understood more than I saw, for I was seeing in a sacred manner the shapes of all things in the spirit, and the shape of all shapes as they must live together like one being. And I saw that the sacred hoop of my people was one of many hoops that made one circle, wide as daylight and as starlight, and in the centre grew one mighty flowering tree to shelter all the children of one mother and one father. And I saw that it was holy.

Then as I stood there, two men were coming from the east, head first like arrows flying, and between them rose the day-break star. They came and gave a herb to me and said: 'With this on earth you shall undertake anything and do it.' It was the daybreak-star herb, the herb of understanding, and they told me to drop it on the earth. I saw it falling far, and when it struck the earth it rooted and grew and flowered, four blos-soms on one stem, a blue, a white, a scarlet, and a yellow; and the rays from these streamed upwards to the heavens so that all creatures saw it and in no place was there darkness.

Then the Voice said: 'Your Six Grandfathers – now you shall go back to them.'

I had not noticed how I was dressed until now, and I saw that I was painted red all over, and my joints were painted black, with white stripes between the joints. My bay had light-ning stripes all over him, and his mane was cloud. And when I breathed, my breath was lightning.

Now two men were leading me, head first like arrows slant-ing upwards – the two that brought me from the earth. And as I followed on the bay, they turned into four flocks of geese that flew in circles, one above each quarter, sending forth a sacred voice as they flew: Br-r-r-p, br-r-r-p, br-r-r-p, br-r-r-p!

Then I saw ahead the rainbow flaming above the tepee of the Six Grandfathers, built and roofed with cloud and sewed with thongs of lightning; and underneath it were all the wings of the air and under them the animals and men. All these were rejoicing, and thunder was like happy laughter.

As I rode in through the rainbow door, there were cheering voices from all over the universe, and I saw the Six Grandfathers sitting in a row, with their arms held towards me and their hands, palms out; and behind them in the cloud were faces thronging, without number, of the people yet to be.

'He has triumphed!' cried the six together, making thunder. And as I passed before them there, each gave again the gift that he had given me before – the cup of water and the bow and arrows, the power to make live and to destroy; the white wing of cleansing and the healing herb; the sacred pipe; the flowering stick. And each one spoke in turn from west to south, explaining what he gave as he had done before, and as each one spoke he melted down into the earth and rose again; and as each did this, I felt nearer to the earth.

Then the oldest of them all said: 'Grandson, all over the universe you have seen. Now you shall go back with power to the place from whence you came, and it shall happen yonder that hundreds shall be sacred, hundreds shall be flames! Behold!'

I looked below and saw my people there, and all were well and happy except one, and he was lying like the dead – and that one was myself. Then the oldest Grandfather sang, and his song was like this:

> There is someone lying on earth in a sacred manner.
> There is someone – on earth he lies.
> In a sacred manner I have made him to walk.

Now the tepee, built and roofed with cloud, began to sway back and forth as in a wind, and the flaming rainbow door was growing dimmer. I could hear voices of all kinds crying from outside: 'Eagle Wing Stretches is coming forth! Behold him!'

When I went through the door, the face of the day of earth

was appearing with the daybreak star upon its forehead; and the sun leaped up and looked upon me, and I was going forth alone.

And as I walked alone, I heard the sun singing as it arose, and it sang like this:

> With visible face I am appearing.
> In a sacred manner I appear.
> For the greening earth a pleasantness I make.
> The centre of the nation's hoop I have made pleasant.
> With visible face, behold me!
> The four-leggeds and two-leggeds, I have made them to walk;
> The wings of the air, I have made them to fly.
> With visible face I appear.
> My day, I have made it holy.

When the singing stopped, I was feeling lost and very lonely. Then a Voice above me said: 'Look back!' It was a spotted eagle that was hovering over me and spoke. I looked, and where the flaming rainbow tepee, built and roofed with cloud, had been, I saw only the tall rock mountain at the centre of the world.

I was all alone on a broad plain now with my feet upon the earth, alone but for the spotted eagle guarding me. I could see my people's village far ahead, and I walked very fast, for I was homesick now. Then I saw my own tepee, and inside I saw my mother and my father bending over a sick boy that was myself. And as I entered the tepee, someone was saying: 'The boy is coming to; you had better give him some water.'

Then I was sitting up; and I was sad because my mother and my father didn't seem to know I had been so far away.

Alice's Adventures in Wonderland

Lewis Carroll

Alice looked all around her at the flowers and the blades of grass, but she could not see anything that looked like the right thing to eat or drink under the circumstances. There was a large mushroom growing near her, about the same height as herself; and when she had looked under it, and on both sides of it, and behind it, it occurred to her that she might as well look and see what was on the top of it.

She stretched herself up on tiptoe, and peeped over the edge of the mushroom, and her eyes immediately met those of a large blue caterpillar, that was sitting on the top with its arms folded, quietly smoking a long hookah, and taking not the smallest notice of her or anything else.

The Caterpillar and Alice looked at each other for some time in silence: at last the Caterpillar took the hookah out of its mouth, and addressed her in a languid, sleepy voice.

'Who are *you*?' said the Caterpillar.

This was not an encouraging opening for a conversation. Alice replied, rather shyly, 'I – I hardly know, sir, just at present – at least I know who I *was* when I got up this morning, but I think I must have been changed several times since then.'

'What do you mean by that?' said the Caterpillar sternly. 'Explain yourself!'

'I can't explain *myself*, I'm afraid, sir,' said Alice, 'because I'm not myself, you see.'

'I don't see,' said the Caterpillar.

'I'm afraid I can't put it more clearly,' Alice replied very politely, 'for I can't understand it myself to begin with; and being so many different sizes in a day is very confusing.'

'It isn't,' said the Caterpillar.

'Well, perhaps you haven't found it so yet,' said Alice; 'but when you have to turn into a chrysalis – you will some day, you know – and then after that into a butterfly, I should think you'll feel it a little queer, won't you?'

'Not a bit,' said the Caterpillar.

'Well, perhaps your feelings may be different,' said Alice; 'all I know is, it would feel very queer to *me*.'

'You!' said the Caterpillar contemptuously. 'Who are *you*?'

Which brought them back again to the beginning of the conversation. Alice felt a little irritated at the Caterpillar's making such *very short* remarks, and she drew herself up and said, very gravely, 'I think you ought to tell me who *you* are, first.'

'Why?' said the Caterpillar.

Here was another puzzling question; and as Alice could not think of any good reason, and as the Caterpillar seemed to be in a *very* unpleasant state of mind, she turned away.

'Come back!' the Caterpillar called after her. 'I've something important to say!'

This sounded promising, certainly: Alice turned and came back again.

'Keep your temper,' said the Caterpillar.

'Is that all?' said Alice, swallowing down her anger as well as she could.

'No,' said the Caterpillar.

Alice thought she might as well wait, as she had nothing else to do, and perhaps after all it might tell her something worth hearing. For some minutes it puffed away without speaking, but at last it unfolded its arms, took the hookah out of its mouth again, and said, 'So you think you're changed, do you?'

'I'm afraid I am, sir,' said Alice; 'I can't remember things as I used – and I don't keep the same size for ten minutes together!'

'Can't remember *what* things?' said the Caterpillar.

'Well, I've tried to say *"How doth the little busy bee"*, but it all came different!' Alice replied in a very melancholy voice.

'Repeat, *"You are old, Father William"*,' said the Caterpillar.

Alice folded her hands, and began: —

'You are old, Father William,' the young man said,
    'And your hair has become very white;
And yet you incessantly stand on your head —
    Do you think, at your age, it is right?'

'In my youth,' Father William replied to his son,
    'I feared it might injure the brain;
But, now that I'm perfectly sure I have none,
    Why, I do it again and again.'

'You are old,' said the youth, 'as I mentioned before,
    And have grown most uncommonly fat;
Yet you turned a back-somersault in at the door —
    Pray, what is the reason of that?'

'In my youth,' said the sage, as he shook his grey locks,
    'I kept all my limbs very supple
By the use of this ointment — one shilling the box —
    Allow me to sell you a couple?'

'You are old,' said the youth, 'and your jaws are too weak
    For anything tougher than suet;
Yet you finished the goose, with the bones and the beak —
    Pray how did you manage to do it?'

'In my youth,' said his father, 'I took to the law,
    And argued each case with my wife;
And the muscular strength, which it gave to my jaw,
    Has lasted the rest of my life.'

'You are old,' said the youth, 'one would hardly suppose
    That your eye was as steady as ever;
Yet you balanced an eel on the end of your nose —
    What made you so awfully clever?'

'I have answered three questions, and that is enough,'
    Said his father; 'don't give yourself airs!

Do you think I can listen all day to such stuff?
   Be off, or I'll kick you down stairs!'

'That is not said right,' said the Caterpillar.

'Not *quite* right, I'm afraid,' said Alice timidly; 'some of the words have got altered.'

'It is wrong from beginning to end,' said the Caterpillar decidedly, and there was silence for some minutes.

The Caterpillar was the first to speak.

'What size do you want to be?' it asked.

'Oh, I'm not particular as to size,' Alice hastily replied; 'only one doesn't like changing so often, you know.'

'I *don't* know,' said the Caterpillar.

Alice said nothing: she had never been so much contradicted in all her life before, and she felt that she was losing her temper.

'Are you content now?' said the Caterpillar.

'Well, I should like to be a *little* larger, sir, if you wouldn't mind,' said Alice: 'three inches is such a wretched height to be.'

'It is a very good height indeed!' said the Caterpillar angrily, rearing itself upright as it spoke (it was exactly three inches high).

'But I'm not used to it!' pleaded poor Alice in a piteous tone. And she thought to herself, 'I wish the creatures wouldn't be so easily offended!'

'You'll get used to it in time,' said the Caterpillar; and it put the hookah into its mouth and began smoking again.

This time Alice waited patiently until it chose to speak again. In a minute or two the Caterpillar took the hookah out of its mouth and yawned once or twice, and shook itself. Then it got down off the mushroom, and crawled away into the grass, merely remarking as it went, 'One side will make you grow taller and the other side will make you grow shorter.'

'One side of *what*? The other side of *what*?' thought Alice to herself.

'Of the mushroom,' said the Caterpillar, just as if she had asked it aloud; and in another moment it was out of sight.

Congo Cult

W. Reininger

The explorer Hermann von Wissmann (1853–1905) visited the Baloubas, a Bantu tribe of the Belgian Congo, as well as the tribes subject to them. He relates that in 1888 Kalamba-Moukenge, the Balouba chief, in order to strengthen the kingdom that he had founded by conquest, and to link together in one cult the diverse subjugated tribes, had the ancient fetishes burned publicly, and replaced the worship of these idols with a new ritual which consisted essentially in the smoking of hashish.

On all important occasions such as holidays, or the conclusion of a treaty or alliance, the Balouba smoke hemp in gourds which may be as much as one metre in circumference. In addition, the men gather each evening in the main square where they solemnly smoke hemp together. But hemp is also used for punishment. The delinquent is compelled to smoke a particularly strong portion until he loses consciousness. The subjects of Kalamba began to smoke hemp with such passion that they ended by calling themselves 'bena-Riamba' (sons of hemp), after the name which this plant has in their language.

A Remedy for the Present

John Addington Symonds

'What is left for us modern men? We cannot be Greek now. The cypress of knowledge springs, and withers when it comes in sight of Troy; the cypress of pleasure likewise, if it has not died already at the root of cankering Calvinism; the cypress of religion is tottering. What is left? Science, for those who are scientific. Art for artists; and all literary men are artists in a way. But science falls not to the lot of all; Art is hardly worth pursuing now. What is left? Hasheesh, I think: Hasheesh of one form or another. We can dull the pangs of the present by living the past again in reveries or learned studies, by illusions of the fancy and a life of self-indulgent dreaming. Take down the perfumed scrolls; open, unroll, peruse, digest, intoxicate your spirit with the flavour. Behold, here is the Athens of Plato in your narcotic visions; Buddha and his anchorites appear; the raptures of St Francis and the fire-oblations of St Dominic; the phantasms of mythologies; the birth-throes of religion, the neurotism of chivalry, the passion of past poems; all pass before you in your Maya world of hasheesh, which is criticism.'

The Herb Dangerous

E. Whineray

Although 'charas' has been properly described as 'a foul and crude drug, the use of which is properly excluded from civilized medicine', it is imported into British India [1909] to the value of 120,000 pounds sterling per annum, a total exceeding the combined value of all the other medicinal imports, so that it is an article which deserves more than passing notice. Indian hemp, when grown in the East, secretes an intoxicating resinous matter on the upper leaves and flowering spikes, the exudation being marked in plants growing throughout the western Himalayas and Turkestan, where charas is prepared as a commercial article. Formerly it was cultivated in fields in Turkestan, but now it is grown as a border around other crops (such as maize), the seeds of both being sown at the same time. A sticky exudation (white when damp and greyish when dry) is found on the upper parts of the plant before the flowers show, and in April and May, when the plants attain a height of four or five feet and the seeds ripen, the cannabis is gathered, after reaping the crops, and stored in a cool, dry place. When dry the powdery resinous substance can be detached by even slight shaking, the dust being collected on a cloth. In some districts the plants are cut close to the roots, suspended head downwards, and the dust or *gard* shaken from them and collected on sheets placed on the floor. The leaves, seeds, etc., are picked out, and sand, etc., separated by passing through a fine sieve, the powder being collected and stored in cloth or skin bags, when it is ready for export. In some villages the charas or extract is made up into small balls, which are collected by the middleman.

On reaching British territory all charas is weighed before the nearest magistrate, by whom it is sealed, a certificate of weight signed by the Deputy Commissioner being given to the owner. The trader, before leaving the district, obtains a permit allowing him to take the drug to a special market. The zamindars of Chinese Turkestan are the vendors of the drug, the importers being Yarkhandis or Ladakhis, who dispose of it at Hoshiapur and Amritsar principally, returning with piece-goods, or Amritsar merchants who trade with Ladakh. The drug in this way reaches the chief cities of the Punjab during September and October. Thence it is distributed over the Central and United Provinces as far as Bombay and Calcutta, and is used everywhere for smoking. Charas, though a drug, plays the part of money to a great extent in the trade that is carried on at Ladakh, the price of the drug depending on the state of the market, and any fluctuations causing a corresponding increase or decrease in the value of the goods for which it is bartered. The exchange price of charas thus gives rise to much gambling. Five years ago the Kashgar growers, encouraged by the high prices, sowed a large crop and reaped a bumper harvest, only to find the market already overstocked and prices on the Leh Exchange fallen from sixty to thirty rupees per maund.

Small quantities of charas are made, chiefly for local consumption, in the Himalayan districts of Nepal, Kumaon, and Garwhal, and in Baluchistan. Samples of Baluchistan charas made in the Sarawan division of the Kalat State have been sent to the Indian Museum by Mr Hughes-Buller.

The following is the mode of preparation:

The female 'bhang' plants are reaped when they are waist high and charged with seed. The leaves and seeds are separated and half-dried. They are then spread on a carpet made of goats' hair, another carpet is spread over them, and slightly rubbed. The dust containing the narcotic principle falls off, and the leaves, etc., are removed to another carpet and again rubbed. The first dust is the best quality, and is known as 'nup'; the dust from the second shaking is called 'tahgalim', and is of inferior quality. A third shaking gives 'gania', of still lower quality. Each kind of dust is made into small balls called 'gabza', and kept in cloth bags. The first quality is recognized by the ease with which it melts.

Small quantities of charas find their way from Tibet into British and Native Garwhal, and a little is prepared in Simla and Kashmir; while other sources are Nepal and the hill districts of Almora and Garwhal. In preparing Nepal charas, the ganja-plant is squeezed between the palms of the hands, and the sticky resinous substance scraped off. 'Momea', black wax-like cakes, valued at ten rupees per seer, and 'Shahjehani', sticks containing portions of leaf, valued at three rupees per seer, are the two kinds of Nepal charas, a few maunds being exported annually to Lucknow and Cawnpore. No charas is made in the plains of India, except a small quantity in Gwalior, the Bengal ganja yielding no charas in all the handling it undergoes in the process of preparation – thus emphasizing the fact that the intoxicating secretion is developed in plants growing where the altitude and climate are suitable, as in the Himalayas and Turkestan.

Adulteration – Aitchison in 1874 stated that no charas of really good quality ever came to Leh, the best charas in the original balls being sent to Bokhara and Kokan. He said the chief adulterant is the mealy covering of the fruits of the wild and cultivated Trebizond date (*Eloeagnus hortensis*). The impression in the United Provinces and the Punjab is that the Yarkhand drug is sophisticated, and a preference is given in some quarters to the Nepal and other Himalayan forms, which command a higher price. The Special Assistant in Kashgar declares there is no advantage in increasing the weight, as when dealers in India buy the drug they test it, otherwise they would pay a heavy duty on the adulterant as well as on the charas itself; so no exporter at present would spoil his charas by adding extraneous substances.

According to Fluckiger and Hanbury, charas yields one fourth to one third of its weight of amorphous resin, and it has been stated that good samples yield 78 per cent of resin. The average yield in the north Indian samples is 40 per cent, the highest being from Kashgar and the lowest from Baluchistan and from Kumaon wild plants, the last-named corresponding to a good sample of ganja.

Captain J. F. Evans, I.M.S., Chemical Examiner to the Government of Bengal, also gave results of his physiological tests in the Indian Hemp Drug Commission's Proceedings for 1893–4. His experiments were made with alcoholic extracts, and only one sample – Amritsar best charas – approached in definite physiological effects the extract, taken as a standard prepared from Bengal ganja. The best Amritsar charas is thirty-two times as potent as the Gwalior product, the latter from plants grown in the plains, while the amount of alcoholic extract bears no relation to the physiological activity of the drug.

Professor Greenish in his well-known work on *Materia Medica* says that *Cannabis indica* is an annual dioecious herb indigenous to central and western Asia, but largely cultivated in temperate countries for its strong fibres (hemp) and its oily seed (hemp-seed) and in tropical countries also for the resinous secretions which it there produces. The secretion possesses very valuable and powerful medicinal properties; but it is not produced in the plant when grown in temperate climates; on the other hand the fibre of the plant under the latter condition is much stronger than that of the tropical plant.

The hemp plant grown in India differs, however, in certain particulars from that grown in Europe; and the plant was formerly considered a distinct species and named *Cannabis indica*, but this opinion is now abandoned.

The cultivation of hemp for its seed and fibre dates from very remote periods. It was used as an intoxicant by the Persians and Arabians in the eleventh and twelfth centuries and probably much earlier, but was not introduced into European medicine until the year 1838. For medicinal use it is grown in the districts of Bogra and Rajshaki to the north of Calcutta and westward, thence through central India to Gujerat. Very good qualities of the drug are purchased in Madras, but the European market is chiefly supplied with inferior grades from Ghalapur.

The pistillate plants by which alone the resin is secreted in any quantity are pruned to produce flowering branches, the tops of these flowering branches are collected, allowed to wilt, and then pressed by treading them under the feet into more or less compact masses. This forms the drug known as 'Aganjah', or (on the London market) Guaza.

The larger leaves are collected separately; when dried they are known as 'bhang'.

During the manipulations to which the plant is subjected in preparing the drug, a certain quantity of the resin is separated; it is collected and forms the drug known as charas. Charas is also prepared by rubbing ganjah between the hands or by men in leather garments brushing against the growing plants, in any case separating part of the active adhesive resin; hence the official description limits the drug to that from which the resin has not been removed.

All these forms of the drug are largely used in India for producing an agreeable form of intoxication; ganjah and charas are smoked, while bhang is used to prepare a drink or sweetmeat.

The drug has a powerful odour, but is almost devoid of taste.

Cannabis indica was formerly used as a hypnotic and anodyne but is uncertain in its action.

It is administered in mania and hysteria as an anodyne and anti-spasmodic.

Mr E. M. Holmes, F.L.S., Curator of the Pharmaceutical Society's Museum, writing on the subject of *Cannabis indica* says 'The Dervishes make a preparation by macerating the resinous type in almond oil and give a small quantity of it in soup to produce prolonged sleep.'

A strong dose of cannabis produces curious hallucinations abolishing temporarily the ideas of time and distance; but the ordinary drug as imported is never the current crop, which the Hindus keep for their own use. The active principle Cannibinol (as far as is known) rapidly oxidizes and loses its properties so that if a really active preparation is required, it is best to get it made in India, using absolute alcohol and the fresh tops, or recently made charas, which, being a solid mass, does not readily oxidize.

Before closing it might be well to notice in detail the final investigations made by Messrs Wood, Spivey, and Easterfield.

The following is reprinted from the *Proceedings of the Chemical Society* for 1897–8, and is to be found on page 66.

'At the beginning of our observations careful search of the literature on the subject was made to determine the toxicity of hemp. Not a single case of fatal poisoning have we been able to find reported, although often alarming symptoms may occur. A dog weighing twenty-five pounds received an injection of two ounces of an active U.S.P. (United States Pharmacopoeia) fluid extract in the jugular vein with the expectation that it would certainly be sufficient to produce death. To our surprise the animal, after being unconscious for about a day and a half, recovered completely. This dog received, not alone the active constituents of the drug, but also the amount of alcohol contained in the fluid extract. Another dog received about seven grammes of solid extract cannabis with the same result. We have never been able to give an animal a sufficient quantity of a U.S.P. or other preparation of the cannabis (indica or americana) to produce death.

'There is some variation in the amount of extractive obtained, as would be expected from the varying amount of stems, seeds, etc., in the different samples. Likewise there is a certain amount of variation in the physiological action, but in every case the administration of 0.01 gramme of the extract per kilo body weight, has elicited the characteristic symptoms in properly selected animals.

'The repeated tests we have made convince us that *Cannabis americana* properly grown and cured is fully as active as the best Indian drug.

'Much has been written relative to the comparative activity of *Cannabis sativa* grown in different climates (*Cannabis indica, mexicana* and *americana*). It has been generally assumed that the American-grown drug was practically worthless therapeutically, and that cannabis grown in India must be used if one would obtain physiologically active preparations.

'Furthermore, it has been claimed that the best Indian drug is that grown especially for medicinal purposes, the part used consisting of the flowering tops of the unfertilized female plants, care being taken during the growth of the drug to weed out the male plants. According to our experience, this is an erroneous notion, as we have repeatedly found that the Indian drug which contains large quantities of seed is fully as active as the drug which consists of the flowering tops only, provided the seed be removed before percolation.

'Several years ago we began a systematic investigation of the American-grown *Cannabis sativa*. Samples from a number of localities were obtained and carefully investigated. From these samples fluid and solid extracts were prepared according to the pharmacopeial method, and carefully tested upon animals for physiological activity, and eventually they were standardized by physiological methods. Repeated tests have convinced us that *Cannabis americana* properly grown and cured is fully as active as the best Indian drug, while on the other hand we have frequently found Indian cannabis to be practically inert.

'Before marketing preparations of *Cannabis americana*, however, we placed specimens of the fluid and solid extracts in the hands of experienced clinicians for practical test; and from these men, all of whom had used large quantities of

Cannabis indica in practice, we have received reports which affirm that they have been unable to determine any therapeutic difference between *Cannabis americana* and *Cannabis indica*. We are, therefore, of the opinion that *Cannabis americana* will be found equally as efficient as, and perhaps more uniformly reliable than *Cannabis indica* obtained from abroad, since it is evident that with a source of supply at our very doors proper precautions can be taken to obtain crude drug of the best quality.

'The proper botanical name of the drug under consideration is *Cannabis sativa*. The Indian plant was formerly supposed to be a distinct species *per se*, but botanists now consider the two plants to be identical. The old name of *Cannabis indica*, however, has been retained in medicine. *Cannabis indica* simply means *Cannabis sativa* grown in the Indies, and *Cannabis americana* means *Cannabis sativa* grown in America. Its introduction into western medicine dates from the beginning of the last century, but it has been used as an intoxicant in Asiatic countries from time immemorial, and under the name of 'hashish', 'bhang', 'ganja', or 'charas' is habitually consumed by upwards of two hundred millions of human beings.

'Cannabis differs from opium in producing no disturbance of digestion and no constipation. The heart is generally accelerated in man when the drug is smoked. Its intravenous injection into animals slows the pulse, partly through inhibitory stimulation and partly through direct action upon the heart muscle. The pupil is generally somewhat dilated. Death from acute poisoning is extremely rare, and recovery has occurred after enormous doses. The continued abuse of hashish by natives of the East sometimes leads to mania and dementia, but does not cause the same disturbance of nutrition that opium does; and the habitual use of small quantities, which is almost universal in some eastern countries, does not appear to be detrimental to health.

'*Cannabis americana* is employed for the same medicinal purposes as *Cannabis indica*, which is frequently used as a hypnotic in cases of sleeplessness, in nervous exhaustion, and as a sedative in patients suffering from pain. Its greatest use has perhaps been in the treatment of various nervous and mental diseases, although it is found as an ingredient in many cough mixtures. In general, *Cannabis americana* can be used when a mild hypnotic or sedative is indicated, as it is said not to disturb digestion, and it produces no subsequent nausea or depression. It is of use in cases of migraine, particularly when opium is contra-indicated. It is recommended in paralysis agitans to quiet the tremors, in spasm of the bladder, and in sexual impotence not the result of organic disease, especially in combinations with nux vomica and ergot.

'The advantages of using carefully prepared solid and fluid extracts of the home-grown drug are apparent when it is considered that every step of the process, from the planting of the drug to the final marketing of the finished product, is under the supervision of experts. The imported drug varies extremely in activity and much of it is inert or flagrantly adulterated.'

The writer desires to acknowledge the able assistance given him in preparing the above notes by Mr E. M. Holmes, F.L.S., and Mr S. Jamieson, M.P.S. (Parke, Davis and Co.).

Part Two

Some High Voices of the Twentieth Century

Each one telling a different story. Multiple versions of a single experience intersect and pinpoint the correspondences, tracing a map of an unknown dimension.

Steppenwolf

Hermann Hesse

'You're ready?' asked Hermine, and her smile fled away like the shadows on her breast. Far up in unknown space rang out that strange and eerie laughter.

I nodded. Oh, yes, I was ready.

At this moment Pablo appeared in the doorway and beamed on us out of his gay eyes that really were animal's eyes except that animal's eyes are always serious, while his always laughed, and this laughter turned them into human eyes. He beckoned to us with his usual friendly cordiality. He had on a gorgeous silk smoking-jacket. His limp collar and tired white face had a withered and pallid look above its red facings; but the impression was erased by his radiant black eyes. So was reality erased, for they too had the witchery.

We joined him when he beckoned and in the doorway he said to me in a low voice: 'Brother Harry, I invite you to a little entertainment. For madmen only, and one price only – your mind. Are you ready?'

Again I nodded.

The dear fellow gave us each an arm with kind solicitude, Hermine his right, me his left, and conducted us upstairs to a small room that was lit from the ceiling with a bluish light and nearly empty. There was nothing in it but a small round table and three easy chairs in which we sat down.

Where were we? Was I asleep? Was I at home? Was I driving in a car? No, I was sitting in a blue light in a round room and a rare atmosphere, in a stratum of reality that had become rarefied in the extreme.

Why then was Hermine so white? Why was Pablo talking so much? Was it not perhaps I who made him talk, spoke, indeed, with his voice? Was it not, too, my own soul that contemplated me out of his black eyes like a lost and frightened bird, just as it had out of Hermine's grey ones?

Pablo looked at us good-naturedly as ever and with something ceremonious in his friendliness; and he talked much and long. He whom I had never heard say two consecutive sentences, whom no discussion nor thesis could interest, whom I had scarcely credited with a single thought, discoursed now in his good-natured warm voice fluently and without a fault.

'My friends, I have invited you to an entertainment that Harry has long wished for and of which he has long dreamed. The hour is a little late and no doubt we are all slightly fatigued. So, first, we will rest and refresh ourselves a little.'

From a recess in the wall he took three glasses, and a quaint little bottle, also a small oriental box inlaid with differently coloured woods. He filled the three glasses from the bottle and taking three long thin yellow cigarettes from the box and a box of matches from the pocket of his silk jacket he gave us a light. And now we all slowly smoked the cigarettes whose smoke was as thick as incense, leaning back in our chairs and slowly sipping the aromatic liquid whose strange taste was so utterly unfamiliar. Its effect was immeasurably enlivening and delightful – as though one were filled with gas and had no longer any gravity. Thus we sat peacefully exhaling small puffs and taking little sips at our glasses, while every moment we felt ourselves growing lighter and more serene.

From far away came Pablo's warm voice.

'It is a pleasure to me, my dear Harry, to have the privilege of being your host in a small way on this occasion. You have often been sorely weary of your life. You were striving, were you not, for escape? You have a longing to forsake this world and its reality and to penetrate to a reality more native to you, to a world beyond time. Now I invite you to do so. You know, of course, where this other world lies hidden. It is the world of your own soul that you seek. Only within yourself exists that other reality for which you long. I can give you nothing that has not already its being within yourself. I can throw open to you no picture-gallery but your own soul. All I can give you is the opportunity, the impulse, the key. I help you to make your own world visible. That is all.'

Again he put his hand into the pocket of his gorgeous jacket and drew out a round looking-glass.

'Look, it is thus that you have so far seen yourself.'

He held the little glass before my eyes (a children's verse came to my mind: 'Little glass, little glass in the hand') and I saw, though indistinctly and cloudily, the reflection of an uneasy, self-tormented, inwardly labouring and seething being – myself, Harry Haller. And within him again I saw the Steppenwolf, a shy, beautiful, dazed wolf with frightened eyes that smouldered now with anger, now with sadness. This shape of a wolf coursed through the other in ceaseless movement, as a tributary pours its cloudy turmoil into a river. In bitter strife, in unfulfilled longing each tried to devour the other so that his shape might prevail. How unutterably sad was the look this fluid inchoate figure of the wolf threw from his beautiful shy eyes.

'This is how you see yourself,' Pablo remarked and put the mirror away in his pocket. I was thankful to close my eyes and take a sip of the elixir.

'And now,' said Pablo, 'we have had our rest. We have had our refreshment and a little talk. If your fatigue has passed off I will conduct you to my peep-show and show you my little theatre. Will you come?'

We got up. With a smile Pablo led. He opened a door, and drew a curtain aside and we found ourselves in the horseshoe-shaped corridor of a theatre, and exactly in the middle. On either side, the curving passage led past a large number, indeed an incredible number, of narrow doors into the boxes.

'This,' explained Pablo, 'is our theatre, an enjoyable theatre. I hope you'll find lots to laugh at.' He laughed aloud as he spoke, a short laugh, but it went through me like a shot. It was the same bright and peculiar laugh that I had heard before from below.

'This little theatre of mine has as many doors into as many boxes as you please, ten or a hundred or a thousand, and behind each door exactly what you seek awaits you. It is a pretty cabinet of pictures, my dear friend; but it would be quite useless for you to go through it as you are. You would be checked and blinded at every turn by what you are pleased to call your personality. You have no doubt guessed long since that the conquest of time and the escape from reality, or however else it may be that you choose to describe your longing, means simply the wish to be relieved of your so-called personality. That is the prison where you lie. And if you were to enter the theatre as you are, you would see everything through the eyes of Harry and the old spectacles of the Steppenwolf. You are therefore requested to lay these spectacles aside and to be so kind as to leave your highly esteemed personality here in the cloak-room where you will find it again when you wish. The pleasant dance from which you have just come, the treatise on the Steppenwolf, and the little stimulant that we have only this moment partaken of may have sufficiently prepared you. You, Harry, after having left behind your valuable personality, will have the left side of the theatre at your disposal, Hermine the right. Once inside, you can meet each other as you please. Hermine will be so kind as to go for a moment behind the curtain. I should like to introduce Harry first.'

Hermine disappeared to the right past a gigantic mirror that covered the rear wall from floor to vaulted ceiling.

'Now, Harry, come along, be as jolly as you can. To make it so and to teach you to laugh is the whole aim of this entertainment – I hope you will make it easy for me. You feel quite well, I trust? Not afraid? That's good, excellent. You will now, without fear and with unfeigned pleasure, enter our visionary world. You will introduce yourself to it by means of a trifling suicide, since this is the custom.'

He took out the pocket-mirror again and held it in front of my face. Again I was confronted by the same indistinct and cloudy reflection, with the wolf's shape encircling it and coursing through it. I knew it too well and disliked it too sincerely for its destruction to cause me any sorrow.

'You will now extinguish this superfluous reflection, my

dear friend. That is all that is necessary. To do so, it will suffice that you greet it, if your mood permits, with a hearty laugh. You are here in a school of humour. You are to learn to laugh. Now, true humour begins when a man ceases to take himself seriously.'

I fixed my eyes on the little mirror, where the man Harry and the wolf were going through their convulsions. For a moment there was a convulsion deep within me too, a faint but painful one like remembrance, or like homesickness, or like remorse. Then the slight oppression gave way to a new feeling like that a man feels when a tooth has been extracted with cocaine, a sense of relief and of letting out a deep breath, and of wonder, at the same time, that it has not hurt in the least. And this feeling was accompanied by a buoyant exhilaration and a desire to laugh so irresistible that I was compelled to give way to it.

The mournful image in the glass gave a final convulsion and vanished. The glass itself turned grey and charred and opaque, as though it had been burnt. With a laugh Pablo threw the thing away and it went rolling down the endless corridor and disappeared.

'Well laughed, Harry,' cried Pablo. 'You will learn to laugh like the immortals yet. You have done with the Steppenwolf at last. It's no good with a razor. Take care that he stays dead. You'll be able to leave the farce of reality behind you directly. At our next meeting we'll drink brotherhood, dear fellow. I never liked you better than I do today. And if you still think it worth your while we can philosophize together and argue and talk about music and Mozart and Gluck and Plato and Goethe to your heart's content. You will understand now why it was so impossible before. I wish you good riddance of the Steppenwolf for today at any rate. For naturally, your suicide is not a final one. We are in a magic theatre; a world of pictures, not realities. See that you pick out beautiful and cheerful ones and show that you really are not in love with your highly questionable personality any longer. Should you still, however, have a hankering after it, you need only have another look in the mirror that I will now show you. But you know the old proverb: "A mirror in the hand is worth two on the wall." Ha! ha!' (again that laugh, beautiful and frightful!) 'And now there only remains one one little ceremony and quite a gay one. You have now to cast aside the spectacles of your personality. So come here and look in a proper looking-glass. It will give you some fun.'

Laughingly with a few droll caresses he turned me about so that I faced the gigantic mirror on the wall. There I saw myself.

I saw myself for a brief instant as my usual self, except that I looked unusually good-humoured, bright and laughing. But I had scarcely had time to recognize myself before the reflection fell to pieces. A second, a third, a tenth, a twentieth figure sprang from it till the whole gigantic mirror was full of nothing but Harrys or bits of him, each of which I saw only for the instant of recognition. Some of these multitudinous Harrys were as old as I, some older, some very old. Others were young. There were youths, boys, schoolboys, scamps, children. Fifty-year-olds and twenty-year-olds played leap frog. Thirty-year-olds and five-year-olds, solemn and merry, worthy and comic, well dressed and unpresentable, and even quite naked, long-haired, and hairless, all were I and all were seen for a flash, recognized and gone. They sprang from each other in all directions, left and right and into the recesses of the mirror and clean out of it. One, an elegant young fellow, leapt laughing into Pablo's arms, embraced him and they went off together. And one who particularly pleased me, a good looking and charming boy of sixteen or seventeen years, sprang like lightning into the corridor and began reading the notices on the doors. I went after him and found him in front of a door on which was inscribed:

ALL GIRLS ARE YOURS
ONE QUARTER IN THE SLOT

The dear boy hurled himself forward, made a leap and, falling head first into the slot himself, disappeared behind the door. Pablo too had vanished. So apparently had the mirror and with it all the countless figures. I realized that I was now left to myself and to the theatre, and I went with curiosity from door to door and read on each its alluring invitation.

Diego Rivera

Errol Flynn

He stood in front of a cactus bush, breathed heavily, remarked that some people wanted him to paint still life. The thought of it provoked more Mexican expletives. He was the most explosive personality I had ever encountered.

'You were talking about the glories of colour. I heard you talking about the colour in my pictures, and you are telling me that colour is more important than what one has to say. What the hell do you know about colour?'

I waited. He asked, 'Can you get emotion out of colour?'

'Yes.'

'More than from music?'

'No.'

'Now, Mr Flynn, I know that you don't know what you're talking about.'

'Señor Rivera, isn't it possible that perhaps I could like both?'

He looked at me as if I were some novice in this area – which I certainly was.

'Now, I will show you something. I want to show you how little you know . . . All right?'

'All right.'

'You see those little potted cacti? You see this one?'

He pointed to where a lovely Mexican flower had closed itself up like a rose with sunset colours, a delicate pastel shade. 'That is how they go to sleep. Amusing, yes?' He said, 'Now watch . . .'

He took the cigarette out of my mouth, put it to the flower.

Sure as hell, the flower opened. 'You see,' he remarked, 'like women. You have to be tough. Rough. Brutal.'

I kept quiet. There was a lot I could still learn about painting, colour, women, and men like Rivera.

'This plant has power,' he said. 'I have carefully cultivated this myself and I take a great deal of pleasure in seeing it growing alongside that convent you keep staring at.'

He seemed to be in a lighter mood as he talked of the plant and he even laughed a bit. He asked, 'Have you ever *heard* a painting?'

'Heard *what*?'

'I said, suppose you looked at a painting and *heard* it play a symphony, would you be surprised?'

I didn't follow.

'Suppose you returned to my studio and you stood in front of one of my paintings and you *heard* it, you heard music coming from the canvas . . .?'

As he talked he moved from one potted plant to the other, fingering them, pressing them fondly, almost caressing them.

He took from a pocket a few sheets of zigzag French paper, the kind of little tissues you use in rolling cigarettes.

'This plant,' he explained, 'will allow you to do both. After smoking this you will see a painting and you will hear it as well.'

It dawned on me that he was rolling in that zigzag paper the 'loco weed' referred to in *The Conquest of Mexico*, the plant called marijuana in Mexico, ganja in Jamaica, anis abiba in other parts of the world, hashish in the Far East.

As he took a puff he said, 'Look, be sure that nobody besides us knows what we are going to do. I will take you up to the storeroom. You will see paintings there I show to nobody else.'

He glanced into the interior of the house, then nudged me in the direction of a side door. We went inside, up a stairs. It was a storeroom for his materials, his paints, canvases, frames. He crossed the room to where there were a couple of big pots of turpentine. He pulled out from under or near them a little can.

The lid opened easily.

I peered in. It contained some brown pulpy material that looked the colour of the bottom end of a cigarette holder.

'You can either chew it or smoke it,' he said. 'This is the same weed the Spanish found here in the fifteenth century. Cortés brought back gold and silver, but he forgot this.'

'I will hear the painting?'

'You will hear the colour!'

The idea of having sounds translated into terms of paintings, and paintings translated into terms of music ... a fascinating idea.

I smoked some of it, ate a little of it.

Diego was talking, observing me. I didn't hear much of what he was saying. I was absorbed, waiting for a reaction.

Suddenly I started to sweat. I could feel my extremities going numb, from the elbow down to the hand, and from the knee down to the foot. Felt a strange sense of touch, yet you wanted to touch things, and if you did there was a numb feeling.

Now I felt paralysed, yet capable of motion.

Over me came the sensation of being suspended in time. All sense of its passage was gone. Everything about me seemed frozen, taut, permanent.

I wasn't certain where we were going, whether among his paintings, or in his garden. Yet we were moving slowly, timelessly. His voice came to me hypnotically. It was getting dark – Mexico – where was I?

I could hear from the convent across the way a girls' choir singing in Latin. Strangely, I could distinguish the peculiar Latin litany. Beyond was the brilliant evening sky, the sun lowering like a great round diver. The pyramids pushed upward into the same red sky. I had the extraordinary feeling that I couldn't cope with this sensation.

Immobile, transfixed, still we were moving, thickly. Once at the studio doorway, looking within, there was a momentary vision: his wife now wore a violently coloured robe off the shoulder, and it swept ankle-length. There was a small red bow at the back of her neck around the fluent length of hair; and then the raven mane dipped downward like a black snake to the cleavage of her buttocks. I stared . . . all was exotic, heightened . . . and Rivera himself stayed close by talking talk that only dimly entered into me.

By now too I lost the sense of balance, which was remarkable for me.

From somewhere came a cry that dinner was ready.

Food! I shouted to the heavens, arms up, singing, imploring, I sip no sup and I crave no cup, while I cry for the love of a ladee!

Rivera was amused at my disabled reactions; he talked on in a Mexicanized English, directing me into a showroom of pictures, his early works, intended, he said, for the Mexican people.

'Here it is quiet,' he suggested. 'Listen to Mexico. Look at my pictures and listen to Mexico . . .'

Whether it was autosuggestion or not, whether it was the suggestive power of a tremendous personality profoundly affecting a young man so much of his time, or whether it was the marihuana – as some will say it was – I heard these pictures singing: the simple Mexican themes, a woman on a mule moving through a field of cacti, the peasants at their labour, in rhythm: illumination and colour and sound in a symphony I could see, feel and hear – but can never translate into words.

No question about it.

Bizarre, I know . . . but I was there.

Island

Aldous Huxley

'What's in a name?' said Dr Robert with a laugh. 'Answer, practically everything. Having had the misfortune to be brought up in Europe, Murugan calls it dope and feels about it all the disapproval that, by conditioned reflex, the dirty word evokes. We, on the contrary, give the stuff good names – the *moksha*-medicine, the reality-revealer, the truth-and-beauty pill. And we know, by direct experience, that the good names are deserved. Whereas our young friend here has no first-hand knowledge of the stuff and can't be persuaded even to give it a try. For him, it's dope and dope is something that, by definition, no decent person ever indulges in.'

'What does His Highness say to that?' Will asked.

Murugan shook his head. 'All it gives you is a lot of illusions,' he muttered. 'Why should I go out of my way to be made a fool of?'

'Why indeed?' said Vijaya with good-humoured irony. 'Seeing that, in your normal condition, you alone of the human race are never made a fool of and never have illusions about anything!'

'I never said that,' Murugan protested. 'All I mean is that I don't want any of your false *samadhi*.'

'How do you know it's false?' Dr Robert inquired.

'Because the real thing only comes to people after years and years of meditation and *tapas* and ... well, you know – not going with women.'

'Murugan,' Vijaya explained to Will, 'is one of the Puritans. He's outraged by the fact that, with four hundred milligrammes of *moksha*-medicine in their bloodstreams, even beginners – yes, and even boys and girls who make love together – can catch a glimpse of the world as it looks to someone who has been liberated from his bondage to the ego.'

'But it isn't real,' Murugan insisted.

'Not real!' Dr Robert repeated. 'You might as well say that the experience of feeling well isn't real.'

'You're begging the question,' Will objected. 'An experience can be real in relation to something going on inside your skull, but completely irrelevant to anything outside.'

'Of course,' Dr Robert agreed.

'Do you know what goes on inside your skull, when you've taken a dose of the mushroom?'

'We know a little.'

'And we're trying all the time to find out more,' Vijaya added.

'For example,' said Dr Robert, 'we've found that the people whose EEG doesn't show any alpha-wave activity when they're relaxed, aren't likely to respond significantly to the *moksha*-medicine. That means that, for about fifteen per cent of the population, we have to find other approaches to liberation.'

'Another thing we're just beginning to understand,' said Vijaya, 'is the neurological correlate of these experiences. What's happening in the brain when you're having a vision? And what's happening when you pass from a pre-mystical to a genuinely mystical state of mind?'

'Do you know?' Will asked.

'"Know" is a big word. Let's say we're in a position to make some plausible guesses. Angels and New Jerusalems and Madonnas and Future Buddhas – they're all related to some kind of unusual stimulation of the brain areas of primary projection – the visual cortex, for example. Just how the *moksha*-medicine produces those unusual stimuli we haven't yet found out. The important fact is that, somehow or other, it does produce them. And somehow or other, it also does something unusual to the silent areas of the brain, the areas not specifically concerned with perceiving, or moving, or feeling.'

'And how do the silent areas respond?' Will inquired.

'Let's start with what they *don't* respond with. They don't respond with visions or auditions, they don't respond with telepathy or clairvoyance or any other kind of parapsychological performance. None of that amusing pre-mystical stuff. Their response is the full-blown mystical experience. You know – One in all and All in one. The basic experience with its corollaries – boundless compassion, fathomless mystery, and meaning.'

'Not to mention joy,' said Dr Robert, 'inexpressible joy.'

'And the whole caboodle is inside your skull,' said Will. 'Strictly private. No reference to any external fact except a toadstool.'

'Not real,' Murugan chimed in. 'That's exactly what I was trying to say.'

'You're assuming,' said Dr Robert, 'that the brain *produces* consciousness. I'm assuming that it transmits consciousness. And my explanation is no more far-fetched than yours. How on earth can a set of events belonging to one order be experienced as a set of events belonging to an entirely different and incommensurable order? Nobody has the faintest idea. All one can do is to accept the facts and concoct hypotheses. And one hypothesis is just about as good, philosophically speaking, as another. You say that the *moksha*-medicine does something to the silent areas of the brain which causes them to produce a set of subjective events to which people have given the name "mystical experience". *I* say that the *moksha*-medicine does something to the silent areas of the brain which opens some kind of neurological sluice and so allows a larger volume of Mind with a large "M" to flow into your mind with a small "m". You can't demonstrate the truth of your hypothesis, and I can't demonstrate the truth of mine. And even if you could prove that I'm wrong, would it make any practical difference?'

'I'd have thought it would make all the difference,' said Will.

'Do you like music?' Dr Robert asked.

'More than most things.'

'And what, may I ask, does Mozart's G Minor Quintet refer to? Does it refer to Allah? Or Tao? Or the second person of the Trinity? Or the Atman-Brahman?'

Will laughed. 'Let's hope not.'

'But that doesn't make the experience of the G Minor Quintet any less rewarding. Well, it's the same with the kind of experience that you get with the *moksha*-medicine, or through prayer and fasting and spiritual exercises. Even if it doesn't refer to anything outside itself, it's still the most important thing that ever happened to you. Like music, only incomparably more so. And if you give the experience a chance, if you're prepared to go along with it, the results are incomparably more therapeutic and transforming. So maybe the whole thing does happen inside one's skull. Maybe it *is* private and there's no unitive knowledge of anything but one's own physiology. Who cares? The fact remains that the experience can open one's eyes and make one blessed and transform one's whole life.' There was a long silence. 'Let me tell you something,' he resumed, turning to Murugan. 'Something I hadn't intended to talk about to anybody. But now I feel that perhaps I have a duty, a duty to the throne, a duty to Pala and all its people – an obligation to tell you about this very private experience. Perhaps the telling may help you to be a little more understanding about your country and its ways.' He was silent for a moment; then in a quietly matter-of-fact tone, 'I suppose you know my wife,' he went on.

His face still averted, Murugan nodded. 'I was sorry,' he mumbled, 'to hear she was so ill.'

'It's a matter of a few days now,' said Dr Robert. 'Four or five at the most. But she's still perfectly lucid, perfectly conscious of what's happening to her. Yesterday she asked me if we could take the *moksha*-medicine together. We'd taken it together,' he added parenthetically, 'once or twice each year for the last thirty-seven years – ever since we decided to get married. And now once more – for the last time, the last, last time. There was a risk involved, because of the damage to the liver. But we decided it was a risk worth taking. And as it turned out, we were right. The *moksha*-medicine – the dope, as you prefer to call it – hardly upset her at all. All that happened to her was the mental transformation.

'Liberation,' Dr Robert began again, 'the ending of sorrow, ceasing to be what you ignorantly think you are and becoming what you are in fact. For a little while, thanks to the *moksha*-medicine, you will know what it's like to be what in fact you are, what in fact you always have been. What a timeless bliss! But, like everything else, this timelessness is transient. Like everything else, it will pass. And when it has passed, what will you do with this experience? What will you do with all the other similar experiences that the *moksha*-medicine will bring you in the years to come? Will you merely enjoy them as you would enjoy an evening at the puppet show, and then go back to business as usual, back to behaving like the silly delinquents you imagine yourselves to be? Or, having glimpsed, will you devote your lives to the business, not at all as usual, of being what you are in fact? All that we older people can do with our teachings, all that Pala can do for you with its social arrangements, is to provide you with techniques and opportunities. And all that the *moksha*-medicine can do is to give you a succession of beatific glimpses, an hour or two, every now and then, of enlightening and liberating grace. It remains for you to decide whether you'll cooperate with the grace and take those opportunities. But that's for the future. Here and now, all you have to do is to follow the mynah bird's advice: Attention! Pay attention and you'll find yourselves, gradually or suddenly, becoming aware of the great primordial facts behind these symbols on the altar.'

Steady Roll

George Andrews

Clint's psyche wriggled through the shining horn. Greet the living jewel of the eye that burns the flesh to ashes, beaming love's light laughter upward to the star where our ancestors dwell. Curves whirl in coils to cluster round the spiral sound that weaves lines of radiant souls into their place in matter. Angels swarm like bees. Drum beats rouse the blood to pulse more freely as the heart pumps wild sounds to the brain. Call down the spirit, gasp for breath, cry out the name. From its nest the eagle comes, its talons clutch my flesh, and we soar into the land of no return. Sing love, sob pain, woe to those who fear. Dance into a trance and see the sun inside the heart, one ray is yours, ride it to the centre of things and stay there, live in it all the time, that spark of light you are born to feed. A rose the colour of the moon sprouts between the eyes, rich in the odour of harmony. I clasp a gold disc in my right hand, a silver crescent in my left, crouched like a cat, coiled like a snake I sit erect, white waves streaming from my skull. Drenched and governed by the source of light, peel off the layers that obscure me, for one glimpse of perfection confers immortality. Liberty in death, a ghost dance for the slave of love who heeds the language of the birds. A phoenix builds its nest of spices. Find the way past the cherubim with the flaming sword and eat of the tree of life. The flower smells of starlight. Orange odours from far away sound very near and shine. The wind fills the bones with thunder. Beyond life and death is the dream. Think all the way back to the egg, not yet touched by sperm, the spirit slumbers in a single cell, unstained by the divisions of desire, both and neither dead nor alive, in need of nothing, alone and passive and infinitely new, pure as the word that makes the worlds, the point in which a circle is a straight line, afloat on the waters of chaos, the source of all my power, before time began and death was born. Dragons are stirring in the night, let us frighten them with toys. I hunt the unicorn, I ride the dolphin's back, I talk with the unborn, have four winds in a sack. Satyr chases nymph around the bowl ancient Greeks drank wine in. Classic beauty eludes the grasp of time. Crouch above the fumes at Delphi, rave to the profane, muse on the fate of mortals. Invoke the spearshaker armed by the gods, tempest-tried inheritor of Merlin's wand. Beneficial rays stream through his eyes, healing ruins, arousing memories of life to come, broadening our knowledge of that ideal world hidden in the imagination. Flee as a bird to the mountain. Voices from the grave show the end of life when the sun goes down and the blood leaves the brain. Make a fog for this trysting hour until the landscape blurs and the dead scamper through our sleep so shamelessly that they are visible to our waking minds. Arise, Osiris! Be thy mouth given unto thee! Triumphant, shout: my heart, my mother! My heart, my coming forth from darkness! The word of a hundred letters resounds in the tomb. The mummy wakes like a bear from its winter sleep.

They walked off the bandstand, got in Can's car, drove to

Gansevoort Street, and walked out to the very end of the pier. They sat with their legs dangling over the water and watched the tugs turn the nose of a tramp steamer downstream as they smoked their atom grass. King had some from the Congo. Euphoria said

– I see a falling star.

Can threw a pebble at a floating grapefruit rind. A liner boomed. There was a fresh breeze. A little vessel beeped. The tramp steamer slipped away in the fog. Clint took a piss off the end of the dock. The river slapped and gurgled against the logs.

– How long must I bear your sewage to the sea?

Clint was somewhat taken aback. As a matter of fact, he was astounded. A talking river? What next? The water sloshed around the wood

– In my depths are too many murdered men.

– River, why do you talk to me?

– The story of the hidden

A sea gull passed between them

– Once my water was clean as the sky. Now I bear the stain of man. In the old days, before they worshipped money, the trout did not turn from my waters in disgust. There were ceremonies performed beside my banks to keep me happy. Henry Hudson should have stayed in bed. Give me back to the Indians. People don't know I have a heart because it beats so fast, almost as fast as stone's.

– I hear my pump, that's the reason I hear yours,

said Clint. The thread thins and frays and breaks, the voice of the water I cease to understand. My flesh is transparent, I see my intestines, my skin is like ice. Clint was incapable of motion as a statue, his body paralysed by the wild flights of his mind. Euphoria snapped her fingers before his eyes, but he was gone. His eyes saw like an X-ray the bones in her fingers and did not respond to them. She caressed his sex and he returned. She danced before him by the light of the moon. It was time to go back to work. As they got out of the car, their extravagant behaviour congealed behind a mask of normalcy. Clint told the doorman

– A Clown is a stone airplane.

A few courageous couples squeezed on to the postage-stamp-sized dance floor. Clint put on his dark glasses. He tried to play his horn and eat a chocolate bar at the same time. He goofed unbearably. There he was, working for a living, an affiliated member of the entertainment industry. The trumpet growled like a lion full of spears. Age-old intensity of jungle heartbreak swims through mud, floundering through turgid depths, all the puzzled pain released in one great thick brooding moan, a snarl gut-full of agony. Play it all night long. Play it for yourself. Do you want to romp, children? Taste these wild oats. Old man grifa. Reefer rising. The Missithinki is in flood. Inhale the paradise plant, exhale the ultimate in absolutes. I and the flow of life are one. I see a flower of marihuana. It is a superb specimen and I am in admiration of its beauty. The flower begins to grow in a strange way: it becomes a face that is neither human nor animal nor insect, yet it resembles all three and is metallic and luminous besides. O God, I am seeing the spirit of the marihuana plant. I see marihuana plants dancing like human beings. Firefoam sceptre, castle in the thunderbolt, treasure of the mountain signals. Spectrum song tastes the odour's touch. Grow insane, feast on the imagination until the reason cracks, shut out entirely the world's intrusion. Beware! Beware! His flashing eyes, his floating hair! Eden exists in each human brain. Awaken the memory of the age of gold. The forbidden tree is the key to the door of the forgotten garden. In the land of the dragon the secret is hidden. Follow the unicorn to its lair. Taste the centre of all suns in this flower from the womb of earth, blossom on the tree of life, fruit forbidden by the jealous god. Seed of endless joy sings euphoria in orgasm. I dissolve into a river of light, swim along the path of the milky way, out the navel of the universe, beyond the stars to my natural home. The flesh of the eater of the sun quivers on a thin point between illumination and annihilation. Deeper than sleep I sink. From far away and with a strange indifference I see my body writhe. I die. My mood changes from black to grey, from grey to purple, turquoise brilliance flares around me, then royal jewel colours in swift snake motion, each scale on the serpent a feathery mountain of diamond purity. All the ordinary objects in my field of vision are aglow with the inhuman and unearthly fire of the endless snake. Blood of other bodies in my bones. I see my dead grandfather. Ancestors awake. Out of a pandemonium of incredible visions Adam comes. Birds the size of trees fly timidly around his head. From me to you is the longest way. In the giant's hand is a dirty egg. There is one spot on the egg that is clean. The voice of the giant thunders that the egg is an image of my soul.

A customer became angry because King refused to play a request number. Clammy Sammy, the boss of the night club, looked up from behind the cash register and frowned.

Clint trumpeted his way back across the border of sanity. Earth's outcast is sky's child. Tearfully I leave this dirty rock, vault through the airless waste to absolute zero, out to regions infernal as a comet's centre, and sink back to the ocean floor where my wounds will heal. A cloud of stars pierces the black wind with a song, each birdnote a crystalline cluster of liquid light, each spark a life, each kiss a cosmic explosion endless as love's rhythm. The priests of Ra go forth in the morning, they wash their hearts with laughter. Burn to find the sound that flings one from the circle. If the eye cannot behold the sun, how can the spirit behold its source, since the brilliance of the sun is only a shadow of the brilliance around which all suns spin. It is said of the perfect that each of his gestures moves all the worlds. A little god made of yellow light comes and sits between the eyes. A great sun with innumerable tiny suns inside, each a different colour spinning in a different direction at a different rate of speed in order to excrete the waste of evil from the system, each little globule an indispensable part of the great organism which will contract into one point composed of what was perfect in each little globule. The little god of yellow light rises from the lotus seat and begins to dance between the eyes. A face without a throat, without a body, the oldest face I have ever seen, no flesh on it, nothing but the skull and skin, never have I seen anything so fragile and so full of life as this Oriental face thousands of years old which flickers on the mental mirror one precious instant and disappears. The brain fills the sky. When East meets West, heaven mates with earth. The nervetree sings of the new flesh, the body made of light that music is the language of. Colours nourishing as mother's milk, not physical but psychic food. Purple flashes on the glimmering green, igniting unscrupulous red and orange rainbows. Wit tweaks the nose of logic. Comedy liberates the inhibited. Candour erases guilt. Elastic egos bounce and recover from the shock of meeting others. Money is the idol it is wiser to die than to worship. Heaven and hell are dreams woven by a lifetime's action in which we are taken like fish in a net. Heaven is the subtlest trap of all because it implies a hell. Light hides the seed of darkness, and darkness hides the seed of light. Find the unity that duality is based on, then find the void that unity is based on. Behind the curtain of fire is the black sun that veils the face of the original light. Chain reaction changes cosmos. A murmur of relief rustles through the marrow of the bones. Bursting stars gem the ocean of silence. The peacock's tail, the leopard skin, the red flower, and the platinum blend into a drop of rain. Night drenches the skull in saffron and musk. A turquoise sun throbs in a golden sky. The heart's tempo smites the temples as I peck my way through the shell of the cosmic egg. Lonelier than the eagle's scream it is to seek the laurel crown. Graveyard lonesome it is to eat of the forbidden tree. Plunge into a trance where the truth that cleaves us to the core and makes us partners is hiding, deep is the chasm into which the mind topples, and the earth closes over me. Dazzling forms ravish the sight, like abstract paintings that not only move but are living creatures. Exquisite shapes there are no words for pass before the eyes. Soak the flesh in wonder. Dissolve back into light. Spectrums expand and contract to the heartbeat. Wild patterns shift in shape to form a gleaming image. Immaculately invulnerable, the multifaced comes from all directions. Lines of clean bright power descend in undulating layers through varying degrees of perfection. Divinity is in humanity like salt is in the sea. Enter vibration, eggborn, become a colour, be a sound, meticulously perform the incredible, connect diverse truths with the thrill of belonging to the one and only tip of the pyramid. The eye that contains all oceans can wash stains from the soul. Concentrate all the energy on a single point, aim that point straight upward, and disappear through it. To die without losing consciousness is to be born wise. The spirit aims for the place in space its actions earned. When the heart is weighed against the feather of truth, one reaps what one has sowed.

They walked off the bandstand. Instead of getting in the car, they strolled over to Washington Square. They sat in the Circle and looked up at the sky. The night was full of drunks festooned in green. One of them leaned against a lamp-post and took a piss. A policeman led him away. Clint got up and walked over to a house near the Square. The others followed him. Clint began throwing gravel at a window.

Pontius Pangloss, the famous psychoanalyst, was deep in his hard-earned slumber. His wife shook him.

– Someone is throwing gravel at our window!

– Oh, no! Not him again!

Light Through Darkness

Henri Michaux

Although written on the subject of mescaline, this also holds true for Indian hemp.

After a brief phase of nausea and discomfort you begin to become particularly aware of light. It proceeds to shine, to strike, to pierce with its rays which suddenly become penetrating. You will perhaps have to shield your eyes under thick layers of fabric, but you yourself are not shielded. The whiteness is in yourself. The sparkling is in your head. A certain part of your head which you can soon feel by its fatigue: the occipital; that is where the white lightning strikes.

Then come visions of crystals, of precious stones, of diamonds or rather their shimmer, their blinding shimmer.

To the excessive stimulation the visual apparatus responds with brilliances, with resplendencies, with excessive colours which shock, harsh, crude colours which form combinations which shock, as your visual cortex is presently shocked and maltreated by the invading poison.

And you come upon multitudes. A host appears, of points, of images, of small forms, which pass very, very very quickly, a too swift passage of *a time which has an enormous crowd of moments*, which streak past prodigiously. *The coexistence of this time* of multiple moments with *normal time*, not wholly vanished, which returns at intervals, only partly obliterated by the attention given to the other, is extraordinary, extraordinarily unreal-izing.

The coexistence, too, of *space having innumerable points* (and all very 'detached') with more or less normal space (the space around you which you look at from time to time), but drowned, as it were, and sub-perceived, is likewise, and, in a parallel way, extraordinary.

And multitude spreads (with speed which is linked to it) in thoughts which nose about dizzyingly, in all directions, in the memory, in the future, in the data of the present, seizing unexpected, luminous, stupefying relationships, which one would like to retain but which the crowd of relationships that follow carries away in hot haste and obliterates from memory.

Multitude in consciousness, a consciousness which spreads until it appears to double, to multiply itself, avid of simultaneous perceptions and knowledge, the better synoptically to observe and embrace the most distant points.

The abnormal excitation radiates. Hyperacuity. The prodigiously present attention, at the height of the possibilities, registers fast and clearly. The separating and evaluating power increases in the eye (which sees the finest reliefs, insignificant lines), in the ear (which hears the slightest sounds from afar, and is hurt by loud ones), in the understanding (observer of unapparent motives, of what lies beneath the surface, of the most remote causes and consequences that ordinarily pass unperceived, of interactions of every kind, too multiple to be grasped simultaneously at other times), finally and above all in the imagination (in which visual images, with unparalleled intensity, crowd out a shrivelled and shrinking reality) and, last but not least, revealing at times to the subject, in the paranormal faculties, the gift of clairvoyance and of divination.

The orchestra of the immense magnified inner life is now prodigious. However agile the mind has become in apprehending on several fronts, you often, all too often, return to the visions which, among all the elusive ones that pass through you, still appear the least elusive. Continuous multitude. Vibratory, zigzagging, in continual transformation. Lines swarm. Here are the cities with a thousand palaces, the palaces with a thousand towers, the halls with a thousand columns about which so much has been said. But the sight is a most trivial one. Tiny columns, much too slender, mere needles which could not support anything. Towers, too many towers, or turrets, rather, graceful, frail, unbelievably slender. Ruins, false trembling ruins. Tangled ornaments (ornaments within the ornament of the ornament) which introduce themselves everywhere even, for example, into a team of runners you were watching and which, unaccountably, forms a ribbon, a serpentine, loops into a series of loops, into endless spirals . . .

At this point of ridiculousness you stop watching the inner show in which nothing corresponds to your tastes. That type of absurdity and a thousand other similar features really do not seem to have their origin in intelligence, even when the latter is turned against itself, even when it is outgoing, but in something which is totally foreign to it, as a piece of mechanism would be. Yet you are seized with a craving to swallow the glue pot, or else the package of steel paper clips, to jump out of the window, to call for help, to kill yourself or to kill someone, but only for a second, and the next again a mad craving, and so the 'yes' and the 'no' pass back and forth, now the one, now the other, without gradations, unpremeditated, with the regularity of a motor piston. You begin to write strings of superlatives which mean nothing. There is a call of the infinite, enormous, all-invading. Why? How? As the wall closes in and recedes rhythmically, and your arm seems to lengthen periodically, there are also gales of unquenchable laughter, which mean nothing either.

Don't forget that you have swallowed poison. Psychological explanations are all too tempting. Tracing everything to psychology is poor psychology.

One phenomenon in mescaline intoxication appears to underline a very large number of what are precisely the most common as well as the most preposterous characteristics.

Ceaselessly, in one form or another, it manifests its presence. This phenomenon is the waves. Is it absurd to think that cerebral waves, which are on the whole slow, become perceptible in certain states of violent nervous hyper-excitation, especially of the visual cortex? New experiments are required in this field, and a more thorough study of encephalograms of subjects in a state of mescaline intoxication.

When people who are unaware of the very existence of cerebral waves speak of waves, of wavelets, of undulations, of oscillations which they see, which they have seen, are we to believe that they are only translating in visual terms an impression of vacillation – an operation which is, in fact, possible, which would not replace the other, but would be additional to it, an example among dozens of parallel, echoing or recall effects which can be observed in drug disturbances?

Why, if they do not have a direct and naked perception of them, could they not experience them obscurely (nearly all mention them; some say they are attacked, submerged by them) and transfer them to different scales and to another frequency, for example to the furniture around them, which they see as shaken by waves. Thus I would sometimes mechanically transfer them to sheets of paper without attaching any great importance to the fact, yet they would nevertheless reflect the oscillatory changes of the various phases of the mescaline disturbance.

So writing, even when it involves taking notes as best 'it' can, also 'renders' the wave and at times produces the very curve of a bristling encephalogram.

As for myself, I perceived slight sinuosities when all went well; great slantwise, whiplash, S-shaped movements when things went badly, before the grave disturbances resembling madness; saw-toothed waves at the beginning of the experiment, when the first violence occurred (at this moment solely in the visual sphere).

Finally I perceived the even, ample, sinusoidal arches and waves, a little before the ecstasies or pseudo-ecstasies.

Here are the different aspects and accidents noticed in the cerebral waves detected up to now, particularly in the alpha waves:

Asymmetry of amplitude, asymmetry of rhythm, total change of rhythm. *High voltage rhythmic paroxysmal outbursts*. Isolated peaks. Multiple peaks. Bifid waves. Sharp waves, strings of waves of *bristling appearance* in the shape of comb-teeth, *saw teeth*. Slow waves. *Slow sinusoidal, hypersynchronous outbursts*.

Laughter. Common to all hallucinogens. The interminable fits of laughter caused by hemp are well known and easily recognizable.

Laughter enables the subject to abandon positions of too great constraint.

With hashish, laughter comes after a kind of sinuosity, extremely relaxed, which is at the same time like a wave, like a tickling and like a shudder and like the steps of a very steep stairway. Sudden releases. The comic comes afterwards. It is not slow in coming. Everything fascinates the imagination. Everything stimulates it, and immediately it begins to embroider, to fabulate, to place and to displace. One thing leading to another, there is then an interminable succession of bursts of laughter, cascades of release which release nothing at all, and the laughter, ever racing, after a moment's halt to get its breath, starts off again, impossible to satiate. Laughter on conveyor belts. Laughter without any subject for laughter. Subjects are found at the beginning. Thereupon the imagination wearies but laughter goes on running.

Like the mad laughter of certain lunatics, it particularly expresses the prodigious absurdity of everything, both metaphysically and (by the tickling) very physically felt, felt in an extraordinary conjunction.

The infinite in mescaline. Its characteristics: Sense of the infinite, *of the presence of the infinite*, of the proximity, of the immediacy, of the penetration of the infinite endlessly passing through the finite. An infinite on the march, with an even step which will never stop, which can never stop. The cessation of the finite, of the mirage of the finite, of the illusory conviction that anything finite, concluded, terminated, arrested exists. The finite, whether prolonged or broken up, taken off guard by a crossing, overflowing, magnificent infinite, annulling and dissipating everything that is 'circumscribed', which can no longer exist. An infinity which no longer allows you to finish with anything whatever, which sets off in infinite series, which is infinity which becomes modulated into an infinization which no finite can escape, where pettiness itself, reobserved, is immediately prolonged, deepened, loses itself and infinizes itself, decircumscribes itself, in which any subject, and mood, emotion or sentiment takes the path of the stupefying and ever so natural infinite. An obsessive, vexatious infinite which rules out everything but itself, return to itself, passage through itself. An infinite which alone is, which rhythm is. If the rhythm is majestic, the infinite will be divine. If the rhythm is hurried, the infinite will be persecution, anguish, fragmentation, maddening, ceaseless re-embarking from here to further on, further, further, further, further, further, further, further, further, forever far from any haven. An infinite infinizing everything, but wonderfully attuned, more than to any other sentiment, to goodness, tolerance, mercifulness, acceptance, equality, pardon, patience, love and universal *compassion*.

Would anyone dare speak here of waves? Yes and even of a certain wave. A genius is after all nourished by vitamins and animal flesh and sustained by hormones. Is it so scandalous that what is most immaterial in matter should contribute to sustaining the sense of the infinite? 'Peyote helps to worship,' one of the addicts has said. The wave that helps to worship. He who has taken mescaline has taken a bowl of vibrations, that is what he has taken and what now possesses him. Helped by his exaltation, may he establish in himself the best wave, the one which by its wonderful inhabitual regularity, and by its fullness, lifts and gives majestic importance, a wave which is a support for the infinite, its sustenance, its litany.

The impression of prolongations, of persistence, of fascination, by inhabitual repetition which you don't get rid of, a certain rambling, the sinuous track of a continuation within yourself which hypnotizes, also appear to come from the sweeping wave. Faith by vibratory path.

Alternation. Oscillation in ideas, desires.

Characteristics of this alternation: First an example: if, in mescaline intoxication, you feel the urge to see someone and no longer to remain alone, no sooner has it appeared than this urge seems to be snapped up by an immaterial grip tugging in opposite directions. Fifty times in a single minute you pass from 'I'm going to call him' to 'No, I won't call him', to 'Yes, I'm calling him,' to 'No, I'm not calling him,' etc.

This alternation is not intellectual. It is not a matter of judgement. You are absolutely no further ahead after fifty about-faces than after the first. Nothing has ripened. You are no closer to a decision. The arguments for or against have had no chance to appear, even less to develop. You have experienced, like so many physical thrusts, fifty impulses in one direction, and as many in the other (or were they cessations of impulses?).

Of these alternate impulses, one is totally 'for' without a trace of 'against' or of 'doubtful' (and always full of impetuosity). Thrusting you into the 'for' and the other perfectly against, or at least cancelling out the other, leaving you without urge, without the slightest trace of an urge, in perfect repose (and, with no reason, absolutely over the urge that was so extreme an instant before).

Only the final result is ambivalent. Never do the two impulses appear together, in a picture containing them both, in a harmonious or unharmonious combination. That seems impossible, contrary to nature. The impulses appear as separate, successive, without the slightest trace of combination.

It is difficult not to think of an oscillatory drive, of an imposed drive ... of a wave strong in amplitude and voltage, whose frequencies rule out an effective functioning of the mind. The least that one can imagine is a periodic phenomenon affecting the nervous cell, like a more rapid succession of polarizations and depolarizations.

Is duality always present, is consciousness an oscillatory state, creating antagonism of which the present state is but the acceleration and the amplification, but such that the system no longer functions, a suitable choice being no longer possible?

The duality is in this case fanatical and its two poles equal in the mind's judgement. At one moment you see the usual aspect, the next moment the bad, perverse, incorrect aspect. The one, and then the other. Without their ever combining. The perverse side, then the pure side, then the perverse one (perverse acts, perverse reflexes, the hidden impulses), then again the pure or the correct, or the normal which is perhaps but the cessation of the perverse. An absolute non-mixing. A diabolical clairvoyance.

By itself alone, the mechanical phenomenon of oscillation (once amplified and accelerated) may be a disaster. The contradictory passages break one's courage to live, break the will. Certain oscillating passages are such as not even to permit an image to form, to subsist, to permit an idea to maintain itself, to come intact. Waves so intolerable that they have led lunatics who were subject to them to jump out of the window, to put an end to that infernal serpent without thickness, which prevented them from thinking and pushed them to thinking, which detached and attached and detached them without end, without end. By committing suicide they put an end to it. Craze-inducing waves.

While the normal state is a combination, an examination and a mastery of antagonistic pulsions and views, while the state created by the drug or by a mental disease is oscillation with total succession and separation of the antagonistic pulsions and opposed points of view, there is a *third state*, which is without alternation, as well as *without combination,* in which consciousness in unparalleled totality reigns *without the slightest antagonism.* Ecstasy (whether cosmic, or of love, or erotic, or diabolic). Without an extreme exaltation one cannot enter into it. Once in it, all variety disappears in what appears an independent universe. Ecstasy and ecstasy alone opens the absolutely without mixture, the absolutely uninterrupted by the slightest opposition or impurity which is the least allusively, other. A pure universe, of a total energizing homogeneity in which the absolutely of the same race, of the same sign, of the same orientation, lives together, and in abundance.

That, and only that is 'the great venture', and little then does it matter whether or not a wave helps this autonomous universe, in which a rapture, comparable to nothing that is of this world, holds you lifted, beyond mental laws, in a sea of felicity.

The animation of the scene under the influence of hemp deserves a special examination. It is not increased in the same proportion as the lighting, the colouring, the smells. No. It stands out among these, even though these have acquired a new and exalted status. Its increase-intensification is incomparable. This vividness itself carries you away into another realm. Almost all who have used hemp have encountered it many, many times. For myself, in the visionary scenes I have experienced, there have occurred thousands of bursts, splashes, explosions, jets, flights. Hemp shoots, hurls, darts, scatters, bursts, erupts, whether in the whole (which is more rare) or, disconcertingly, in only a small part of the vision where its filiform dash is all the more surprising, more vehement, more ardent. With stupefaction you witness those sporadic eruptions, thin, mad fountains, those jets of water, more jet than water, bursts primarily, punctiform excesses of forces, delirious spectacle of inner geyserization, signs of the prodigious increase in the potential of the neurons, of their sudden nervous discharges, signs of hurried releases, of micro-movements, of beginnings of movements, of 'budding movements' and of incoercible, incessant micro-impulses, which in the case of some subjects end up by provoking a maniacal agitation.

Hashish is the travel of the poor. You are particularly offered the 'materials'. By their rejuvenation I was often able to recognize the first sign of the effect of hashish, by their sudden importance emphasized without apparent reason, almost detaching themselves from vision. Sandstone, schist (which I ordinarily pay no attention to), slag, skin, a bacon rind, would appear as they would to a geologist or a craftsman. Deep-napped carpets, horse's or sheep's hooves, and also the granular, the prickly, the bumpy, the woody, the wrinkled, the porous, the knotty, the moist also and the hollow, the elbowed, all this comes to you 'as in nature'. Hashish is a paradise by sensations, by the 'elementaries'.

Unlike mescaline, which provides solely visual visions, or thoughts which are translated into pure visualizations, much more intense it is true, corresponding to a view of specialists (landscape painters, or portraitists), hashish furnishes, better even than reality, the casing of impressions concomitant to sight, furnishes a feast of them.

The garden which appears to you in inner vision will not be solely composed of touches of colour, far from it.

This garden will be before you, or around you, with its potentialities, its proposals of movements, of pleasures. With your tactile imagination overexcited, you are there as though ready to pluck, to walk, to turn, to stoop down, to slide, to climb a hummock, to approach a terrace, to move away from it and, though motionless, you are at the feast of 'participation'. The garden – a real garden, therefore, and not a coloured residue of a garden – exhales its temptations for you. You are surrounded by them.

Isolated sensations are at times furiously revived. Holding the photograph of a street in Rotterdam in my hand, all at once I had to fling it away from me, as I was suddenly overcome by the reek of herring, and the detested, unendurable taste of *rollmops* forgotten for thirty-five years was there again intact in my mouth and I could not get rid of it. I would not have tasted it better if I had really had a piece on my tongue.

> *Am lifted*
> *elevation*
> *extreme elevation.*

The impression of one's body lifting is one of those which everywhere and by all have been the most generally felt. And odd levitation, by spurts, but so marked that from time to time one verifies if one is not up in the air. The first nomads who in the Persian or Arabian deserts used hemp, stretched out on carpets, felt themselves lifted, unable to get down, carried afar. How many of those flying carpets have taken to the air in the course of luminous oriental nights! This illusion is not for us; nevertheless ascension remains one of the adventures of the hemp smoker. This power establishes itself so discreetly, however, so outside the range of consciousness (quite different from the impression of lightness, more mental, more abstract) that it can happen that one notices it only through the intermediary of a photograph, in which one suddenly finds oneself *en rapport* with what appears most elevated in it, by virtue of a wholly new preference for peaks, summits, roofs, the tops of trees, the tallest chimneys, the rocks from which, having (mentally) alighted on them inadvertently, one has the greatest difficulty getting down, caught by the malice of the hemp which has lifted you and keeps you there.

Having taken some one day, on the beach of Arcachon, to see what would happen out in the open, I found myself all at once at a good altitude, climbing, fast, fast, fast, behind a football which had been sent sky-high by an athlete's powerful kick. I followed behind, in swift ascent, having clung to it as soon as I had perceived it, like iron to a magnet. It was altogether extraordinary. I had become a strange aeronaut of a new kind. The descent was far from being as remarkable. The other beach games did not strike me as being greatly modified. The beach was swarming with people without being really transformed for me, except here and there, by those sudden rises 'behind' balls which periodically pulled me up into the air.

Those instantaneous altitudes always take one by surprise. One ought to be able to foresee them better. One rarely succeeds.

The modulations, indeed, which 'hemp' is able to achieve from such neutral beginnings are so astounding, so wondrous, so demonstrative of its superhuman power, so luminous, that no metaphysical brain, even with the most magnificent idea, could equal them. Meaning either contrasting or coupled almost to infinity and in a minute space of time, lightning parentheses: there is no greater miracle of the 'grasping' intellect. Thus it is not surprising that these prodigious 'exchanges' have given many a drug addict, even among the most mediocre, a somewhat exalted idea of his intelligence. No one, in fact, has a greater density of ideas than they do at certain moments, nor is capable of more unexpected associations of ideas – of which they subsequently have not the slightest recollection.

NOW LED BY THE HEMP NOW LEADING IT

The session of intimacy

It had been three years or more since I had experimented with hemp, going back to it reluctantly at long intervals, convinced that I was missing something, when one day, perhaps a little less impatient than usual, I discovered what thousands upon thousands of persons, in the Orient, have known and more or less practised for ages. It was quite simple, and it *is* quite simple, and it can be taught in five minutes to a novice. I was, then, looking at some reproductions of paintings and at some photographs. One of these was a portrait of a woman. I was about to pass on to another when she ... became alive. Yes, she was alive. In my home. There beside me. She stayed. I had just discovered the hashish paradise, about which so much has been written, which has relations with Mohammed's paradise for the use of the simple-minded, father relations. There must of course have been something other than hallucinations or visions for people of all kinds to have enjoyed it for so long, in all countries.

The woman, then, showed no sign of leaving, developed her life before me, a vibrant life, an immediate life, a life linked to my company. The impossible *living together* was becoming a reality on the spot with miraculous ease. This secret of secrets was an open secret, in which any number of men in several countries of Asia and Africa had found bliss, of which they had made a habit, their paradise on earth. With perfumes, bells, with crudely suggestive daubings the absent one could be made to appear surrounded by birds in enchanting gardens, she could be made to dance, and the sordid shack or the ill-smelling tent became filled with the grace of the houris, of their arms, their bosoms, their utterly natural presence. They came to the tryst. They arrived irresistibly, accepting *to be with* — with anyone, so long as he used the powder that has power.

Ah! if I had had this faculty in the natural state! If the capacity had been given to me to bring persons to life instantly before me at the mere sight of their photograph!

This present power I needed to verify. One has all too great a tendency to illusion, when it comes to women. I must therefore now try a man. Let's see this photo. A prolonged gaze ... and the man comes. Neither faster nor less fast than the woman. Let us increase the difficulty. This group of three now. I look. It works. The first, the second, the third. They are there. No, they are here. I go from one to another. They continue to live, to communicate among themselves, with me present. Not too fascinating, the company of those three fellows, moulded by politics and vulgar ambition. Out with them! A few more tests on groups, a few others on isolated individuals, on men of different appearance, of different ages, of different types and, having established the proof, I come back to the first person observed.

I look at her. She comes back. She comes back without any reluctance. She comes back automatically. I find her again. She hardly moves. And does she even move? She moves on the spot. She vibrates. Her eye, her mouth, this or that part of her face which I look at, as if caught up in an imponderable, almost psychic haze, or oscillation, or subtle balancing, becomes animated, not really moving, but able to move, having perhaps just moved, having been able to take advantage of a moment of inattention to move. You feel ever on the point of catching her having moved, having frankly smiled, having markedly bowed her head to one side to cast a sidelong glance, having really turned round to burst out laughing. An extraordinary and indefinable animation, of which no actress on this planet is capable. A kind of psychic trembling, so fine it is, so perfectly does fineness suit it (this is why women's faces, the most beautiful, the most harmonious, are so completely pre-adapted to it), incapable of leading to crudeness, attuned only to the vibrant, the radiant, gradations of fineness which would be lost in the theatre and are meant for intimacy. The same minute variation, endless and mysterious, which produces visions of fabulous cities with slender towers and the iridescent palaces of Kubla Khan, indefinitely different and alike, makes this moving face vary, indefinitely, makes it reform and become other.

How many expressions the infinitely variant can convert into life! If the woman has a simple, naïve face, she will radiate simplicity, if her face is mocking, she will be ravishingly mocking, if witty, she will radiate wit, if it expresses goodness, her goodness will radiate, will be convincing, if it is sensual, her sensual impregnation will be magnetizing, if she is pure, she will be adorable, angelic, yes, she will be an angel perhaps better than anything, for she irradiates. The beyond, in her, radiant, transpires . . . and renews itself.

For modulation is probably the most extraordinary character. This face is in movement, in fluid movements, an admirable screen on which inscriptions of sentiments appear and vanish, on which new inscriptions tirelessly recur. She is in movement. Her life, her soul, a miraculous company. The stream of moments, the stream of emotions with its alterations, its micro-alterations (for an emotion, a sentiment, is but an average, an average of outpourings, of impulses, of impressions, of inclinations or of distastes felt, drops and particles of the emotional flow that is in you, vibrant, trembling, with multiple currents and eddies), this stream, then, which constantly turns, which changes affectively every second, which you are unable to see in yourself, this stream you do see in those paradisiacal moments, before you, on the moving face, in unbelievably delicate alterations, which lovers would like to and cannot make out on the loved faces. There they are, the variations are no longer concealed from you, pass under her skin, like a naked body beneath a transparent chiffon. An endless screw. A life continued continuously, whose instants, however, are 'distinguished', detached, like words spelled out by a child but fast, fast, fast, following lovingly in a vertigo of passionate attention.

Deciphering faces

Deliberately leaving aside faces capable of seduction, those women's faces unfailingly transmuted by a yearning which definitely persists in us for a lifetime to the day of our death, I began to look at the faces of men, and of unprepossessing men. Faces which I have no desire to be surrounded by or to have turn up in my house, faces which I want to understand, to penetrate. No more closed faces which tell me nothing, or very little. I enter them. They would ordinarily be hostile to me. Perfect. I have to exert myself for three or four seconds and then . . . I penetrate and I am inside them. I seem to know them. If I were to meet them later in a gathering I should, it seems to me, make no psychological blunder with them. I already know them. I have entered their capital, whence they direct and feel and practise their lives. When I am affected by hashish, and by this investigating mood, I aim at them, I aim at their centre.

Nothing vague subsists before me. They have become expressive. I open them. I explore them. When I can make no further substantial progress in the understanding of a head (at times of a body), I put it aside, I draw aside and pass to another, to which I force entry in a few seconds and at once make for the essential, for what then manifestly appears his centre of strength, of control, the centre from which his decisions and his actions spring. I am in his current. Everyone has certain areas on which his body more particularly balances and which he uses as take-off points for a leap, energy-distribution centres, crossroads of force components, bases of confidence, of assurance, of certainty, locus of the dominants of his constitution, all of which form a point of departure for his impulses to action and his releases of tension. This is it with which I am in syntony – for the moment (which explains why no one then can be antipathetic to me, since in his force, with his force, I feel and sense his impulses which I must inevitably at least excuse).

I think I have found his focal point. But on becoming normal again, hesitant and somewhat resistant, I have lost it. Yet I thought I had found it so completely that it would remain unforgettable to me. I was wrong. I can no longer find it. I therefore took to marking those centres with a cross or several crosses, as best I could, during the observation under the effect of the hashish, with the directions and the approximate depth (for these psychic axes and these lines of departure must be apprehended in depth). More or less in vain. Sober, I was confronted with the discovery that each head had again become an obstacle, an enigma, an uncertainty, his present inner self no longer superimposing itself upon his previously divined inner self had become a head which I now opposed. To be sure, this very opposition, special and appropriate to each, enlightened me in its own way as to the person, as to the possible relations between him and me, a not negligible but reduced understanding, with which I had to content myself. There would be no penetration for me before the next dose of hashish. What was this clairvoyance worth, if such it was? Others, more gifted, could study it with greater profit.

Reading while under the influence of hashish

After an average dose of hashish one is unfit for reading. This is well known. Even a literary text can be followed only with difficulty ... followed at the same pace line after line. Nevertheless I have found hashish to be an admirable detector. Some of the greatest authors of literature and of mystical theology have not resisted its 'penetration' for a minute. You can hear the authors in person, they are no longer imposing, or ever so little. You met them as certain cool-headed men, meeting them during their lifetime, must have gauged them and estimated them. You have them in their natural state. Words no longer play any part. The man who is behind them comes out in front. You immediately perceive his limitless conformity, his tepidity, and his tiny audacities, his prudence, the slightness of his ventures into imprudence, the enormous pocket of his ignorance, on which was applied a thin film of personality and of personal reflection. Everything or nearly everything about the man is unconsciousness, surface efforts and self-satisfaction. A highly revered saint is suddenly shown me. What a disappointment! No doubt she has devoted herself, worked, made progress. She still had a long way to go. Garrulous dame that she was, she proved to be nothing but a lightweight. I shall never be taken in by her again. Others, rare wonders, have something to say to you, are really behind their words, which are true, without emphasis. What a joy (of too short duration)! Ramana Maharshi was one of these surprises.

There is matter here for future study. The text, at whatever point you pick it up, becomes a voice, the very voice that suits it, and the man speaks behind this voice. The one who wrote it is there, of little substance as he was, no longer given solidity by the printed character, he is there again, immediately engaged in thinking, in expressing himself, finding his way among his ideas. He begins over again. An end of abstractness, of vagueness. The man behind his name comes with his weight, his lack of weight.

Treacherous hashish, hashish as hunting dog, instructive hashish. It sees quicker than we do, pointing to what we have not yet understood. At the outset, and each time, there is an effort to be made. Which is the reason why it has not been used to this end. It is doing violence to the hashish-smoker to call upon him to make an effort just when by letting himself go he can experience so many wonders. He has to force himself to make the contact, to maintain it, to pierce through. But once the contact has been made in depth, what an experience!

One day when during one of these moments I was looking at a study in a review having a very limited, almost secret, circulation, the study by an erudite young philosopher, I heard something that sounded like the murmur of crowds gathered to listen to these words! Well, well! The sentence, even when later I read it cold, philosophic though it appeared, was a model of the kind of false thinking that is trying for effect, a sentence that could never come from the pen of one who had not caressed the idea of multiple approbations and ... of appearing on a platform.

Thus, by virtue of a succession of short circuits, I heard the applause with which this writer had felt himself surrounded, having without the slightest doubt sought it. The rest of the article showed in several places that he was not a man to content himself solely with ideas (ideas thereby invalidated despite their metaphysical and difficult appearance). Presently, though he was still soft-pedalling this ambition, his projects, it was clear that it was acclaim which would interest him in ten years, having an audience right up in front and reacting immediately. Hashish opens the inner space of sentences, and the concealed preoccupations come out, it pierces them at once. It is curious that this hashish, when I used it to test a few authors, never proved vain, or eccentric. Set at the quarry, it never faltered. It was diligent as a falcon. The author thus unmasked never altogether recovered his mantle or his former retreat.

Marihuana and Sex

Alexander Trocchi

Experts agree that marihuana has no aphrodisiac effect, and in this as in a large percentage of their judgements they are entirely wrong. If one is sexually bent, if it occurs to one that it would be pleasant to make love, the judicious use of the drug will stimulate the desire and heighten the pleasure immeasurably, for it is perhaps the principal effect of marihuana to take one more intensely into whatever experience. I should recommend its use in schools to make the pleasures of poetry, art, and music available to pupils who, to the common detriment of our civilization, are congenitally or by infection insensitive to symbolic expression. It provokes a more sensual (or aesthetic) kind of concentration, a detailed articulation of minute areas, an ability to adopt play postures. What can be more relevant in the act of love?

Kif – Prologue and Compendium of Terms

Paul Bowles

One of the great phenomena of the century is the unquestioning world-wide acceptance of the accessories of Judaeo-Christian civilization, regardless of whether or not these trappings have any relevance to the peoples adopting them. The United Nations, like a philanthropical society devoted to reclaiming and educating young delinquents, points the way grandly for the little nations just recruited, assuring them that they too one day may be important and respected members of world society. Political schisms do not really exist. Whether the new ones study Marx or Jefferson, the destructive impact on the original culture is identical. It would seem that the important task is to get them into the parade, now that they have been convinced that there is only the one direction in which they can go. Once they are marching too, they will appreciate more fully how far ahead of them we are. These are *faits accomplis*; in the future it will be fascinating to watch the annihilation of the entire structure of Judaeo-Christian culture by these 'underprivileged' groups which, having had only the most superficial contacts with that culture, nevertheless will have learned enough thereby to do a thorough job of destroying it.

If you are going to sit at table with the grown-ups, you have to be willing to give up certain childish habits that the grown-ups don't like: cannibalism, magic, and all the other facets of 'irrational' religious observances. You must eat, drink, relax and make love the way the grown-ups do, otherwise your heart won't really be in it; you won't truly be disciplining yourself to become like them. One of the first things you must accept when you join the grown-ups' club is the fact that the Judaeo-Christians approve of only one out of all the substances capable of effecting a quick psychic change in the human organism – and that one is alcohol. The liquid is sacred in the ceremonies of both branches of the Judaeo-Christian religion. Therefore all other such substances are taboo. But since you are forsaking your own culture in any case, you won't mind giving up the traditional prescriptions for relaxation it provided for you; enthusiastically you will accept alcohol along with democratic (or communist) ideology and the gadgets that go with it, since the sooner you learn to use these things, the sooner you can expect to be patted on the head, granted special privileges, and told that you are growing up – fulfilling your destiny, I think they sometimes call it. This news, presumably, you find particularly exciting.

And so the last strongholds fashioned around the use of substances other than alcohol are being flushed out, to make everything clean and in readiness for the great alcoholic future. In Africa particularly, the dagga, the ganja, the bangui, the kif, as well as the dawamesk, the sammit, the majoun and the hashish, are all on their way to the bonfires of progressivism. They just don't go with pretending to be European. The young fanatics of the four corners of the continent are furiously aware of that. They are, incidentally, also aware that a population of satisfied smokers or eaters offers no foothold to an ambitious demagogue. The crowd pleasantly heated by alcohol behaves in a classical and foreseeable fashion, but you can't even get together a crowd of smokers : each man is alone and happy to stay that way. (Then, too, there is the fact to be considered that once one gets power, one can regulate the revenue on alcohol, and sit back to count one's take. The other substances don't lend themselves so easily to efficient governmental racketeering.)

Cannabis, the only serious world-wide rival to alcohol, reckoned in millions of users, is always described in alcoholic countries as a 'social menace'. And the grown-ups mean just that. They don't infer that it's detrimental to the health or welfare of the individual who uses it, since for them the individual separated from his social context is an irregularity to be remedied, in any case. No, they mean that the user of cannabis is all too likely to see the truth where it exists, and to fail to see it where it does not. Obviously few things are potentially more dangerous to those interested in prolonging the *status quo* of organized society. If people refuse to play the game of society at all, of what use are they? How can they be enticed or threatened, save by the ultimately unsatisfactory device of brute force? No, no, there are no two ways about it: society has got to go on being played (and quietly directed); alcohol is the only safe substance to allow human beings, and everything else must go.

In spite of the Madison Avenue techniques being applied to the launching of campaigns in praise of the new millennium, old cultures do not lie down and die merely because they are told to. They have to be methodically killed, and that takes a certain time. Deculturizing programmes have to be arranged, resettlement projects undertaken, rehabilitation camps set up and filled, and all this in each place before the party in power is superseded by an enemy party, which in Africa often means very soon indeed. It is not astonishing, then, that the drive to standardization should have proven to be a bumpy one and that, now, there should be geographical pockets on the continent where all kinds of anachronisms are the temporary norm. There is still bangui in the Congo precisely because the region has not yet been successfully unified and steam-rollered by the grown-ups' pets; the hillsides of South Africa are still covered with dagga because no organized group has had the time to uproot it; kif is still widely smoked in Morocco because the forces which would otherwise be being used to suppress the practice are too busy tracking down illicit arms and black-market currency. There is so much the African progressives find themselves unable to do that this complaint might almost seem premature, were it not for the fact that their eventual success is guaranteed: they are implemented by all the technology of the Judaeo-Christian world.

The terms expounded below have nothing esoteric about them; they are as much a part of the everyday vocabulary in North Africa as words like chaser, neat or soda are in the United States, with the difference that over the centuries cannabis has played a far more important part in shaping the local culture than alcohol has with us. The music, the literature, and even certain aspects of the architecture, have evolved with cannabis-directed appreciation in mind.

In the wintertime a family will often have a 'hashish evening': father, mother, children and relatives shut themselves in, eat the jam prepared by the womenfolk of the household, and enjoy several hours of stories, song, dance and laughter in complete intimacy. 'To hear this music you must have kif first', you are sometimes told, or: 'This is a kif room. Everything in it is meant to be looked at through kif.' The typical kif story is an endless, proliferated tale of intrigue and fantasy in which the unexpected turns of the narrative line play a far more decisive role than the development of character or plot.

Quite apart from the intimate relationship that exists between cannabis and the cultural and religious manifestations of both Moslem and animist Africa, there exists also the explicit proscription of alcohol in the Koran's accompanying Hadith. The moral (and often the legal) codes of Moslem countries are based solely upon Koranic law. The advocated switch to alcohol can cause only moral confusion in the mind of the average Moslem citizen, and further lower his respect for the authorities responsible for it.

CHQAF (plural chqofa). The L-shaped bowl, generally made of baked clay, which fits the end of the pipe-stem and holds the kif. The diameter of the bowl's opening is about a quarter of an inch. In the throat, at the angle, is a tiny uvula upon which the chqaf's efficacy depends. In order to avoid damaging this, smokers never clean their chqofa when they get clogged with tar, but put them into the fire until they are burned out. The chqaf breaks with great ease, usually as it is being fitted on to the stem. Attempts have been made to obviate this by fashioning chqofa of metal (a failure, since no one will use them) and of stone. In Taroudant there are artisans who carve excellent ones out of a translucent soapstone; these have the advantage of enabling the smoker to see just how far down his ash has burned in the bowl. The only objection to these is that they cost roughly twenty times as much as the clay ones.

CORREDOR (northern Morocco). A small-time kif retailer who sells to cafés and acquaintances. Never has a large quantity on hand.

DJIBLI. Third-grade kif, grown in the lowlands. The plant attains a great height, but is short on cannabin. There are two categories of djibli kif: hameimoun, considered slightly better because it is at least able to cause hunger, and the ordinary – the harsh, cheap kif sold to tourists.

HACHICH. The word has various meanings. First, it is a

blanket term for all parts of the kif plant save the small top
leaves. In the preparation of good smoking kif, these small
leaves are the only part used. At least two thirds of the plant
is discarded. Large, dried or damaged leaves, flowers, seeds
and stalks are all rejected. The term is also used to refer to
candy made by boiling these unusable parts with water and
sugar. This is the poor man's majoun. You can buy two pounds
of it for a quarter of a dollar. (Xauen, 1960.) True hashish,
made with the pollen of the flower, is not commercially available in North Africa. The word *m'hachiyich* indicates the state
of mind induced by having eaten the candy.

JDUQ JMEL (known in northern Morocco as QOQA). Tiny
snail-shaped seeds, available at the magic stalls of Marrakech
and other cities, which are sometimes used to intensify the
active properties of edible kif preparations, and even on occasion in kif for smoking. Popular belief holds that too many
seeds can cause permanent mental derangement.

KETAMI. Adjective derived from the place-name Ketama,
a town in the western Rif, centre of a large kif-growing district.
It is still legal to grow the plant here, since it is the only crop
that can be grown on the steep mountainsides. In other words,
it can be grown but not transported. As soon as it leaves the
vicinity of Ketama the chase is on; if the shipment gets through
the blockade, it reaches the consumer directly, by the normal
channels. If it is captured by the authorities, the route to the
consumer is of necessity more circuitous. Fines are levied according to quantity seized. Several thousand people of the
area depend for their livelihood upon its cultivation. Ketama,
at an altitude of about five thousand feet, supplies all of Morocco with its first-grade kif, and the word ketami is a synonym
of the best.

KHALDI. Second-grade kif, grown in the mountains around
Beni Khaled, which although in the Rif lies at a lower altitude
and thus produces a somewhat inferior smoking leaf.

KIF. The *Cannabis sativa* plant of northern Africa and the
Middle East. (The cannabis of east Africa, south-east Asia and
the Americas is of a stronger and less subtle flavour.) Also the

small leaves of the plant, chopped to a coarse, slightly greasy, greyish-green powder for smoking.

KSESS. The cutting of the kif. No matter how good the quality of the raw material, if the cutter does not know his business, the result cannot be the desired one. It takes roughly eight hours of steady hard work for a professional to cut a pound of finished kif properly. The cutter has the marks of his trade emblazoned in callouses on his fingers.

MAJOUN. Literally, jam, but universally understood to be jam containing cannabis. There are almost as many procedures for making majoun as there are people who make it, but the ingredients are more or less standard: kif, honey, nuts, fruit and spices in varying proportions.

MKIYIF. The state of the individual who has smoked enough kif to feel its effect clearly. (Usually followed by the phrase *ma ras* plus the proper pronomial suffix.)

MOTTOUI. Leather pouch for kif. There are always at least two compartments in a mottoui, and sometimes as many as four. A different grade goes into each compartment. If you know A well and watch him offer kif to B, you can tell the degree of his esteem for B by the kif he gives him to smoke. The ceremonial facets of kif smoking are fast disappearing as persecution of the custom increases. Good mottouis are no longer made, and the average worker now carries his kif in a small tin box, or, even more abject, in the paper in which he purchased it.

MSOUSS. Kif which has not a sufficient quantity of tobacco blended with it is described by this adjective (as are unsweetened or partially sweetened tea or coffee). Kif is never smoked neat, the popular belief being that kif msouss is bound to give the smoker a headache.

NABOULA. A cured sheep's bladder for storing kif. Glass and metal are not considered as efficacious for preserving the highly volatile preparation. The naboula, tightly tied at the neck, is truly hermetic, and the kif kept in it remains as fresh as the day it was packed.

NCHAIOUI. A man whose entire life is devoted to the preparation, smoking and appreciation of kif.

RHAITA. The datura flower. A square inch of the petal dropped into the teapot is enough to paralyse five or six people, particularly in combination with kif. (Generally added by the host without the knowledge of his guests.)

SBOULA. The unit by which kif is sold wholesale. A sboula comprises a dozen or more stalks tightly tied together. Stalks are about eight inches long.

SEBSI (plural SBASSA). The stem of the kif pipe. A few decades ago the sebsi was commonly, anywhere, from sixteen to twenty-four inches long, and usually came in two parts that could be coupled to make the pipe. The recent tendency has been to make them increasingly shorter, so that they can be pocketed as swiftly as possible under adverse conditions. The elaborately carved sebsi is becoming a thing of the past; nowadays they are often simple wooden tubes. The variety of wood determines the quality of the sebsi. Olive and walnut are considered good, run-of-the-mill materials, although there are still numerous recherché varieties to be found by the connoisseur in the interior of Morocco. There are sebsi stalls in the public markets of most towns.

SMINN. Rancid butter, preferably aged for a year or longer, which when mixed with kif makes an unpleasant-tasting but powerful and cheap substitute for majoun.

ZBIL. The residue of stalks, leaves, seeds and flowers which is thrown out after the small leaves have been extracted. The foreigner is always appalled the first time he sees this great quantity of what elsewhere would be considered perfectly good material being tossed into the fire. In cafés it is chopped up and used by unscrupulous corredores to hoodwink the ingenuous foreigner. Moslems refuse to smoke it.

ZREYA. The uncrushed seeds of the kif plant, sold until recently in pharmacies and apothecary shops as a culinary adjunct.

He of the Assembly

Paul Bowles

*He salutes all parts of the sky and the earth where it is bright.
He thinks the colour of the amethysts of Aguelmous will be
dark if it has rained in the valley of Zerekten. The eye wants to
sleep, he says, but the head is no mattress. When it rained for
three days and water covered the flat-lands outside the ramparts, he slept by the bamboo fence at the Café of the Two
Bridges.*

It seems there was a man named Ben Tajah who went to Fez
to visit his cousin. The day he came back he was walking in the
Djemaa el Fna, and he saw a letter lying on the pavement. He
picked it up and found that his name was written on the envelope. He went to the Café of the Two Bridges with the letter
in his hand, sat down on a mat and opened the envelope. Inside was a paper which read: 'The sky trembles and the earth
is afraid, and the two eyes are not brothers.' Ben Tajah did not
understand, and he was very unhappy because his name was on
the envelope. It made him think that Satan was near by. He of
the Assembly was sitting in the same part of the café. He was
listening to the wind in the telephone wires. The sky was almost
empty of daytime light. 'The eye wants to sleep,' he thought,
'but the head is no mattress. I know what that is, but I have
forgotten it.' Three days is a long time for rain to keep falling
on flat bare ground. 'If I got up and ran down the street,' he
thought, 'a policeman would follow me and call to me to stop.
I would run faster, and he would run after me. When he shot at
me, I'd duck around the corners of houses.' He felt the rough
dried mud of the wall under his fingertips. 'And I'd be running
through the streets looking for a place to hide, but no door
would be open, until finally I came to one door that was open,

and I'd go in through the rooms and courtyards until finally I came to the kitchen. The old woman would be there.' He stopped and wondered for a moment why an old woman should be there alone in the kitchen at that hour. She was stirring a big kettle of soup on the stove. 'And I'd look for a place to hide there in the kitchen, and there'd be no place. And I'd be waiting to hear the policeman's footsteps, because he wouldn't miss the open door. And I'd look in the dark corner of the room where she kept the charcoal, but it wouldn't be dark enough. And the old woman would turn and look at me and say: "If you're trying to get away, my boy, I can help you. Jump into the soup-kettle."' The wind sighed in the telephone wires. Men came into the Café of the Two Bridges with their garments flapping. Ben Tajah sat on his mat. He had put the letter away, but first he had stared at it a long time. He of the Assembly leaned back and looked at the sky. 'The old woman,' he said to himself. 'What is she trying to do? The soup is hot. It may be a trap. I may find there's no way out, once I get down there.' He wanted a pipe of kif, but he was afraid the policeman would run into the kitchen before he was able to smoke it. He said to the old woman: 'How can I get in? Tell me.' And it seemed to him that he heard footsteps in the street, or perhaps even in one of the rooms of the house. He leaned over the stove and looked down into the kettle. It was dark and very hot down in there. Steam was coming up in clouds, and there was a thick smell in the air that made it hard to breathe. 'Quick!' said the old woman, and she unrolled a rope ladder and hung it over the edge of the kettle. He began to climb down, and she leaned over and looked after him. 'Until the other world!' he shouted. And he climbed all the way down. There was a rowboat below. When he was in it he tugged on the ladder and the old woman began to pull it up. And at that instant the policeman ran in, and two more were with him, and the old woman had just the time to throw the ladder down into the soup. 'Now they are going to take her to the commissariat,' he thought, 'and the poor woman only did me a favour.' He rowed around in the dark for a few minutes, and it was very hot. Soon he took off his clothes. For a while he could see the round top of the kettle up above, like a port-hole in the side of a ship, with the heads of the policemen look-ing down in, but then it grew smaller as he rowed, until it was only a light. Sometimes he could find it and sometimes he lost it, and finally it was gone. He was worried about the old woman, and he thought he must find a way to help her. No policeman can go into the Café of the Two Bridges because it belongs to the Sultan's sister. This is why there is so much kif smoke inside that a berrada can't fall over even if it is pushed, and why most customers like to sit outside, and even there keep one hand on their money. As long as the thieves stay inside and their friends bring them food and kif, they are all right. One day police headquarters will forget to send a man to watch the café, or one man will leave five minutes before the other gets there to take his place. Outside everyone smokes kif too, but only for an hour or two – not all day and night like the ones inside. He of the Assembly had forgotten to light his sebsi. He was in a café where no policeman could come, and he wanted to go away to a kif world where the police were chasing him. 'This is the way we are now,' he thought. 'We work back-wards. If we have something good, we look for something bad instead.' He lighted the sebsi and smoked it. Then he blew the hard ash out of the chqaf. It landed in the brook beside the second bridge. 'The world is too good. We can only work forward if we make it bad again first.' This made him sad, so he stopped thinking, and filled his sebsi. While he was smoking it, Ben Tajah looked in his direction, and although they were facing each other, He of the Assembly did not notice Ben Tajah until he got up and paid for his tea. Then he looked at him because he took such a long time getting up off the floor. He saw his face and he thought: 'That man has no one in the world.' The idea made him feel cold. He filled his sebsi again and lighted it. He saw the man as he was going to go out of the café and walk alone down the long road outside the ramparts. In a little while he himself would have to go out to the souks to try and borrow money for dinner. When he smoked a lot of

kif he did not like his aunt to see him, and he did not want to
see her. 'Soup and bread. No one can want more than that.
Will thirty francs be enough the fourth time? The qahaouaji
wasn't satisfied last night. But he took it. And he went away
and let me sleep. A Moslem, even in the city, can't refuse his
brother shelter.' He was not convinced, because he had been
born in the mountains, and so he kept thinking back and forth
in this way. He smoked many chqofa, and when he got up to
go into the street he found that the world had changed.

Ben Tajah was not a rich man. He lived alone in a room near
Bab Doukkala, and he had a stall in the bazaars where he sold
coat-hangers and chests. Often he did not open the shop because he was in bed with a liver attack. At such times he poun-
ded on the floor of his bed, using a brass pestle, and the postman who lived downstairs brought him up some food. Sometimes he stayed in bed for a week at a time. Each morning and
night the postman came in with a tray. The food was not very
good because the postman's wife did not understand much
about cooking. But he was glad to have it. Twice he had
brought the postman a new chest to keep clothes and blankets
in. One of the postman's wives a few years before had taken
a chest with her when she had left him and gone back to her
family in Kasba Tadla. Ben Tajah himself had tried having a
wife for a while because he needed someone to get him regular
meals and to wash his clothes, but the girl was from the mountains, and was wild. No matter how much he beat her she
would not be tamed. Everything in the room got broken, and
finally he had to put her out into the street. 'No more women
will get into my house,' he told his friends in the bazaars, and
they laughed. He took home many women, and one day he
found that he had en noua. He knew that was a bad disease,
because it stays in the blood and eats the nose from inside.
'A man loses his nose only long after he has already lost his
head.' He asked a doctor for medicine. The doctor gave him a
paper and told him to take it to the Pharmacie de l'Étoile.
There he bought six vials of penicillin in a box. He took them

home and tied each little bottle with a silk thread, stringing them so that they made a necklace. He wore this always around his neck, taking care that the glass vials touched his skin. He thought it likely that by now he was cured, but his cousin in Fez had just told him that he must go on wearing the medicine for another three months, or at least until the beginning of the moon of Chouwal. He had thought about this now and then on the way home, sitting in the bus for two days, and he had decided that his cousin was too cautious. He stood in the Djemaa el Fna a minute watching the trained monkeys, but the crowd pushed too much, so he walked on. When he got home he shut the door and put his hand in his pocket to pull out the envelope, because he wanted to look at it again inside his own room, and be sure that the name written on it was beyond a doubt his. But the letter was gone. He remembered the jostling in the Djemaa el Fna. Someone had reached into his pocket and imagined his hand was feeling money, and taken it. Yet Ben Tajah did not truly believe this. He was convinced that he would have known such a theft was happening. There had been a letter in his pocket. He was not even sure of that. He sat down on the cushions. 'Two days in the bus,' he thought. 'Probably I'm tired. I found no letter.' He searched in his pocket again, and it seemed to him he could still remember how the fold of the envelope had felt. 'Why would it have my name on it? I never found any letter at all.' Then he wondered if anyone had seen him in the café with the envelope in one hand and the sheet of paper in the other, looking at them both for such a long time. He stood up. He wanted to go back to the Café of the Two Bridges and ask the qahaouaji: 'Did you see me an hour ago? Was I looking at a letter?' If the qahaouaji said: 'Yes,' then the letter was real. He repeated the words aloud. 'The sky trembles, and the earth is afraid, and the two eyes are not brothers.' In the silence afterwards the memory of the sound of the words frightened him. 'If there was no letter, where are these words from?' And he shivered because the answer to that was: 'From Satan.' He was about to open the door when a new fear stopped him. The qahaouaji might say: 'No,' and this would be still worse, because it would mean that the words had been put directly into his head by Satan, that Satan had chosen him to reveal Himself to. In that case He might appear at any moment. 'Ach haddou laillaha ill'Allah ...' he prayed, holding his two forefingers up, one on each side of him. He sat down again and did not move. In the streets the children were crying. He did not want to hear the qahaouaji say: 'No. You had no letter.' If he knew that Satan was coming to tempt him, he would have that much less power to keep him away with his prayers, because he would be more afraid.

He of the Assembly stood. Behind him was a wall. In his hand was the sebsi. Over his head was the sky, which he felt was about to burst into light. He was leaning back looking at it. It was dark on the earth, but there was still light up there behind the stars. Ahead of him was the pissoir of the Carpenters' Souk which the French had put there. People said only Jews used it. It was made of tin, and there was a puddle in front of it that reflected the sky and the top of the pissoir. It looked like a boat in the water. Or like a pier where boats land. Without moving from where he stood, He of the Assembly saw it approaching slowly. He was going toward it. And he remembered he was naked, and put his hand over his sex. In a minute the rowboat would be bumping against the pier. He steadied himself on his legs and waited. But at that moment a large cat ran out of the shadow of the wall and stopped in the middle of the street to turn and look at him with an evil face. He saw its two eyes and for a while could not take his own eyes away. Then the cat ran across the street and was gone. He was not sure what had happened, and he stood very still looking at the ground. He looked back at the pissoir reflected in the puddle and thought: 'It was a cat on the shore, nothing else.' But the cat's eyes had frightened him. Instead of being like cat's eyes, they had looked like the eyes of a person who was interested in him. He made himself forget he had had this thought. He was still waiting for the rowboat to touch the landing pier, but nothing had happened. It was going to stay where it was, that near the shore but not near enough to touch. He stood still a long time, waiting for something to happen. Then he began to walk very fast down the street toward the bazaars. He had just remembered that the old woman was in the police station. He wanted to help her, but first he had to find out where they had taken her. 'I'll have to go to every police station in the Medina,' he thought, and he was not hungry any more. It was one thing to promise himself he would help her when he was far from land, and another when he was a few doors from a commissariat. He walked by the entrance. Two policemen stood in the doorway. He kept walking. The street curved and he was alone. 'This night is going to be a jewel in my crown,' he said, and he turned quickly to the left and went along a dark passageway. At the end he saw flames, and he knew that Mustapha would be there tending the fire of the bakery. He crawled into the mud hut where the oven was. 'Ah, the jackal has come back from the forest!' said Mustapha. He of the Assembly shook his head. 'This is a bad world,' he told Mustapha. 'I've got no money,' Mustapha said. He of the Assembly did not understand. 'Everything goes backwards,' he said. 'It's bad now, and we have to make it still worse if we want to go forwards.' Mustapha saw that He of the Assembly was nkiyif ma rassou and was not interested in money. He looked at him in a more friendly way and said: 'Secrets are not between friends. Talk.' He of the Assembly told him that an old woman had done him a great favour, and because of that three policemen had arrested her and taken her to the police station. 'You must go for me to the commissariat and ask them if they have an old woman there.' He pulled out his sebsi and took a very long time filling it. When he finished it he smoked it himself and did not offer any to Mustapha, because Mustapha never offered him any of his. 'You see how full of kif my head is,' he said laughing. 'I can't go.' Mustapha laughed too and said it would not be a good idea, and that he would go for him.

'I was there, and I heard him going away for a long time, so long that he had to be gone, and yet he was still there, and his footsteps were still going away. He went away and there was nobody. There was the fire and I moved away from it. I wanted to hear a sound like a muezzin crying Allah akbar! or a French plane from the Pilot Base flying over the Medina, or news on the radio. It wasn't there. And when the wind came in the door it was made of dust high as a man. A night to be chased by dogs in the Mellah. I looked in the fire and I saw an eye in there, like the eye that's left when you burn chibb and you knew there was a djinn in the house. I got up and stood. The fire was making a noise like a voice. I think it was talking. I went out and walked along the street. I walked a long time and I came to Bab el Khemiss. It was dark there and the wind was cold. I went to the wall where the camels were lying and stood there. Sometimes the men have fires and play songs on their aouadas. But they were asleep. All snoring. I walked again and went to the gate and looked out. The big trucks went by full of vegetables and I thought I would like to be on a truck and ride all night. Then in another city I would be a soldier and go to Algeria. Everything would be good if we had a war. I thought a long time. Then I was so cold I turned around and walked again. It was as cold as the belly of the oldest goat of Ijoukak. I thought I heard a muezzin and I stopped and listened. The only thing I heard was the water running in the seguia that carries the water out to the gardens. It was near the mçid of Moulay Boujemaa. I heard the water running by and I felt cold. Then I knew I was cold because I was afraid. In my head I was thinking: if something should happen that never happened before, what would I do? You want to laugh? Hashish in your heart and wind in your head. You think it's like your grandmother's prayer-mat. This is the truth. This isn't a dream brought back from another world past the customs like a teapot from Mecca. I heard the water and I was afraid. There were some trees by the path ahead of me. You know at night sometimes it's good to pull out the sebsi and smoke. I smoked and I started to walk. And then I heard something. Not a muezzin. Something that sounded like my name. But it came up from below, from the seguia, Allah istir! And I walked with my head down. I heard it again saying my name, a voice like water, like the wind moving the leaves in the trees, a woman. It was a woman calling me. The wind was in the trees and the water was running, but there was a woman too. You think it's kif. No, she was calling my name. Now and then, not very loud. When I was under the trees it was louder, and I heard that the voice was my mother's. I heard that the way I can hear you. Then I knew the cat was not a cat, and I knew that Aïcha Qandicha wanted me. I thought of other nights when perhaps she had been watching me from the eyes of a cat or a donkey. I knew she was not going to catch me. Nothing in the seven skies could make me turn around. But I was cold and afraid and when I licked my lips my tongue had no spit on it. I was under the safsaf trees and I thought: she's going to reach down and try to touch me. But she can't touch me from the front and I won't turn around, not even if I hear a pistol. I remembered how the policeman had fired at me and how I'd found only one door open. I began to yell: "You threw me the ladder and told me to climb down! You brought me here! The filthiest whore in the Mellah, with the pus coming out of her, is a thousand times cleaner than you, daughter of all the padronas and dogs in seven worlds!" I got past the trees and I began to run. I called up to the sky so she could hear my voice behind: "I hope the police put a hose in your mouth and pump you full of salt water until you crack open!" I thought: tomorrow I'm going to buy fasoukh and tib and nidd and hasalouba and mska and all the bakhour in the Djemaa, and put them in the mijmah and burn them, and walk back and forth over the mijmah ten times slowly, so the smoke can clean out all my clothes. Then I'll see if there's an eye in the ashes afterwards. If there is, I'll do it all over again right away. And every Thursday I'll buy the bakhour and every Friday I'll burn it. That will be strong enough to keep her away. If I could find a window and look through and see what they're doing to the old woman! If only they could kill her! I kept running. There were a few people in the streets. I didn't look to see where I was going, but I went to the street near Mustapha's oven where the commissariat was. I stopped running before I got to the door. The one standing there saw me before that. He stepped out and raised his arm. He said: "Come here."'

He of the Assembly ran. He felt as though he were on horseback. He did not feel his legs moving. He saw the road coming toward him and the doors going by. The policeman had not shot at him yet, but it was worse than the other time because he was very close behind and he was blowing his whistle. 'The policeman is old. At least thirty-five. I can run faster.' But from any street others could come. It was dangerous and he did not want to think about danger. He of the Assembly let songs come into his head. When it rains in the valley of Zerekten the amethysts are darker in Aguelmous. The eye wants to sleep but the head is no mattress. It was a song. Ah, my brother, the ink on the paper is like smoke in the air. What words are there to tell how long a night can be? Drunk with love, I wander in the dark. He was running through the dye-souk, and he splashed into a puddle. The whistle blew again behind him, like a crazy bird screaming. The sound made him feel like laughing, but that did not mean he was not afraid. He thought: 'If I'm seventeen I can run faster. That has to be true.' It was very dark ahead. He had to slow his running. There was no time for his eyes to get used to the dark. He nearly ran into the wall of the shop at the end of the street. He turned to the right and saw the narrow alley ahead of him. The police had tied the old woman naked to a table with her thin legs wide apart and were sliding electrodes up inside her. He ran ahead. He could see the course of the alley now even in the dark. Then he stopped dead, moved to the wall, and stood still. He heard the footsteps slowing down. 'He's going to turn to the left.' And he whispered aloud: 'It ends that way.' The footsteps stopped and there was silence. The policeman was looking into the silence and listening into the dark to the left and to the right. He of the Assembly could not see him or hear him, but he knew that was what he was doing. He did not move. When it rains in the valley of Zerekten. A hand seized his shoulder. He opened his mouth and swiftly turned, but the man had moved and was

pushing him from the side. He felt the wool of the man's djellaba against the back of his hand. He had gone through a door
and the man had shut it without making any noise. Now they
both stood still in the dark, listening to the policeman walking
quickly by outside the door. Then the man struck a match. He
was facing the other way, and there was a flight of stairs ahead.
The man did not turn around, but he said: 'Come up,' and
they both climbed the stairs. At the top the man took out a key
and opened a door. He of the Assembly stood in the doorway
while the man lit a candle. He liked the room because it had
many mattresses and cushions and a white sheepskin under
the tea-tray in a corner on the floor. The man turned around
and said: 'Sit down.' His face looked serious and kind and
unhappy. He of the Assembly had never seen it before, but he
knew it was not the face of a policeman. He of the Assembly
pulled out his sebsi.

Ben Tajah looked at the boy and asked him: 'What did you
mean when you said down there: "It ends that way"? I heard
you say it.' The boy was embarrassed. He smiled and looked
at the floor. Ben Tajah felt happy to have him there. He had
been standing outside the door downstairs in the dark for a
long time, trying to make himself go to the Café of the Two
Bridges and talk to the qahaouaji. In his mind it was almost as
though he already had been there and spoken with him. He
had heard the qahaouaji telling him that he had seen no letter,
and he had felt his own dismay. He had not wanted to believe
that, but he would be willing to say yes, I made a mistake and
there was no letter, if only he could find out where the words
had come from. For the words were certainly in his head.
'. . . and the two eyes are not brothers.' That was like the
footprint found in the garden the morning after a bad dream,
the proof that there had been a reason for the dream, that
something had been there after all. Ben Tajah had not been
able to go or to stay. He had started and stopped so many
times that now, although he did not know it, he was very tired.
When a man is tired he mistakes the hopes of children for the
knowledge of men. It seemed to him that He of the Assembly's

words had a meaning all for him. Even though the boy might not know it, he could have been sent by Allah to help him at that minute. In a nearby street a police whistle blew. The boy looked at him. Ben Tajah did not care very much what the answer would be, but he said: 'Why are they looking for you?' The boy held out his lighted sebsi and his mottoui fat with kif. He did not want to talk because he was listening. Ben Tajah smoked kif only when a friend offered it to him, but he understood that the police had begun once more to try to enforce their law against kif. Each year they arrested people for a few weeks, and then stopped arresting them. He looked at the boy, and decided that probably he smoked too much. With the sebsi in his hand he was sitting very still listening to the voices of some passers-by in the street below. 'I know who he is,' one said. 'I've got his name from Mustapha.' 'The baker?' 'That's the one.' They walked on. The boy's expression was so intense that Ben Tajah said to him: 'It's nobody. Just people.' He was feeling happy because he was certain that Satan would not appear before him as long as the boy was with him. He said quietly: 'Still you haven't told me why you said: "It ends that way".' The boy filled his sebsi slowly and smoked all the kif in it. 'I meant,' he said, 'thanks to Allah. Praise the sky and the earth where it is bright. What else can you mean when something ends?' Ben Tajah nodded his head. Pious thoughts can be of as much use for keeping Satan at a distance as camphor or bakhour dropped on to hot coals. Each holy word is worth a high column of smoke, and the eyelids do not smart afterwards. 'He has a good heart,' thought Ben Tajah, 'even though he is probably a guide for the Nazarenes.' And he asked himself why it would not be possible for the boy to have been sent to protect him from Satan. 'Probably not. But it could be.' The boy offered him the sebsi. He took it and smoked it. After that Ben Tajah began to think that he would like to go to the Café of the Two Bridges and speak to the qahaouaji about the letter. He felt that if the boy went with him the qahaouaji might say there had been a letter, and that even if the man could not remember, he would not mind so much because he would be less afraid. He waited until he thought the boy was not nervous about going into the street, and then he said: 'Let's go out and get some tea.' 'Good,' said the boy. He was not afraid of the police if he was with Ben Tajah. They went through the empty streets, crossed the Djemaa el Fna and the garden beyond. When they were near the café, Ben Tajah said to the boy: 'Do you know the Café of the Two Bridges?' The boy said he always sat there, and Ben Tajah was not surprised. It seemed to him that perhaps he had even seen him there. He seized the boy's arm. 'Were you there today?' he asked him. The boy said 'Yes,' and turned to look at him. He let go of the arm. 'Nothing,' he said. 'Did you ever see me there?' They came to the gate of the café and Ben Tajah stopped walking. 'No,' the boy said. They went across the first bridge and then the second bridge, and sat down in a corner. Not many people were left outside. Those inside were making a great noise. The qahaouaji brought the tea and went away again. Ben Tajah did not say anything to him about the letter. He wanted to drink the tea quietly and leave trouble until later.

When the muezzin called from the minaret of the Koutoubia, He of the Assembly thought of being in the Agdal. The great mountains were ahead of him and the olive trees stood in rows on each side of him. Then he heard the trickle of water and he remembered the seguia that is there in the Agdal, and he swiftly came back to the Café of the Two Bridges. Aïcha Qandicha can be only where there are trees by running water. 'She comes only for single men by trees and fresh moving water. Her arms are gold and she calls in the voice of the most cherished one.' Ben Tajah gave him the sebsi. He filled it and smoked it. 'When a man sees her face he will never see another woman's face. He will make love with her all the night, and every night, and in the sunlight by the walls, before the eyes of children. Soon he will be an empty pod and he will leave this world for his home in Jehennem.' The last carriage went by, taking the last tourists down the road beside the ramparts to their rooms in the Mamounia. He of the Assembly thought: the eye wants to sleep. But this man is alone in the world. He wants to talk all night. He wants to tell me about his wife and how he beat her and how she broke everything. Why do I want to know all those things? He is a good man but he has no head. Ben Tajah was sad. He said: 'What have I done? Why does Satan choose me?' Then at last he told the boy about the letter, about how he wondered if it had had his name on the envelope and how he was not even sure there had been a letter. When he finished he looked sadly at the boy. 'And you didn't see me.' He of the Assembly shut his eyes and kept them shut for a while. When he opened them again he said: 'Are you alone in the world?' Ben Tajah stared at him and did not speak. The boy laughed. 'I did see you,' he said, 'but you had no letter. I saw you when you were getting up and I thought you were old. Then I saw you were not old. That's all I saw.' 'No, it isn't,' Ben Tajah said. 'You saw I was alone.' He of the Assembly shrugged. 'Who knows?' He filled the sebsi and handed it to Ben Tajah. The kif was in Ben Tajah's head. His eyes were small. He of the Assembly listened to the wind in the telephone wires, took back the sebsi and filled it again. Then he said: 'You think Satan is coming to make trouble for you because you're alone in the world. I see that. Get a wife or somebody to be with you always, and you won't think about it any more. That's true. Because Satan doesn't come to men like you.' He of the Assembly did not believe this himself. He knew that Father Satan can come for anyone in the world, but he hoped to live with Ben Tajah, so he would not have to borrow money in the souks to buy food. Ben Tajah drank some tea. He did not want the boy to see that his face was happy. He felt that the boy was right, and that there never had been a letter. 'Two days on a bus is a long time. A man can get very tired,' he said. Then he called the qahaouaji and told him to bring two more glasses of tea. He of the Assembly gave him the sebsi. He knew that Ben Tajah wanted to stay as long as possible in the Café of the Two Bridges. He put his finger into the mottoui. The kif was almost gone. 'We can talk,' he said. 'Not much kif is in the mottoui.' The qahaouaji brought the tea. They talked for an hour or more. The qahaouaji slept and snored. They talked about Satan and the bad thing it is to live alone, to wake up in the dark and know that there is no one else near by. Many times He of the Assembly told Ben Tajah that he must not worry. The kif was all gone. He held his empty mottoui in his hand. He did not understand how he had got back to the town without climbing up out of the soup-kettle. Once he said to Ben Tajah: 'I never climbed back up.' Ben Tajah looked at him and said he did not understand. He of the Assembly told him the story. Ben Tajah laughed. He said: 'You smoke too much kif, brother.' He of the Assembly put his sebsi into his pocket. 'And you don't smoke and you're afraid of Satan,' he told Ben Tajah. 'No!' Ben Tajah shouted. 'By Allah! No more! But one thing is in my head, and I can't put it out. The sky trembles and the earth is afraid, and the two eyes are not brothers. Did you ever hear those words? Where did they come from?' Ben Tajah looked hard at the boy. He of the Assembly understood that these had been the words on the paper, and he felt cold in the middle of his back because he had never heard them before and they sounded evil. He knew, too, that he must not let Ben Tajah know this. He began to laugh. Ben Tajah took hold of his knee and shook it. His face was troubled. 'Did you ever hear them?' He of the Assembly went on laughing. Ben Tajah shook his leg so hard that he stopped and said: 'Yes!' When Ben Tajah waited and he said nothing more, he saw the man's face growing angry, and so he said: 'Yes, I've heard them. But will you tell me what happened to me and how I got out of the soup-kettle if I tell you about those words?' Ben Tajah understood that the kif was going away from the boy's head. But he saw that it had not all gone, or he would not have been asking that question. And he said: 'Wait a while for the answer to that question.' He of the Assembly woke the qahaouaji and Ben Tajah paid him, and they went out of the café. They did not talk while they walked. When they got to the Mouassine mosque, Ben Tajah held out his hand to say good night, but He of the Assembly said: 'I'm looking in my head for the place I heard your words. I'll walk to your door with you. Maybe I'll remember.' Ben Tajah said:

'May Allah help you find it.' And he took his arm and they walked to Ben Tajah's door while He of the Assembly said nothing. They stood outside the door in the dark. 'Have you found it?' said Ben Tajah. 'Almost,' said He of the Assembly. Ben Tajah thought that perhaps when the kif had gone out of the boy's head he might be able to tell him about the words. He wanted to know how the boy's head was, and so he said: 'Do you still want to know how you got out of the soup-kettle?' He of the Assembly laughed. 'You said you would tell me later,' he told Ben Tajah. 'I will,' said Ben Tajah. 'Come upstairs. Since we have to wait, we can sit down.' Ben Tajah opened the door and they went upstairs. This time He of the Assembly sat down on Ben Tajah's bed. He yawned and stretched. It was a good bed. He was glad it was not the mat by the bamboo fence at the Café of the Two Bridges. 'And so, tell me how I got out of the soup-kettle,' he said laughing. Ben Tajah said: 'You're still asking me that? Have you thought of the words?' 'I know the words,' the boy said. 'The sky trembles. . . .' Ben Tajah did not want him to say them again. 'Where did you hear them? What are they? That's what I want to know.' The boy shook his head. Then he sat up very straight and looked beyond Ben Tajah, beyond the wall of the room, beyond the streets of the Medina, beyond the gardens, toward the mountains where the people speak Tachelhait. He remembered being a little boy. 'This night is a jewel in my crown,' he thought. 'It went this way.' And he began to sing, making up a melody for the words Ben Tajah had told him. When he had finished '. . . and the two eyes are not brothers,' he added a few more words of his own and stopped singing. 'That's all I remember of the song,' he said. Ben Tajah clapped his hands together hard. 'A song!' he cried. 'I must have heard it on the radio.' He of the Assembly shrugged. 'They play it sometimes,' he said. 'I've made him happy,' he thought. 'But I won't ever tell him another lie. That's the only one. What I'm going to do now is not the same as lying.' He got up off the bed and went to the window. The muezzins were calling the fjer. 'It's almost morning,' he said to Ben Tajah. 'I still have kif in my head.'

'Sit down,' said Ben Tajah. He was sure now there had been no letter. He of the Assembly took off his djellaba and got into the bed. Ben Tajah looked at him in surprise. Then he undressed and got into bed beside him. He left the candle burning on the floor beside the bed. He meant to stay awake, but he went to sleep because he was not used to smoking kif and the kif was in his head. He of the Assembly did not believe he was asleep. He lay for a long time without moving. He listened to the voices of the muezzins, and he thought that the man beside him would speak or move. When he saw that Ben Tajah was surely asleep, he was angry. 'This is how he treats a friend who has made him happy. He forgets his trouble and his friend too.' He thought about it more and he was angrier. The muezzins were still calling the fjer. 'Before they stop, or he will hear.' Very slowly he got out of the bed. He put on his djellaba and opened the door. Then he went back and took all the money out of Ben Tajah's pockets. In with the banknotes was an envelope that was folded. It had Ben Tajah's name written across it. He pulled out the piece of paper inside and held it near the candle, and then he looked at it as he would have looked at a snake. The words were written there. Ben Tajah's face was turned toward the wall and he was snoring. He of the Assembly held the paper above the flame and burned it, and then he burned the envelope. He blew the black paper-ashes across the floor. Without making any noise he ran downstairs and let himself out into the street. He shut the door. The money was in his pocket and he walked fast to his aunt's house. His aunt awoke and was angry for a while. Finally he said: 'It was raining. How could I come home? Let me sleep.' He had a little kif hidden under his pillow. He smoked a pipe. Then he looked across his sleep to the morning and thought: 'A pipe of kif before breakfast gives a man the strength of a hundred camels in the courtyard.'

The Three Alis

Mohammed Ben Abdullah Yussufi
(*Translated by Irving Rosenthal*)

The author died at the age of twenty-one in the prison hospital of Tangier, after having been beaten during questioning.

A man had three sons. All three were named Ali. When the man was on his deathbed, he said 'I leave half of my land to my son Ali and the other half to my son Ali.' And then he died. The three Alis fought among themselves as to which two of them would inherit their father's land, and then they decided to take their dispute to the Sultan. They set out for the Alcazar or Sultan's Palace with a donkey laden with their belongings. One night while they were asleep, a one-eyed man led away their donkey. In the morning they discovered the theft, and so they sat down and began to smoke kif. The first Ali took a few puffs on his sebsi, expelled the burning ash, and said, 'The thief has one eye.' The second Ali took a few puffs on his sebsi, expelled the burning ash, and said 'The thief's name is Amar.' The third Ali took a few puffs on his sebsi, expelled the burning ash, and said 'The thief lives in the Alcazar.' So the three Alis completed their journey to the Sultan's Palace, and once there began looking for Amar the one-eyed. When they found him they accused him of stealing their donkey. He denied it, and so the three Alis decided to complain about Amar to the Sultan at the same time they were asking him to settle their dispute about their father's land. When the Sultan had heard their story, he said to them 'You did not see Amar steal your donkey. How can I believe the ideas you had while you were smoking kif?' The three Alis asked the Sultan to test them, and so he ordered a covered bowl to be brought into the room. He asked them what was in the bowl. The three Alis took out their sebsis and began to smoke kif. The first Ali took a few puffs on his sebsi, expelled the burning ash, and said 'It is round.' The second Ali took a few puffs on his sebsi, expelled the burning ash, and said 'It is orange.' The third Ali took a few puffs on his sebsi, expelled the burning ash, and said 'It is a tangerine.' The Sultan removed the cover of the bowl and lo! there was a tangerine. But the Sultan demanded one more proof. He ordered another covered bowl to be brought in and asked the three men what it contained. The three Alis refilled their sebsis with kif and began to smoke. The first Ali took a few puffs on his sebsi, expelled the burning ash, and said 'It is couscous made from wheat which is unfit to eat.' The second Ali took a few puffs on his sebsi, expelled the burning ash, and said 'It is couscous made from lamb which is unfit to eat.' The third Ali took a few puffs on his sebsi, expelled the burning ash, and said 'It is couscous made for a Sultan who is unfit to rule.' The Sultan removed the cover of the second bowl and lo! it was filled with couscous. The Sultan asked the three Alis to appear before him on the following day when he would give them a decision about their inheritance. Then he ordered the chief cook to appear and taste the couscous. The cook did so and immediately became violently ill. Then the Sultan sent for the man who had ground the wheat for the couscous. Under threat of torture this man revealed that he had been violently ill the day before, and that just before grinding the wheat he had taken a shit and had not washed his hands afterwards. Then the Sultan sent for the man who had prepared the meat for the couscous. This man was in perfect health, and so the Sultan asked him whom he had bought the lamb from. This man answered 'From a peasant woman who brought it to the Alcazar.' The Sultan sent for the peasant woman, and she confessed that the lamb's mother had died, and the lamb had been put to suckle with a bitch. Finally the Sultan went to his own mother and said 'Who was my father?' His mother answered 'Your father was my husband the Sultan before you.' The Sultan pulled out his sword, held it to his mother's throat, and said 'I will kill you if you do not tell me who my father is.' The woman trembled and confessed that his father was a wool merchant in the market place. On the next day the three Alis returned for their audience with the Sultan. The Sultan took them for a walk in the Alcazar and led them to a room with three doors. He turned to the first Ali and said 'You told me the wheat in my couscous was unfit to eat. In return I give you everything behind this door.' The Sultan opened the first door on a roomful of gold. Then he turned to the second Ali and said 'You told me the lamb in my couscous was unfit to eat. In return I give you everything behind this door.' The Sultan opened the second door on a roomful of jewels. Then he turned to the third Ali and said 'You told me my couscous was made for a Sultan unfit to rule. In return I give you everything behind this door.' The Sultan opened the third door on a roomful of rocks. Then he said 'Those who see what is base deserve what is base. Moreover you are the Ali your father left without an inheritance – unfit to inherit – for you saw that I was unfit to inherit the kingdom. We recognized each other.'

In Morocco the smokers of kif have a patron saint. According to legend, Sidi Hidi was the man who first brought the seeds of the plant to Morocco from Asia. His prehistoric tomb is a shrine to which pilgrimages are still being made.

Night at the Burning Ghat

Allen Ginsberg

Night at the burning ghat – 25 np. two triangle paper packets of ganja at Nimtallah St pipe shop – Long-haired scruffy orange robe sadhu with thin nose and long droopy hip face, chattering animatedly in broken English – from Gauhati, his ashram – we go there? – Benares? – Pranayam – On main Ganges waterfront street, the cymbal chorus in the brick shed – 'men from Bihar' – chain clashes and chanting all night? – A body burning in the first ash pit – pile of wood and the head slowly bubbling up around mouth and nose – cheeks blackened with sheets of flame clasping the volume of the face – splitting, and pink underskin sizzling open – Sat on the bench and watched five minutes, staring at the head – feet painted red sticking out the other end of the wood structure bed –

In the mandir, the handsome naked torso with big strong face, and red bushy-curled hair – sitting with red robed wanderer, black faced beard with little eyes who exchanged amicable glance, full eyed stare at me – my strained back against the marble door post – sharing a pipe I coughed and so began roll my own cigarette – staring at thc handsome sadhu whose chest glistened with oil, muscular shining breasts and happy smile – he massaged his thin sadhu friend, rubbing down the belly – and beamed with joy when in return the thin sadhu anointed him, a hand passed round and round his chest from nipple to nipple rubbing in the heated oil – Then burned a pan of ghee, and one pea of prasad for ceremony – then lay down to sleep on a thin piece of white cloth in the corner – 'You're a beautiful man' I said to him thru sadhu Broken English – he brought out a big handful of prasad, smiled like a child at me – 'Healthy he smoke all day people come sit down make him smoke smoke all day all night – he just sleep an hour – lay down head with all that in it' – I lay and snoozed next to him a while, sleepy Darshan. Then walked out for tea – gave bhog tea and leaf of chapatties and potato curry to another looney sadhu I seen dance jazzy burlesk to Kirtan music that nite – he smiled too – a boy next to him stole his cigarette off table. I watched secretly – said 'I ate it' and gave him another – he all ash smeared and a hump-backed rump at base of his spine and spidery arms, with dusty tantrik red loincloth and a white worn spread over his shoulder. Back to ghat from tea, sat at fire by old babu with Kailash-pile of hair on his head who slept greyly on his side – In front of burning ground gate an old ashy unshaven fellow in pants followed me for an anna – I said no, irritably – touched his feet – he begged again – I touched his feet he reached for mine and I slipped away – listening at 2.30 a.m. last chant crisis of Bihari boys – Returning saw him squatting on step of sleeping mandir, chanting ram hari bolsong alone in froggy beautiful lone voice – long long, as I passed I placed 25 np. at his feet and he reached out and touched my foot – I lay down awhile along side handsome sadhu's corner, near his charcoal brazier still glowing with a new chunk taken from the burning pits – But the priests came and sloshed water and opened gates and turned on lites so I left and went wandering back to the burning pits again – Now all the groups had gathered, silent and grey, crying a suave together round several pit fires they cared for warmth – one half-naked sadhu stretched on ground with his loincloth slipped off his buttock looking like one of the dead corpses beside the all nite fire of the old man whose head I saw adorn the woodpile earlier that even (now all ash in the Ganges spreading out near the steps on the brown muddy surface like huge inkstain) – a few kids at another fire with a gentle round-faced bald saffron Pop. And my singing beggar now squatting over a red pit, lucidly chanting away god's name – I thought perhaps this be master-sign since I been earlier so rejectful to him and he turning out to be such a simple holy sustained all night praying fellow like this in front of my eyes – I sat on bench near his fire and he talked to me in a loud voice, a speech I couldn't follow, sounded like he complaining my being so selfish waving his arms at me from his little brush-wood hot flamy pyre – I moved away, just in case he get further noisy and mad – Back to the handsome sadhu's side in the mandir – A stranger sadhu in orange robe squatted down nearby and made us a pipe. I blasted enough till my throat dry and panicky – Then walked up and down my body trembling my neck constricted till I peed and still the trembling came on me, as if I vomit soon or Ramakrishna appear in the river – or Krishna in every animal eye all around, each of the beggars – lay down to sleep finally on marble bench in inner waiting room – Baul singers and rags and sadhu buttocks sheeted on the floor – left my rubber sandals below my bench – when I awoke – I had drifted to sleep as earlier nites before on ganja seeing a sort of crystal cabinet Krishna beribboned and jewelled in mind's eye – thru universes of feet and skulls and fire and wars and firesides – crystal cabinets a-million – Found my foot rubbers disappeared from their place on the floor. Walked out gleaned around each old spot of the night – where ash pit men were smearing their morning skin – I had wakened, thinking it all a cartoon dream, no longer trembling, as the temple bell-gong shout rose to a noisy Bong climax like the end of a laughing-gas movie – Shoes gone like Donald Duck – went barefoot for tea and puries and potatoes. Tram car 19 home all the way to Dharamtala 8 a.m.

'High Season'

Simon Vinkenoog

Theun got his cigarette paper from his pocket and started making sticks. One, two, three, four went around ... Immediately the full blast of the stuff hit me. Thousands of words and thoughts stumbled for priority and formation within me. I didn't say a thing, looked inside and listened outside, only an ear until I found that Klaas was asking for my attention. I performed violently gesticulating pantomimes with him, then fell silent in great astonishment when he began talking, quietly and deliberately, with a vocabulary I hadn't thought him capable of, he who always stutters with the one hundred words normally at his disposal.

Suddenly he appeared to be a new Einstein, enunciating clearly a new cosmic law, fitting in all the details. He, whom I had always considered almost an imbecile, had been thinking over a problem for centuries, an enormously important problem (I have forgotten which), and now at this exact moment he had found the precise words for it, which made his speech as correct as could be. Not one word too many. Each sentence supported by gestures was a detail of the great closely-knit story, towering erect over us sitting listeners.

I followed his story step by step, surprised that I was able to follow his complex arguments, happy that I had been privileged to witness this moment. And the others? I looked at them, they smiled at me, sunk within their own worlds.

'Do you want to write it all down?' Klaas asked me at the end of his lecture. With a broad and elegant gesture he drew our attention to Cecile, who had been listening sunk in the deep sofa, delighted and astonished, almost crying from compassion. I had become the disciple of Mad Klaas, forever I was turned to him, and would have cried too if I'd had the tears at my disposal. I tried to press them into existence, but they wouldn't come, my tear-glands stayed dry even though my eyes were moist from the sweet and silly smoke. The laws were meant not only for our misty party, but for a completely new world, hardly discovered and not yet mapped at all, still without dates. We were floating between heaven and earth, loosened from all the others yet at one with everything. I felt for an indivisible moment as sad as could be because people who have something to say these days are hardly able to articulate.

Low-toned gramophone music hammered against my temples, spread clickety clack through my body. Benevolently languid, I had settled on the bed with the others, who didn't move. As I pulled up my knees, tremors of emotion rolled through me. I was aware of the fact that I was being looked at. The first words from far behind my consciousness began to come out, and I listened to them just as the others did. Slowly I started paying attention to my own words, listening to my greedy voice, somersaulting sounds which were not to be overtaken nor to be repeated, volatized like the ether Klaas used to sniff, hanging in the air, déjà vu, waiting for a command from my fingers to be magically snapped into existence again.

Impossible, it can't be done.

I was no longer talking aloud. Without will I drifted back into a pre-natal state, my head grew heavier and heavier, larger than my body. A few more difficult swimming motions brought me into the realm of the archetypes, eternally renewed. After an endless silence: 'The more people fill the room, the more the silence grows.'

The first words groped their way to us, searching for our ears. The clumsiness left our legs. Whispering we discussed the high, almost respectfully. We got up and went downstairs slowly.

Dope Dealer – New Robin Hood

Timothy Leary

There are three groups who are bringing about the great evolution of the new age that we are going through now. They are the DOPE DEALERS, the ROCK MUSICIANS and the underground ARTISTS and WRITERS.

Of these three heroes, mythic groups. I think the dealers are the most essential and important. In the years to come the television dramas and movies will be making a big thing of the dope dealer of the sixties. He is going to be the Robin Hood, spiritual guerilla, mysterious agent who will take the place of the cowboy hero or the cops and robbers hero. There is nothing really new about this. Throughout human history the shadowy figure of the alchemist, the shaman, the herbalist, the smiling wise man who has the key to turn you on and make you feel good, has always been the centre of the religious, aesthetic, revolutionary impulse. I think that this is the noblest of all human professions and certainly would like to urge any creative young person sincerely interested in evolving himself and helping society grow to consider this ancient and honourable profession. The paradoxical thing about the righteous dealer is that he is selling you the celestial dream. He is very different from any other merchant because the commodity he is peddling is freedom and joy. You expect your car dealer to drive a good car and you want your clothier to be well dressed and so it logically holds that you expect your righteous dope dealer to radiate exactly that joy and freedom that you seek in his product. So therefore the challenge to the dealer is that not only must his product be pure and spiritual but that he himself must reflect the human light that he represents. Therefore never buy dope, never purchase sacrament from a person that hasn't got the qualities you aspire for.

Rosemary and I just came back from a trip to the Middle East. Naturally we spent most of our time with Sufis, cannabis alchemists, and magicians. It was a great joy for us to see that the Arab dope dealers that we contacted actually did shine forth as the grooviest people you could find. I recall the night we wandered out into the native quarter and found ourselves in a little Bazaar shop in the Souk talking to a dude named Mohamed who had the reputation among the international set as being the finest dealer in town. We walked into Mohamed's shop and immediately realized that we were stepping into a psychedelic stage.

Beautiful costumes, gold embroidered vests, dangling, shining jewelry, silver bracelets and what not. The room was a retinal orgasm. Mohamed was standing behind his little desk and he himself, in his grooming and dress, was telling you that he was a turned on cat. He was wearing an outrageous shirt. His hair, instead of being close clipped as most Arabs have it, was in soul brother natural style and he had a spectacular fluorescent scarf around his neck. I knew that I had seen him in the market place earlier, weaving his way through the crowd. You knew right away that here was a magician. Here was a guy who was announcing with his mere presence that he was a flipped-out dealer in some sort of wondrous magic.

As he sat down, the first thing he did was rummage around in his beautiful leather pouches and started to fill a hash pipe with great skill and dexterity. At the same time he was laying the typical Owsley alchemist rap on us. He was telling us that he was not a businessman but sent by God to turn people on. His product was not to intoxicate you but to give you what you were looking for – freedom and joy and that indeed his kif and hashish were the best in the world. He had different varieties that would turn one on to food, turn you on erotically and give you visual and musical enhancement. All this time his eyes were twinkling and even before partaking of the sacrament one became turned on by the man himself. Your trust in his product is therefore greatly enhanced.

The paradox of the dealer is that he must be pure. He must be straight and he must be radiant. The socio-economics of dealing psychedelic dope is extremely curious. Here we have this enormous, billion dollar industry going on in the United States, all of which is essentially run by amateurs. I know no one who had dealt psychedelic drugs over a period of months and survived without being busted or being freaked out who wasn't pure. You have to be pure. You can't be doing it for the money or the power and you can't do it on your own. Most, if not all, righteous dealers work in groups or brotherhoods. This again is the ancient message of the Middle East. The brotherhoods or groups of men who are engaged in this spiritual journey together, which is always, of course, against the law, always has to be illegal and always has to be the object of persecution by Caesar, the Sultan or by the police.

I have spent a lot of my time in the last eight years looking for turned-on people, holy men to find out where they were at and to learn from them. I have been in India, Japan, all through the Middle East and Europe. I have talked to the Swamis, the Rishis, the Maharishis and I can say flatly that the holiest, handsomest, healthiest, horniest, humorest, most saintly group of men that I have met in my life are the righteous dope dealers. They have got to be that way because they have to continue to use their own product. That is one of the interesting psychopharmacological aspects of dope dealing. A dealer has to know his product. He has to know what these different dopes do to his head, otherwise he doesn't know what he is selling. This means that your righteous dope dealer has to know about the effects of acid, mescaline, DMT, grass and hashish. He has to be able to break off a little lump of Nepalese hash, smell it, chew it and light it up and then decide whether it is grade A, B, or C. He has got to take an acid tab, swallow it and observe on his own detecting instruments whether it is acid, whether it is good acid and roughly what the microgram quantity is. This means that he has got to be a master Sufi. The dealer has got to be a completely accurate, straight spiritual detective. He has got to be free of his own hangups. He can't be riddled with paranoias or he is going to take a puff and scream for the psychiatrist. This means by definition that your righteous dealer must have a pure head and a holy heart. Otherwise he is going to be freaked out by his own product. It was of great interest for Rosemary and me to discover, after ten years in the psychedelic medicine-man business, that increasingly most of our friends turned out to be dealers, which we now see is not accidental but indeed inevitable.

There is a great deal of hypocrisy throughout all levels of the establishment as well as the underground about the dealer. There are many psychedelic liberals who say: 'Well, it's OK for young people to experiment with grass and acid. We don't want to have laws against them, but we should have laws punishing the dealers.'

Somehow the dealer is in a lower moral or sociological category. THIS IS PLAIN BUNK. Let's be straight and honest about it. The thirty million people in the United States who are turned on to psychedelic drugs – anyone of them has been a passive collaborator in an illegal act and everyone of the 30 million people who have used grass or acid in this country in the last few years has got to face up to the fact that it was a righteous and courageous person who took great risks to make the acid or smuggle in the cannabis. Not only does it take courage and dedication but it takes skill. After all the amateur LSD chemist has to have the knowhow to spin the molecules together. He had to have the efficiency and organizational ability to bring together a laboratory in secret and perform a minor chemical miracle. This requires a heavy, together sort of person. I think it is a moral exercise that everyone of the 30 million who are using psychedelic drugs should take a turn at dealing. I think it is almost symbolically necessary that sometimes in your spiritual psychedelic career that you do DEAL. Not for the money but simply to pay tribute to this most honourable profession.

I remember talking recently to a group of clear-eyed, smiling beautiful dealers. They were young men in their twenties, as all dealers have to be young. At that time their life situation was close to perfect. They were living together with their families in nature and there was no reason for them to leave the country on one of these thrilling missions. They were planning another scam. I asked them 'Why are you doing it? You know that at this particular time, with the Nixon administration waging all out war on turned-on kids, with all aid of border guards, secret agents, it's just not a cool time to do it. You have got all the land and dope to centre your own lives. Why take chances?' They thought for a minute and their answer was interesting. 'We deal because that's our thing. We believe that dope is the hope of the human race, it is a way to make people free and happy. We wouldn't feel good just sitting here smoking the dope we have and saving our souls knowing that there are 30 million kids that need dope to centre themselves. Our lives have been saved from the plastic nightmare because of dope and we would feel selfish if we just stayed here in our beautiful utopia. Our brothers and sisters out there should be as liberated and loving as we are.' As far as the police network that is being built up against them, they just laughed. 'We are smarter and wiser than the FBI, the CIA and the Narcotics Bureau put together. We have to be. We just can't admit defeat just because they have more and more equipment against us.'

There was no use for me to argue with that point of view and then they took off for the Middle East with my blessings.

I think of the most remarkable acid chemists. Ones who arranged their laboratories like shrines. They pray constantly while performing their chemical miracle, that the acid they are making will bring freedom and liberation to the people who will take it. Praying that there will be no bad trips and paranoias in the mysterious molecules that they were brewing.

The acid chemist is in a particularly vulnerable position because you can't make acid without being constantly exposed to this powerful molecule. You have to get high. They are floating on 10,000 mikes while performing their magic. They have got to be pure. They have got to be centred to accomplish their technical achievement. I don't know of one successful psychedelic chemist who doesn't have a feeling about how he does it. None who doesn't attempt to purify his mind of negative thinking and who doesn't believe that the acid is influenced by the spiritual and psychic status of those who make it and distribute it.

I don't know one righteous and successful dealer who doesn't. Don't ever buy grass or acid from a dealer who doesn't lay a prayer on you while he takes your money.

IT'S POWERFUL MEDICINE. IT'S MAGIC. AND IT HAS GOT TO BE TREATED THAT WAY.

Part Three
Medical Opinions

Doctors define the properties of the plant within the limits of their knowledge. The literature on the subject abounds in contradictory statements. Praised by one, damned by another, it is astonishing how little is actually known about it.

Concerning Cannabis Indica

Victor Robinson, M.D.

The habitat of the hemp-plant is extensive: not by the hand of man were the seeds sown that gave it birth near the Caspian Sea, where it wildly flourishes on the banks of the immense Volga; it climbs the Altai range and thrives where the Himalaya rears its stony head ten thousand feet on high; it extends to Persia, and China knows it; the Congo River and the hot Zambesi bathe it in Africa, it is not a stranger in sunny France, and how well it thrives in Kentucky the numerous readers of the *Reign of Law* will ever remember.

In the seventeenth century Rumphius noticed that there were differences between the hemp grown in India and the hemp grown in Europe. In the nineteenth century Lamarck accepted these distinctions, and believing the Indian hemp to be a separate species, agreed in calling it *Cannabis indica,* as distinct from the *Cannabis sativa* of Linnaeus and Wildenow. But it is now conceded that from a botanical standpoint the variations are by no means certain or important enough to warrant the maintenance of Indian hemp as a species distinct from common hemp. And as the greater includes the lesser, in botany as well as in geometry, its botanical name is *Cannabis sativa,* with *Cannabis indica* as one variety, just as *Cannabis americana* is another variety.

The plant is cultivated for its seeds, which contain a large quantity of oil, and is therefore used in pharmacy for emulsions, and in the domestic arts because of its drying properties. But the seeds are chiefly used as a favourite food for birds. In fact, some birds consume them to excess, which should lead us to suspect that these seeds, though they cannot intoxicate us, have a narcotic effect on them. The seeds also contain sugar and considerable albumen, making them very nutritious; rabbits eat them readily.

The medicinal hemp; the hemp with the potent narcotic principles – is *Cannabis indica*. In this case we have an example of compensation that would have made Emerson's eyes glisten, for although the fibrous texture of hemp disappears under a southern sun, to make up for the loss there is secreted a resin – Churrus. This resin is collected in a most singular manner. During the hot season, according to Dr O'Shaughnessy, men clothed in leather run violently through the hemp-fields and brush forcibly against the plants. The soft, sticky resin adheres to the garments, and is later scraped off and kneaded into balls. Dr McKinnon informed Dr O'Shaughnessy that in the province of Nepal even the leather attire is dispensed with, and that the natives run naked through the hemp-fields, gathering the resin on their bare bodies.

When the larger leaves turn brown and fall to the ground, it is an indication of the approach of maturity. The flowering tops are then cut off, and subjected to a process of rolling and treading by trained human feet. The hemp is placed on a hard floor surrounded by a rail; the natives take hold of a revolving post, march around and around, singing the while, and press the plants in a technical manner. Whether the perspiration which drips from their unshod organs of locomotion works any chemical change in the composition of cannabis has not yet been determined by E. M. Holmes or E. W. Dixon.

It is not surprising to learn that dealing in hashish is a government monopoly, and that heavy punishment is meted out to those offenders who buy or sell it without permission. 'The importation of it into Egypt is so strongly interdicted,' explains the *Dispensatory of the United States*, 'that the mere possession of it is a penal offence; we found it, however, readily procurable. It is said to be brought into the country in pigs' bladders, in the Indo-European steamers, and thrown out at night during the passage into the Suez Canal, to be picked up by the boats of confederates.'

Cannabis sativa is a member of the *Moracae* or Mulberry family, which family was formerly an order of apetalous dicotyledonous trees or shrubs, but is now reduced to a tribe of the

Urticaceae or Nettle family which embraces 110 genera and 1,500 species.

Cannabis is an annual herb, and thus endures but one year, because instead of storing away nutritious matter in underground bulbs and tubers like the industrious biennials or perennials, it exultingly expends its new-born energy in the production of beautiful blossoms and the maturation of fruit and seed. 'This completed,' says Asa Gray, 'the exhausted and not at all replenished individual perishes.'

Sexually, hemp is dioecious, which means that its staminate and pistillate organs are not on the same plant. When cultivated for its narcotic properties, only the flowering tops of the unfertilized female plants are used, and the male plants are eradicated with great care, as it is claimed that a single one can spoil an entire field. The process of weeding out the males is performed by an expert called a *poddar,* who brings to his work a conscious technical skill, and an unconscious but interesting argument in illustration of what Lester F. Ward has described as the Androcentric World View, for the *poddar* deliberately reverses the names of the sexes, and designates the useful females as males, and calls the rejected males the females.

Cannabis is from four to twelve feet in height; its stem is angular, branching, and covered with matted hairs; its leaves are palmate and, therefore, roughly resemble an open hand; its leaflets are lance-shaped, possessing margins dentated with saw-like teeth; its flowers are yellow and axillary, the male cluster being a raceme and therefore pedicelled, and the female a spike and consequently sessile or stemless; the five male organs or stamens contain pendulous double-celled sacs or anthers; the two female organs or pistils have glandular stigmas, the stigma being the spot where fertilization occurs; the fruit is a grey nut or achene, each containing a single oily seed; the whole plant is covered with a scarcely visible down; the roughness of the leaves and stem is due to the silica, which is a characteristic of the plants of the *Moraceae*.

Not much need be said of the microscopical characteristics

of hemp, for although the powder contains several histological elements, as pollen grains, glands, crystals, resin, fibres, vessels, stone cells, epidermis, parenchyma – indicating presence of stem, leaf, flower, seed – its characteristic hairs or trichomes with their cystolith deposits are of sufficient diagnostic value to make it readily recognizable.

Unfortunately, when we come to the chemical constituents of cannabis, certainty is at an end. As Dorvoult's *L'Officine* says, '*La composition chimique du cannabis indica est mal connue.*'

As to the physiological action of cannabis: It primarily stimulates the brain, slightly accelerates the pulse, sometimes quickens and sometimes retards breathing, produces a ravenous appetite, and augments the contractions of the uterus. In other words, it has an effect on the nervous, respiratory, circulatory, digestive, and genito-urinary systems.

As a therapeutic agent hashish has its eulogizers, though like many other drugs it has been replaced by later remedies in various disorders for which it was formerly used.

In medicinal doses cannabis has been used as an aphrodisiac, for neuralgia, to quiet maniacs, for the cure of chronic alcoholism and morphine and chloral addiction, for mental depression, hysteria, nervous vomiting, for distressing cough, for St Vitus' dance, and for the falling sickness so successfully simulated by Kipling's Sleary – epileptic fits of a most appalling kind. It is used in spasm of the bladder, in migraine, and when the dreaded *Bacillus tetanus* makes the muscles rigid. It is a uterine tonic, and a remedy in the headaches and haemorrhages occurring at the final cessation of the menses. It has been pressed into the service of the diseases that mankind has named in honour of Venus. According to Osler, cannabis is sometimes useful in locomotor ataxia. Christison reports a case in which cannabis entirely cured the intense itching of eczema, while the patient was enjoying the delightful slumber which the hemp induced. It is sometimes employed as a hypnotic in those cases where opium, because of long-continued use, has lost its efficiency. As a specific in hydrophobia it was once claimed to be marvellous, for Dr J. W. Palmer wrote that he himself had seen a sepoy, an hour before furiously hydrophobic, under the influence of cannabis drinking water freely and pleasantly washing his face and hands! Despite the value of personal observation, it is not hashish that has caused mankind to cease to fear Montaigne's terrible line: 'The saliva of a wretched dog touching the hand of Socrates, might disturb and destroy his intellect.' Frankly, if hashish depended solely on its therapeutic potency for its reputation, it would be resting in the pharmacologic graveyards of the past. *Cannabis indica* need not be included in the restricted list of 'Useful Drugs'.

Pharmacopoeia of India (1868)

E. J. Waring, M.D.

Cannabis Sativa, Linn. Indian hemp.
Properties – Primarily stimulant; secondary anodyne, sedative, and antispasmodic.
Narcotic, diuretic, and parturifacient properties have been assigned to it; but these require confirmation.

Therapeutic Uses. – In tetanus, hydrophobia, delirium tremens, ebriatas, infantile convulsions, various forms of neuralgia and other nervous affections, its use has been attended with benefit. Amongst other diseases in which it has been employed are cholera, menorrhagia, and uterine haemorrhage, rheumatism, hay fever, asthma, cardiac functional derangement, and skin diseases attended with much pain and pruritis. It has likewise been employed in lingering and protracted labours depending on atony of the uterus, with the view of producing uterine contractions.

With reference to the therapeutic applications of Indian hemp, Professor Christison offers the following valuable remarks, derived from his personal experience with the drug: 'I have for some years,' he observes,

used a very good alcoholic Extract, sent to me from Calcutta twenty years ago, and still as powerful as ever to subdue pain, obtain sleep, and put an end to spasm in circumstances under which Morphia either did not suit or was objected to by the patient; and after wide experience with it, I am quite satisfied that it is an excellent substitute for it, if given in sufficient doses. The difficulty is, to be always sure of the quality of the Extract, or rather of the Ganja from which the Extract is obtained. I have known two grains of my alcoholic Extract, given in the form of Tincture, to put an end, promptly and permanently, to the agonizing pain caused by biliary calculus impacted in the ducts; and there can be no more unequivocal test than this of the potency of an anodyne. I have long been convinced, and new experience confirms the conviction, that for energy, certainty, and convenience, Indian hemp is the next anodyne, hypnotic, and anti-spasmodic to opium and its derivatives, and often equal to it.

He considers that a well-prepared alcoholic Extract is the best of all forms for use, but it requires to be prepared from Ganja, not too old, collected in the right district, and at the right season. The ordinary resin (Churrus) is generally very impure and untrustworthy.

Hemp Drugs Commission Report (1894)

British Army in India

Question 45a: Does the habitual moderate use of any of these drugs (varieties of hemp) produce any noxious effects – physical, mental or moral?

Answer (by Surgeon-Major R. Cobb, Civil Surgeon and Superintendent, Lunatic Asylum, Dacca): No.

Answer (by Asst-Surgeon Bosonto Kumar Sen, in Civil Medical Charge, Bogra) (v.4, p. 314): Yes, the use of ganja and bhang produces noxious effects. They weaken the constitution and produce loss of appetite. They generally produce dysentery, asthma and bronchitis. They impair the moral sense, induce laziness or habits of immorality or debauchery. A ganja-smoker never talks on any important moral, social or religious subject, nor does he mix with good people. He has got a circle of his own where he indulges in loathesome conversation. Ganja produces insanity (mania) both temporary and permanent.

Answer (by Asst-Surgeon Preonath Bose, Teacher of Materia Medica and Practical Pharmacy, Dacca): Evidence on these points is conflicting.

Answer to Question 41. (a) I have heard it is a digestive; (b) Yes, decidedly so. It helps a man travel long distances without food. I had a syce who went sixty miles in eighteen consecutive hours merely smoking ganja and was quite fit the next day.

(c) and (d) No information. Travellers and others who have to undergo fatigue use it in moderation habitually.

Answer to Question 42. I consider it harmless. I know of no cases where its moderate use has done harm.

Evidence of Mr J. J. S. Driberg, Commissioner of Excise and Inspector-General of Police and Jails.

Answer to Question 45. As a rule, a lunatic is sent in (say) by a planter with a letter telling of his violence. The man is put in jail for observation, and the police are ordered to make an inquiry. They do so, and submit information in a prescribed form. The cause is a point they have to inquire into. If a man does not enter a cause, I know by experience that the District Superintendent of Police gets a slip telling him to send a more experienced man, or fine this man for carelessness. The man must, therefore, look out for a cause. The readiest is ganja. There is another difficulty here, viz., that many of the lunatics are from other provinces, and nothing is known of them. The safest thing to say is 'ganja'. The police know that no further inquiry will be made, so they stick it down. I think also that a policeman would naturally tend to think rather of physical causes than moral causes ... I think that this consideration may also, to a certain extent, explain the popular idea. Ignorant people would look most naturally for physical causes. I think the causes assigned by the police are generally incorrect (1) because I do not think the police have the ability required to make this inquiry; and (2) because they so seldom see people who are able to give them information. We have similarly unreliable information about vital statistics. There is no popular idea among the Assamese that ganja causes insanity. But among planters and others there is. This is due, I think, to the old official idea, which is due to custom.

551. Of these twenty-three cases then, the records in not less than eighteen show that the crimes cannot be connected with hemp drugs. There is one case on which doubt is thrown by subsequent discoveries. The connection between hemp drugs and crime is only established in the remaining four. It is astonishing to find how defective and misleading are the recollections which many witnesses retain even of cases with which they have had special opportunities of being well acquainted. It is instructive to see how preconceived notions based on rumour and tradition tend to preserve the impression of certain particulars, while the impressions of far more important features of the case are completely forgotten. In some cases these preconceived notions seem to prevail to distort the incident altogether and to create a picture in the mind of the witness quite different from the recorded facts. Some of the witnesses whose memories have thus failed them are men who might have been expected to be careful and accurate. Their failure must tend to increase the distrust with which similar evidence, which there has been no opportunity of testing, must be received.

552. The Commission have now examined all the evidence before them regarding the effects attributed to hemp drugs. It will be well to summarize briefly the conclusions to which they come. It has been clearly established that the occasional use of hemp in moderate doses may be beneficial; but this use may be regarded as medicinal in character. It is rather to the popu-

lar and common use of the drugs that the Commission will now
confine their attention. It is convenient to consider the effects
separately as affecting the physical, mental, or moral nature.
In regard to the physical effects, the Commission have come to
the conclusion that the moderate use of hemp drugs is practically attended by no evil results at all. There may be exceptional cases in which, owing to idiosyncrasies of constitution,
the drugs in even moderate use may be injurious. There is
probably nothing the use of which may not possibly be injurious in cases of exceptional intolerance. There are also many
cases where in tracts with a specially malarious climate, or in
circumstances of hard work and exposure, the people attribute
beneficial effects to the habitual moderate use of these drugs;
and there is evidence to show that the popular impression may
have some basis in fact. Speaking generally, the Commission
are of opinion that the moderate use of hemp drugs appears
to cause no appreciable physical injury of any kind. The excessive use does cause injury. As in the case of other intoxicants,
excessive use tends to weaken the constitution and to render
the consumer more susceptible to disease. In respect to the
particular diseases which according to a considerable number
of witnesses should be associated directly with hemp drugs, it
appears to be reasonably established that the excessive use of
these drugs does not cause asthma; that it may indirectly cause
dysentery by weakening the constitution as above indicated;
and that it may cause bronchitis mainly through the action of
the inhaled smoke on the bronchial tubes.

In respect to the alleged mental effects of the drugs, the
Commission have come to the conclusion that the moderate
use of hemp drugs produces no injurious effects on the mind.
It may indeed be accepted that in the case of specially marked
neurotic diathesis, even the moderate use may produce mental
injury. For the slightest mental stimulation or excitement may
have that effect in such cases. But putting aside these quite
exceptional cases, the moderate use of these drugs produces
no mental injury. It is otherwise with the excessive use. Excessive use indicates and intensifies mental instability. It tends

to weaken the mind. It may even lead to insanity. It has been said by Dr Blanford that 'two factors only are necessary for the causation of insanity, which are complementary, hereditary, and stress. Both enter into every case: the stronger the influence of one factor, the less of the other factor is requisite to produce the result. Insanity, therefore, needs for its production a certain instability of nerve tissue and the incidents of a certain disturbance.' It appears that the excessive use of hemp drugs may, especially in cases where there is any weakness or hereditary predisposition, induce insanity. It has been shown that the effect of hemp drugs in this respect has hitherto been greatly exaggerated, but that they do sometimes produce insanity seems beyond question.

In regard to the moral effects of the drugs, the Commission are of opinion that their moderate use produces no moral injury whatever. There is no adequate ground for believing that it injuriously affects the character of the consumer. Excessive consumption, on the other hand, both indicates and intensifies moral weakness or depravity. Manifest excess leads directly to loss of self-respect, and thus to moral degradation. In respect to his relations with society, however, even the excessive consumer of hemp drugs is ordinarily inoffensive. His excesses may indeed bring him to degraded poverty which may lead him to dishonest practices; and occasionally, but apparently very rarely indeed, excessive indulgence in hemp drugs may lead to violent crime. But for all practical purposes it may be laid down that there is little or no connection between the use of hemp drugs and crime.

Viewing the subject generally, it may be added that the moderate use of these drugs is the rule, and that the excessive use is comparatively exceptional. The moderate use practically produces no ill effects. In all but the most exceptional cases, the injury from habitual moderate use is not appreciable. The excessive use may certainly be accepted as very injurious, though it must be admitted that in many excessive consumers the injury is not clearly marked. The injury done by the excessive use is, however, confined almost exclusively to the consumer himself; the effect on society is rarely appreciable. It has been the most striking feature in this inquiry to find how little the effects of hemp drugs have obtruded themselves on observation. The large number of witnesses of all classes who professed never to have seen these effects, the vague statements made by many who professed to have observed them, the very few witnesses who could so recall a case as to give any definite account of it, and the manner in which a large proportion of these cases broke down on the first attempt to examine them, are facts which combine to show most clearly how little injury society has hitherto sustained from hemp drugs.

A Dictionary of Malayan Medicine (1939)

Gimlette and Thomson

Seeds of *Hydnocarpus anthelmintica* ... form the basis of the Tai Foong Chee treatment of leprosy. After crushing and sieving, they are mixed with *Cannabis indica* in the proportion of two parts of the seeds to one of Indian hemp. This Chinese treatment was introduced into the Leper Asylum, Selangor, a few years ago by Dr E. A. O. Travers with signal success in his hands.

Medicinal and Poisonous Plants of Southern and Eastern Africa (1962)

J. M. Watt and M. G. Breyer-Brandwijk

In South Africa various species of Leonotis are miscalled dagga, a name which really appertains to *Cannabis sativa* ... Very little work has been done on the genus and chemical, pharmacological and clinical investigation of these plants is urgently required ... Which states that the plant has properties similar to those of *Cannabis sativa* ... The active principle is not really known but Marloth has isolated a dark green resin to which he ascribes the 'narcotic' property of the plant ... Leonitis Leonurus has been used since early times by the African ... Pappe mentions that the Hottentot was particularly fond of smoking it instead of tobacco ... Pappe states also that the early colonist employed a decoction in the treatment of chronic cutaneous eruptions, possibly even in leprosy, and that the preparation produces narcotic effects if used incautiously ... According to Pijper a decoction of 'dagga' tops is taken by the European in the Transvaal for the relief of cardiac asthma ... and the plant is smoked for the relief of epilepsy.

The leaf of *Cineraria aspera* is smoked by the southern Sotho for asthma and tuberculosis. It is said to be as intoxicating as *Cannabis sativa*.

Cannabis sativa: The Mfengu use the leaf as a snake-bite remedy and the Xhosa as part of the treatment for bots in the horse. The 'oil' from a dagga pipe has been used as an external application by European 'cancer curers' and others. In Southern Rhodesia the African uses the plant, among others, as a remedy for malaria, blackwater fever, blood-poisoning, anthrax and dysentery, and as a 'war-medicine'. The Sotho administer the ground-up seed with bread or mealie-pap to children during weaning. Sotho women smoke cannabis to stupefy themselves during childbirth ... Speight is of the opinion that the Hottentot not only used the plant as a snake-bite remedy but also for centuries as an intoxicant.

Smoking seems to give a much finer gradation of effect than does oral administration ... The electro-encephalogram remains unchanged under the effects of cannabis even with high dosage ... In our opinion, the ill effects of the dagga [hashish] habit are negligible compared with those of opium ... Bourhill states that the African smoker begins very young and rarely leaves off ... One African puts it thus: 'We forget all our troubles, we forget we are working and so work very much.' This type of smoker brightens visibly after a smoke but looks tired and worn out between times.

Médicaments Végétaux (1923)

Drs Pic and Bonnamour

Physiological Action: It provokes hallucinations and a special type of intoxication without loss of consciousness ... All the impressions are perceived in gigantic proportions, and the cerebral reaction is in proportion to the illusion.

Bouquet has described hashish intoxication very well:

Half an hour or an hour after eating a sufficient dose of a hemp preparation, the first effect is felt, and it is a feeling of physical and moral well-being, as Moreau du Tours says, of intense joy; well-being, contentment, indefinable joy which you try in vain to understand, to analyse, of which you cannot seize the cause. You feel happy, you say it, you proclaim it with exaltation, you try to express it by all the means which are in your power, you repeat it over and over; but to say why or in what you are happy, you cannot find words to express it, to make it clear to yourself.

You feel strong, agile, elegant, capable of extraordinary feats; you feel an intense desire for movement. The intelligence remains calm during this period. Then suddenly a certain hilarity, absurd but irresistible, bursts out over an insignificant incident: a banal phrase, a very natural act, the sight of someone is enough to start this laughter. The period of the dissociation of ideas begins at the same time as a need for conversation, for outpouring, is felt. The dialogues become more and more incoherent, the ideas crowd more and more upon each other, they follow each other with dizzying rapidity, but with an exaggeration, a fantastic hypertrophy. Without your noticing it, the disorder of the faculties increases; the lucid moments become shorter and shorter, and you abandon yourself without reservations to subjective impressions; to boisterous joy, agitated at the beginning, succeeds an agreeable state of physical and moral lassitude; the least effort becomes a colossal labour, and the spirit lets itself go with delight into a sort of apathy, of unconsciousness, of complete calm. There is at the same time complete alteration of the notions of space and time, joined to an excessive sharpening of all the senses, especially sight and hearing: the colours of objects are changed; a painting or some flowers become marvellous landscapes, enchanted places; a naked wall becomes covered with the fantastic and brilliant flowering of extraordinary vegetations, strange animals, flamboyant designs. All is animated, surging, shining, evolving to the will of the exalted imagination, then diminishes, fades out to make way for new apparitions just as seductive. The slightest musical sound produces the effect of an ineffable harmony. The memory and the affective faculties are also very excited: scenes long forgotten reappear before the eyes, unroll in their most minute details; the memory of loved ones comes forth with intensity, with insistence; on the other hand, the slightest dislike is transformed into savage hatred.

Finally at the end of a certain time, which varies according to the individual, the extreme excitement of the imaginative faculties calms down bit by bit: the haze which surrounds all objects thickens more and more. The weary brain no longer seems to have the strength to follow imagination and memory in their runaway race: one abandons one's self then to a sort of calm and tranquil ecstasy, which is still crossed by flashes, a few fleeting dreams. Finally a deep absolute sleep terminates the session, and one wakes up fresh and rested, with no other ill effects than a ferocious appetite and a slight depression.

Thus hashish intoxication can be divided into four distinct phases:

(a) Period of motor and sense excitation.
(b) Period of intellectual incoordination.
(c) Period of ecstasy.
(d) Period of sleep.

The voluptuous form of hashish intoxication is not as frequent as is commonly believed; it seems to be most frequent among Orientals, and is probably due to other substances being mixed with it, particularly cantharides. Hemp by itself has no aphrodisiac effect.

Therapeutic Indications: The calming and hypnagogic properties of Indian hemp have been tried out on a large number of diseases.

1. Against troubles of psychic origin: melancholia, delirium, hysteria, painful facial tics, chorea, delirium tremens, migraine headaches, neuralgia, sciatica, insomnia with delirium and nightmares, neurasthenia (Maurice de Fleury).
2. Against certain genito-urinary troubles: gonorrhea, prostatitis, cystitis, dysmenorrhea.
3. Against troubles of the respiratory system: in the form of cigarettes, vapour, and inhalations against chronic catarrh, emphysema, asthma, whooping cough.
4. Against painful troubles of the stomach and intestine: cancer, ulcer, anorexy.
5. Against certain skin diseases: eruptions, herpes, chronic itching (Gillibert).
6. Against infectious diseases; tetanus, cholera, pest, erysipelas, eruptive fevers (Michaud and Deydier).

However, the results have been extremely variable and inconsistent, which is probably because of the disconcerting unreliability of the preparation used and to the addition of foreign substances in drugs of Oriental origin: henbane, datura, opium, *nux vomica*, cantharides, etc. The study of the therapeutic action of Indian hemp should be taken up again, being careful, as Bouquet insists, to use only hemp, its extract or purified resin, without addition of other substances, and to use only preparations containing a determined proportion by dosage of purified resin. Then perhaps hemp will be able, as Trousseau predicted, to make a victorious entry into the domain of medicine, and there occupy the place that it deserves.

Materia Medica (1928)
(A dictionary of homeopathic substances)

Boericke

Cannabis indica (Hashish): Inhibits the higher faculties and stimulates the imagination to a remarkable degree without any marked stimulation of the lower or animal instinct. A condition of intense exaltation, in which all perceptions and conceptions, all sensations and emotions are exaggerated to the utmost degree. Subconscious or dual nature state. Apparently under the control of the second self, but the original self prevents the performance of acts which are under the domination of the second self. Apparently the two selves cannot act independently, one acting as a check upon the other.

Effects of one dram doses by Dr Schneider: The experimenter feels ever and anon that he is distinct from the subject of the hashish dream and can think rationally. Produces the most remarkable hallucinations and imaginations, exaggeration of the duration of time and extent of space being most characteristic. Conception of time, space, and place is gone. Extremely happy and contented, nothing troubles. Ideas crowd upon each other.

Has great soothing influence in many nervous disorders like epilepsy, mania, dementia, delirium tremens, and irritable reflexes. Exopthalmic goitre. Catalepsy.

Marihuana
Roger Adams

The author is on the staff of the Noyes Chemical Laboratory, University of Illinois, the Department of Pharmacology of Cornell University Medical College, and the Welfare Island

Hospital. The following is taken from a lecture delivered on 19 February 1942.

The clarification of the chemical and medical aspects of hemp extracts has been extraordinarily slow for a material known as long and used as frequently as marihuana. The reasons have been several – the failure of chemists to isolate a pure active principle, the unsuccessful attempts of the pharmacologist to find an animal test which paralleled the activity in humans, and finally the lack of controlled clinical experiments.

The recorded medical literature is most confusing. The reports are contradictory, and the description of the drug varies from one which is habit-forming and which with constant use is as harmful to the system as morphine, to one which is almost completely innocuous with a stimulation not far remote from that of alcohol.

Clinical tests revealed that marihuana produces no signicant changes in basal metabolic rates, blood chemistry, hematological picture, liver function, kidney function or cardiac electric conduction. Marihuana delays somewhat gastric and intestinal motility as gauged by the Carlson apparatus and X-ray studies; it produces definite increase in the frequency of the alpha wave in electroencephalographic recordings, thus indicating increased relaxation.

After the Welfare Island study of every phase of the action of marihuana and the synthetic drugs and after finding no discernible evidence of any permanent deleterious effects, either mental, or physical, Dr Allentuck considered the question of the possible therapeutic value of these substances. The potential availability of pure synthetics of standard potency invites such a study, for hitherto merely hemp extracts were accessible, the clinical activity of which must be determined for each batch of extracted material. Since the outstanding manifestation of the marihuana action is the euphoria which makes its user feel 'high', consideration was given to its possible employment as a drug for individuals in various stages of mental depression such as cyclothymics, involutionals, reactives, or those with organic conditions in which dysphoria is a dominant factor. The invariable characteristic of the drugs to stimulate the appetite suggests they might be applicable in psychoneurosis in which a lack of desire for food exists. Many subjects show an alcohol-like picture of intoxication following the use of marihuana. The idea of using these drugs in the treatment of chronic alcoholic addiction was considered and preliminary experiments by Dr Allentuck on private patients and colleagues were sufficiently encouraging to merit investigation on a larger scale and over a longer period of time.

The euphoria produced by marihuana is in many ways comparable to that achieved by the use of opium derivatives. This suggested the possibility of use in the treatment of opiate derivative addictions to eliminate or ameliorate the withdrawal symptoms commonly experienced during previously attempted so-called 'cures'. To clarify this question Dr Allentuck selected a series of cases among drug addicts undergoing treatment. One group of thirteen received 15 mg. of tetrahydrocannibinol orally three times daily at five a.m., two p.m. and ten p.m. and a sterile hypodermic injection; another group of fourteen received the same treatment without the sterile injection. Subjective and objective findings were recorded. In general the consensus of subjective opinions favoured the new treatment as compared to previous cures and the established routine taken by some of these patients. They felt happier, had a better appetite and wanted to return to activity sooner. These results served as a basis for further study of fifty cases in which quantitative criteria were employed.

Two groups of twenty subjects were selected, one group receiving the tetrahydrocannibinol treatment up to a maximum of ten days and the others receiving none. Members of each group were observed throughout the day. Each morning they were interviewed and any complaints recorded on a chart. Thus an attempt was made to arrive at a quantitative comparison of the withdrawal symptoms. It was found that the tetrahydrocannibinol treatment was useful in alleviation or elimination of withdrawal symptoms and in diminishing or eliminating the accompanying discomfort which follows cessation of narcotic indulgence. Any withdrawal symptoms under the tetrahydrocannibinol treatment were of a mild character and occurred within the first three or four days following which the patient began to feel better. The chief complaints were restlessness, headache and dryness of the throat. They had an increased appetite and desire for food which diminished or eliminated such withdrawal symptoms as nausea, diarrhoea, perspiration, etc. They felt physically stronger and showed psychomotor activity. The feeling of euphoria produced by the tetrahydrocannibinol helped in rehabilitating the physical condition and in facilitating social reorientation. An outstanding result is a subjective feeling of relaxation. The sleep induced by the drug, likewise contributes to the general improvement in the patients' health. These results are in contrast to those from the use of Magendie's solution which produces in the patients contentment for the first three or four days, after which signs of marked discomfort or withdrawal effects appear. The patients, after this treatment, upon their discharge, were shaky and generally in poor physical condition. These preliminary results with tetrahydrocannibinol justify a more exhaustive study of its possibilities as a means of relieving the withdrawal symptoms in narcotic addicts.

The Pharmacological Basis of Therapeutics (1955)

Louis S. Goldman and Alfred Gilman

Cannabis has been considered as a breeder of crime, especially in psychopathic individuals, a concept supported by the acts of violence presumably committed while under the acute influence of the drug. Suicide, homicide, and sexual assaults have been blamed on marihuana. It has been contended that inhibitions are removed and personality traits exaggerated, and that the criminal is thereby emboldened to do violence. Evidence on which the above view is based is not always of the most acceptable variety. The sociological, psychiatric and criminological aspects of marihuana were studied and reviewed by Bromberg (1939) and Shoenfield (1944), and no positive relation could be found between violent crime and the use of the drug. Marihuana is no more an aphrodisiac than is alcohol, and the drug apparently is not used for sexual stimulation. No cases of murder or sexual crimes due to marihuana were established, and Shoenfield concluded that the smoking of marihuana was not associated with juvenile delinquency. Marihuana habituation does not lead to the use of morphine, heroin, cocaine, or alcohol, and the associated use of marihuana and narcotic drugs is rare. Indeed, strong alcoholic beverages counteract the psychic effects of marihuana and are avoided by the habitué.

Drugs and the Mind (1957)

Robert S. De Ropp

The preparation of these active materials represented a prodigious amount of work on the part of the chemists, but for some strange reason practically all work on the drug has now been abandoned. We have no idea what happens to this potent substance, tetrahydrocannibinol, after it enters the body. We cannot tell in what form it enters the brain or in what manner it affects the chemistry of the brain cells. Despite the tremendous recent interest in psychochemistry this important group of compounds has been ignored and we know as little about the mode of action of the hemp drug on the brain as did Hasan-i-Sabbah when he fed it to his followers a thousand years ago.

The Medical Use of Cannabis Sativa

R. Polderman

The author, who lives in Baarn, Holland, has made a wide study of Oriental medical systems.

The plant is a narcotic inebriant. In some countries it is reputed to be a remedy for malaria, blackwater fever, blood poisoning, anthrax, and dysentery. A poultice of the plant is beneficial in local inflammation, erysipelas, neuralgia, etc.

The leaves are sedative, anodyne, narcotic, antispasmodic, diuretic, digestive, and astringent. They are given in doses of forty grains as a sedative or anodyne. Half a drachm of the dried leaves are given with a little sugar and black pepper as a household remedy for dysentery and diarrhoea. The powdered leaves are administered as a stomachic and for relieving flatulence. In cases where it is not advisable to use opium, the leaves are given to induce sleep. They are also used in tetanus and for relieving pain in dysmenorrhoea. Some practitioners consider it preferable to boil the leaves before use. The leaves are also used externally. A cataplasm of fresh leaves is applied to tumours as an aid in resolving them. The fresh juice of the plant is used for removing dandruff and vermin from the scalp, and for allaying pain in the ear. A powder of the leaves is useful for dressing fresh wounds and sores, as it promotes granulation. A poultice of the fresh leaves is used in diseases of the eye with photophobia, in piles, and in orchitis.

Bhang or hashish is prepared from the dried leaves and flowers of both male and female plants, wild or cultivated, by infusing them with milk and other ingredients. It is given in dyspepsia, gonorrhea, bowel complaints, and also as an appetizer and a nerve stimulant. The dose of the dried leaves is one-fourth to two grains, and they may be used even without infusing them.

Ganja is the dried pistillate flowering top of the cultivated plant, which is coated with a resinous exudation. It contains an oily principle, cannabinol. As an antidote to orpiment poisoning, Ganja smoke is swallowed through the mouth. In cases of strangulated hernia and the griping pains of dysentery, Ganja smoke is passed through the rectum. It is classed as one of the best of the anodyne, hypnotic, and anti-spasmodic drugs. It is administered with advantage for inducing sleep in those suffering from hallucinations. It is applied locally to relieve pain and itching in eczema, pruritis, etc. Ganja is given in doses from one fourth to two grains.

Charas is the resinous exudation that collects on the leaves and flowering tops of the plants. It is the most active part of the plant and is a valuable narcotic, especially in cases where opium cannot be used. It is of great value in malaria, chronic headache, migraine, acute mania, whooping cough, asthma, anaemia of the brain, nervous vomiting, tetanic convulsion, insanity, delirium, dysuria and nervous exhaustion. It is also used as an anaesthetic in dysmenorrhoea, as an appetizer and aphrodisiac, as an anodyne in the itching of eczema, in neuralgia, in pain from the various kinds of corns, etc Homoeopathically it is a wonderful remedy for stuttering, yielding remarkable results. In the lower potencies, it is used against bladder troubles with urine retention and painful urges. It has been known to relieve the symptoms in cases of oppressed breathing and palpitation. It is also given against nightmares. Charas is given in doses from one sixth to one fourth of a grain, and is also widely used in veterinary practice.

The Psychological Significance of the Soma Ritual

Esther Harding

In the legend of the soma we find records of a gift, namely, inspiration or ecstasy, which leads on to the final initiation of the moon, that is into a higher stage of consciousness. This new condition comes, however, not from the Logos, the brightness of mind, or intellect, but from the unconscious.

For the inspiration of the moon comes, the myths relate, from the dark moon and from the soma drink brewed from the moon tree. It is not embodied in rational thought but in dark obscure movements, in thoughts and impulses of darkness, intoxicating like the soma drink, producing an enthusiasm which may even lead to madness. To eat the soma, or to drink the soma drink was to partake of the food of the gods, to become godlike and to share in those attributes which distinguish the gods from the mortals. These attributes are the power to transcend death, to be immortal, and the power to create, to make that which had not being before. These two gifts are bestowed by the soma drink.

In the Hindu teachings about the soma it is said: '... the moon. That is Soma, the king. They are food of the gods. The gods do eat it.' (Khandogya Upanishad 5, 10, 4.) In another translation this text reads: 'King Soma, he is the food of the Gods that Gods eat ... But they who conquer the worlds (future states) by means of sacrifice, charity, and austerity, go to smoke, from smoke to night, from night to the decreasing half of the moon, from the decreasing half of the moon ... to the world of the fathers, from the world of the fathers to the moon. Having reached the moon they become food, and then the Devas (the gods) feed on them there, as sacrificers feed on Soma, as it increases and decreases.' (Brihadaranyaka Upanishad 6, 2, 16.) Another rendering reads: 'Just as one eats the

King Soma with the words "swell and decrease" so they are eaten by the gods ... This moon is the honey (nectar) of all beings, and all beings are the honey of this moon. Likewise this bright immortal person in this moon, and that bright immortal person existing as mind in the body both are (madhu) (soul). He is indeed the same as that Self, that Immortal, that Brahman, that All.' (Brihadaranyaka Upanishad 2, 5, 7.) 'The person or spirit that is in the moon on him I meditate ... I meditate on him as Soma, the king, the self (Atman) (source) of all food. Who so meditates on him thus, becomes the self (source) of all food.' (Kaushitaki Upanishad 4, 4.) Or as another translation renders it, 'becomes the Self of Nourishment'.

The soma is nourishment of the gods, and man, too, can partake of it, thereby becoming part of the Self, the Atman. This is a mystical way of expressing the belief that through this ritual there develops within the worshipper a self which is not his personal ego, but is non-personal, partaking of the qualities of the divine self or Atman. This self is unique, it is said to be 'free from all the pairs of opposites', 'it never bends the head to anyone', 'it is immovable and homeless'. (Mahabharata, Anugita XLIII). Jung has called this nonpersonal, non-ego self the individuality, and I must refer the reader to his works for most illuminating discussions of the whole subject.

The ancient teachings about the moon state that this 'self' develops in that individual who has undergone the required initiations to the moon deity, or, as we might say in psychological terms, who has related himself to the feminine principle. The 'self' possesses those qualities which alone can stand against the inflooding of the chaotic unconscious. For it is said that the self is immovable, it is homeless, that is to say it is not dependent on being established or conditioned, its strength is in itself; one might also say its strength lies in its being itself. It is that which it is, and nothing else. 'It never bends the head to anyone.' The ritual of the soma drink was believed to have power to put the worshipper in touch with this aspect of his psyche, the eternal, immovable, reality of Self.

In drinking the soma the initiant gave himself up to be filled with the god. He knew that he would lose his personal, conscious control. He would become the prey of whatever thoughts or inspirations came to him out of the unknown. His mind would be the playground of strange thoughts, of inexplicable feelings and impulses. He would experience an intoxication, an ecstasy, which he believed to be a possession by God. Even those who think of God as all-good, a loving father, a beneficent spiritual being, might still hesitate before handing themselves over to His power in this way and renouncing their personal self-control through the influence of the soma drink. Even the boon of the renewal of life, which the soma is believed to give, might not be sufficient to induce them so to lay aside their personal autonomy. How much greater a sacrifice was demanded of those worshippers who believed that God, like the moon, was black as well as white, destructive as well as creative, cruel as well as kind. How great an act of devotion was needed can be sensed only when we contemplate giving ourselves up to the daemonic influence which arises within our own psyches. For in actual fact we find that the belief in the unity of the one good God is little more than an intellectual formula, counterbalanced by the theory that man is the victim of original sin which will arise spontaneously within him if he relaxes his control for a moment.

What it means, psychologically, to drink the soma and allow the inner voice of the daemon to speak within and take over the control for a space, Jung has discussed in his essay on the *Becoming of the Personality*. To dare to listen to that inspiration from within which voices the ultimate reality of one's own being requires an act of faith which is rare indeed. When the conviction is borne in upon one that anything which is put together, or made up, has no ultimate reality and so is certain to disintegrate, one turns to one's own final reality in the faith that it and it alone can have any virtue or any value. Jung has used the Greek word *pistis* to express the kind of faith in, or devotion to, the rightness, the wisdom of that inner spark which speaks and functions of itself, quite apart from our conscious control. This wisdom was called the Divine Sophia. The Greek word *sophos* means wisdom and Sophia is a personification of wisdom, the Lady Wisdom, or the Goddess Wisdom. She is the highest incarnation of the feminine principle, the Moon Goddess in her function of spirit, divine knowledge. The moon goddesses were, in the majority of cases, considered to be the source of knowledge and wisdom. The words used for mental activity are associated in many languages, it will be recalled, with the names of the moon or of the moon deities, while in many cases the name for the moon deity meant far more than mental activity. Plato, for instance, says that the ancients signified the Holy Lady by calling her Isia and also Mental Perception and Prudence, for the Greeks believed that the name Isis was cognate with *Isia* which means knowledge. The etymology is probably incorrect but the comment shows that to the Greeks of Plato's time the goddess Isis was goddess of knowledge. The robe of Isis, Goddess of Wisdom, concealed, it will be recalled, the deepest revelation, and Shing Moo, the Chinese moon goddess, is called Perfect Intelligence, while the Virgin Mary, Moon of our Church, is also the bearer of Perfect Wisdom. To the Gnostics of Greece and Egypt, Sophia was the Divine Wisdom, the female form of the Holy Spirit. Devotion to, or faith in, this wisdom is the one motive which can make it possible for a human being, whether man or woman, to listen to his inner voice, relinquishing his own autonomy and resigning himself to the inflow of the dark powers of the moon, through partaking of the drink of soma.

The ritual of the soma drink was, however, highly prized by the initiants and brought them the priceless gifts of which we have been speaking. Their confession was:

> We've quaffed the Soma bright,
> And have immortal grown;
> We've entered into light,
> And all the Gods have known.

The soma drink was believed to bring not only immortality but also inspiration and wisdom. The wisdom it brought was not the outcome of wide knowledge, or great erudition, or of worldly experience, but was rather the wisdom of nature. It is the wisdom that knows without knowing how. A gull, for instance, can soar as no modern glider can. This unconscious bird can utilize the winds with their varying currents and velocities, it knows all about areas of high pressure and areas of low pressure without, however, knowing anything about them at all. The bird's unknowing knowledge is a picture of the moon wisdom, which we human beings have so largely bartered for our conscious rationale and exact information. Our information is a priceless achievement but it is after all only a tool of the mind and not the real content of wisdom. Again, to quote from one of the sacred books of India, in the Mahabharata it is said: 'The Supreme Lord creates all creatures ... his mind is in the moon, his understanding dwells always in knowledge.' 'When the understanding, of its own motion, forms ideas within itself, it then comes to be called Mind.' This text agrees with primitive concepts that one of the chief characteristics of the moon is her ability to give men thoughts, ideas, and inspiration 'of its own motion'. For the moon, *mens*, is mind, not only in the language of many peoples, but in the underlying concept as well. In Hindu thought, moon is King Soma, and soma *is* manas, mind.

The ideas which the moon gives, however, are far from academic thinking, with its power to dissect, organize, and formulate. These aspects of thinking belong to the sun, while from the moon come phantasies, intuitions, and strange ideas, or so primitive men and the cultured people of antiquity as well, believed.

The moon, it was thought, insinuates into man's mind ideas and intuitions which are not at all in accordance with intellectual standards but are strange and bizarre, and, because of the profound truth hidden beneath their unusual form, they may be creatively new. These ideas are filled with a peculiar emotion or with intoxicating delight, like the ecstasy of the soma drink.

Thus the moon stands for that strange kind of thinking

which comes and goes apparently with complete autonomy; man's rational laws have no more power to control it than his wishes control the moon's movements high in the heavens. A man can of his own will sit down and think logical thoughts. He can say: 'Now I will work on this mathematical problem, or draw up a plan for this or that' and his thinking obeys him. But 'moon' thinking goes of itself. It is not under the sway of logic. It will not come when he bids it. It will not go at his command. It does not originate in his head. It rises rather from the lower depths of his being and befuddles his mind, like the intoxicating drink, soma.

Thinking of this kind is despised among us, but it has been highly esteemed in many ages and many civilizations. It is thought to be due to a possession by a divine power. Even in extreme form, as in the case of lunacy (*lune* is moon), primitives and the ancients thought that a god spoke through the man's delirium. Today in modern art we find again the cult of that which goes of itself. Our artists seek, painstakingly, to express that which is *not* rational and indeed unfolds of its own volition. There is to us, in this twentieth century, undoubtedly a value concealed in the irrational, in that which is not controlled by rational laws. It will be recalled that the wisdom of Isis, when searching for the lost body of the dead Osiris, was represented as coming to her in quite irrational ways. She was first guided by the babbling of little children, then by the instinct of the dog, and lastly by the word of her own daemon voice. These three stages represent ways through which men and women, today, may listen to the voice of the moon wisdom, much as Isis did. The babbling of little children represents, perhaps, taking note of the irresponsible phantasy which flits by beneath the contents to which conscious attention is directed; the instinct of the dog will represent those things that the body, the animal part of the human being, tells one. These intimations are also disregarded in large measure, by the average person, as being too trivial for serious consideration. And thirdly, the inner voice still speaks, although it is usually drowned out by the clamour of personal interest and the insistent demands of the world, during the daytime. It is more easily heard in the dreams and visions of the night.

To pay attention to these things is by no means easy, to do so requires the renouncing of personal autonomy over one's own thoughts for the time being and allowing dark, unknown ideas to take possession of one's mind. Usually a man in whom 'moon thinking' arises feels that there is something inferior about the whole process, something uncanny, something not quite clean, by which he is besmirched. He feels that such thinking is not a masculine but a 'womanish' sort of thinking; and he may add that women think in that confused way most of the time. But certain women, if they were asked, would say that the thoughts and inspirations which come to them from the depths of their being are likely to be right, can be relied on, and can be acted on with confidence. When a woman thinks in her head as a man thinks, she is often wrong; she is very apt to be deceived by ready-made opinions, to spend her time on side issues; and her thinking, when of this kind, is usually unproductive and uncreative. Ideas formed under the moon, inferior though they may seem to be, yet have a power and compelling quality which ideas originating in the head rarely have. They are like the moon in that they grow of themselves. They demand an outlet; if a suitable one is not provided they may become obsessive and produce, as the primitives would say, 'moon madness'. For the children of the moon must come to birth just as surely as physical children. And furthermore as the Hindus have said, only when the Understanding of its own motion forms ideas within itself can it be called Mind. When written in this way with the capital letter the Mind refers to the Atman, supreme consciousness, the Self. In other words when one listens to the voice of that non-personal factor within one's own psyche one comes into touch with that unique factor with oneself, which the Hindus felt to be part of the Atman, the Self. Through such an experience it is said that the individual's life is renewed by partaking of the ever-renewed life of the moon.

What this may mean to us when the symbols are recognized

as symbols and the whole is translated into psychological terms, is hard to say with any certainty. It surely does *not* mean that to give oneself over to the guidance of the unconscious, renouncing all the achievements of consciousness, will give one eternal life. Such a course of action could produce nothing but disintegration, the loss of individuality and, in extreme form, mental unbalance or insanity. To us the ravings of the lunatic certainly do not voice the oracles of divine wisdom. If the strange thoughts and images arising from the unconscious are to have any value at all for us, they have to be interpreted, made available for life, through the mediation of the human understanding. One must ask with the Knight of the Grail legends, 'What does it mean?'

Cannabis Intoxication and Its Similarity to that of Peyote and LSD

William H. McGlothlin

Pharmacology texts invariably classify cannabis as a hallucinogen, along with LSD, mescaline and psilocybin. Recent interest, however, has concentrated on the last three, probably because the 'model psychosis' hypothesis grew out of work with these more potent hallucinogens. Also, those interested in examining possible therapeutic effects of these agents have preferred to avoid the stigma attached to marihuana. On examining descriptions of cannabis intoxication, however, it is clear that virtually all of the phenomena associated with LSD are, or can, also be produced with cannabis.[1, 2, 3] The wavelike aspect of the experience is almost invariably reported for

1. Ames, F., 'A Clinical and Metabolic Study of Acute Intoxication with Cannabis Sativa and Its Role in the Model Psychoses', *Journal of Mental Science*, 104, 1958, pp. 972–99.

2. Bouquet, R. J., 'Cannabis, Part III-V', *Bulletin on Narcotics*, 3, No. 1, 1951, pp. 22–43.

3. Walton, R. P., *Marihuana, America's New Drug Problem*, Lippincott, New York, 1938.

cannabis as well as for all the other hallucinogens. Reports of perceiving various parts of the body as distorted, and depersonalization, or 'double consciousness', are very frequent, as well as spatial and temporal distortion. Visual hallucinations, seeing faces as grotesque, increased sensitivity to sound and merging of senses (synaesthesia) are also common. Heightened suggestibility, perception of thinking more clearly and deeper awareness of the meaning of things are characteristic. Anxiety and paranoid reactions may also occur. Walton writes:

> The acute intoxication with hashish probably more nearly resembles that with mescaline than any of the other well-known drugs. Comparison with cocaine and the opiates does not bring out a very striking parallelism. With mescaline and hashish there are numerous common features which seem to differ only in degree.[3]

Similarly, De Ropp states:

> We have no reason to suppose that Gautier had ever heard of peyote but his descriptions of his experience under the influence of hashish are so like those of other investigators under the spell of the sacred cactus that one is tempted to suppose that the two drugs must produce within the brain a similar reaction, despite the chemical dissimilarity of their active principles.[4]

The difference between cannabis and the other hallucinogens must be understood in terms of the motivation of the user as well as the strength of the reaction. This is not to say that the set of the user is not very important for the others as well, but cannabis is especially amenable to control and direction so that the desired effects can usually be obtained at will. Michaux, a French writer, has repeatedly explored his own reactions to the various hallucinogens and writes, 'Compared to other hallucinogenic drugs, hashish is feeble, without great range, but easy to handle, convenient, repeatable without immediate danger.'[5] It is these features, plus the fact that

4. De Ropp, R. S., *Drugs and the Mind*, St Martin's Press, New York, 1957.

5. Michaux, H., *Light Through Darkness*, trans. by H. Chevalier, The Orion Press, New York, 1963.

consumption by smoking enables the experienced user to accurately control the amount absorbed, that makes cannabis a dependable producer of the desired euphoria and sense of well-being. This aspect is pointed up in the study by the New York Mayor's Committee which examined the reaction of experienced users to smoking and ingesting marihuana extract.[6] When smoking, the effect was almost immediate, and the subjects carefully limited the intake to produce the desired 'high' feeling. They had no difficulty maintaining a 'euphoric state with its feeling of well-being, contentment, sociability, mental and physical relaxation, which usually ended in a feeling of drowsiness'. When ingested, the effect could not be accurately controlled and, although the most common experience was still euphoria, users also frequently showed anxiety, irritability, and antagonism. It is common knowledge among marihuana users that one must LEARN to use the drug effectively, and that beginners are often disappointed in the effect.[7]

With the much stronger and longer lasting hallucinogens, LSD and mescaline, there is much less control and direction possible, and even the experienced user may find himself plunged into an agonizing hell, instead of experiencing satori. In summary, it appears that the reaction to cannabis is on a continuum with the other hallucinogens and, given the same motivation on the part of the user, will produce some of the same effects. On the other hand, cannabis permits a dependable controlled usage that is very difficult if not impossible with LSD and mescaline.

One distinct difference that does exist between cannabis and the other hallucinogens is its tendency to act as a true narcotic and produce sleep, whereas LSD and mescaline cause a long period of wakefulness. One other very important difference from the sociological standpoint is the lack of rapid onset of tolerance that occurs with the other hallucinogens. The can-

6. *Mayor's Committee on Marihuana*, New York City, Cattell Press, Lancaster, Pa., 1944.
7. Becker, H. S., 'Becoming a Marihuana User', *American Journal of Sociology*, 59, 1953, pp. 235–42.

nabis intoxication may be maintained continuously through repeated doses, whereas the intake of LSD and mescaline must be spaced over several days to be effective. In addition, the evidence on the use of these drugs indicates that, although the mild euphoria obtained from cannabis may be desirable daily, or even more frequently, the overwhelming impact of the peyote and LSD experience generally results in a psychological satiation that lasts much longer than the tolerance effect.

MOTIVATION

In this country marihuana users almost invariably report the motivation is to attain a 'high' feeling which is generally described as 'a feeling of adequacy and efficiency' in which mental conflicts are allayed. The experienced user is able to achieve consistently a state of self-confidence, satisfaction and relaxation, and he much prefers a congenial group setting to experiencing the effects alone. Unlike the reasons the Indian gives for taking peyote, the marihuana user typically does not claim any lasting benefits beyond the immediate pleasure obtained.

In India and the Middle East, cannabis is apparently taken under a much wider range of circumstances and motivations. The long history, wide range of amount used, and the fact that legal restrictions do not require its concealment permits investigation under a variety of conditions. Most eastern investigators draw a clear distinction between the occasional or moderate regular user and those who indulge to excess. Chopra states that cannabis is still used fairly extensively in Indian indigenous medicine, and that it is also frequently taken in small quantities by labourers to alleviate fatigue and sometimes hunger.[8] In certain parts of India this results in a 50 per cent increase in consumption during the harvest season. Chopra writes:

A common practice among labourers engaged on building or excavation work is to have a few pulls at a ganja pipe or to drink a glass of bhang towards the evening. This produces a sense of well-

8. Chopra, I. C. and R. N. Chopra, 'The Use of Cannabis Drugs in India', *Bulletin on Narcotics*, 9, No. 1, 1957, pp. 4–29.

being, relieves fatigue, stimulates the appetite, and induces a feeling of mild stimulation, which enables the worker to bear more cheerfully the strain and perhaps the monotony of the daily routine of life.

Similarly, Benabud found moderate use of kif by the country people in Morocco to 'keep spirits up'. The need for moderation is expressed in the folk saying, 'Kif is like fire; a little warms, a lot burns'.[9] Bhang is also frequently used as a cooling drink or food supplement.

Cannabis also has a long history of religious use in India, being taken at various ceremonies and for 'clearing the head and stimulating the brain to think' in meditation.[8] It also plays a central role in the religions of certain primitive African and South American tribes.[10] In India, the religious use of cannabis is by no means always moderate. Chopra writes, 'The deliberate abuse of bhang is met with almost entirely among certain classes of religious mendicants.'[8]

Whatever aphrodisiac qualities cannabis may possess, virtually all investigators agree these are cerebral in nature and due to the reduction of inhibition and increased suggestibility. It is probable that it is little, if any, more effective than alcohol in this respect. In fact, Chopra writes, 'Amongst profligate women and prostitutes bhang-sherbet used to be a popular drink in the course of the evening when their paramours visited them. This practice has, however, been largely replaced by the drinking of alcohol which is much more harmful.'[11] Chopra also mentions that certain 'saintly people who wish to renounce world pleasure use cannabis drugs for suppressing sexual desires.'

One final motivation should be mentioned – that of musici-

9. Benabud, A., 'Psycho-pathological Aspects of the Cannabis Situation in Morocco: Statistical Data for 1956', *Bulletin on Narcotics*, 9, No. 4, 1957, pp. 1–16.

10. Murphy, H. B. M., 'The Cannabis Habit: A Review of Recent Psychiatric Literature', *Bulletin on Narcotics*, 15, No. 1, 1963, pp. 15–23.

11. Chopra, R. N. and G. S. Chopra, 'The Present Position of Hemp-Drug Addiction in India', *Indian Journal of Medical Research Memoirs*, No. 31, 1939, pp. 1–119.

ans who feel marihuana improves their ability. Walton writes, 'The habit is so common among this professional group that it may properly be considered a special occupational hazard.' He grants that the release of inhibitions may intensify the 'emotional character of the performance' for certain audiences, but doubts that technical performance is improved.

Benabud stresses that the major problems with cannabis in Morocco exist among the urban slum dwellers, especially among those who have newly come from the country and are 'no longer buttressed by traditional customs'. By contrast, he points out that although kif is widely used among the country people, there is no sign of compulsive need, such as exists 'among the uprooted, and poverty-stricken proletariat of the large town'.

FREQUENCY OF USE AND THE QUESTION OF ADDICTION

The confirmed user takes cannabis at least once per day; however, many others indulge only occasionally. There are no statistics on the ratio of regular to occasional users, but Bromberg found that only a small proportion of those who smoked marihuana in New York used it regularly.[12] Of those who use it regularly in the United States, most report they have voluntarily or involuntarily discontinued the habit from time to time without difficulty.

Regarding the question of addiction to cannabis, most investigators agree there is generally no physiological dependence developed and only slight tolerance. This applies particularly to the moderate use observed in the United States. In the Mayor's Committee study, the officers who posed as marihuana habitués found no evidence of compulsion on the part of the user – there was no particular sign of frustration or compulsive seeking of a source of marihuana when it was not immediately available. In the studies mentioned above, where experienced

12. Bromberg, W., 'Marihuana Intoxication', *American Journal of Psychiatry*, 91, 1934, pp. 303–30.

subjects were allowed to smoke marihuana at will, no behavioral evidence of discomfort was observed when it was abruptly withdrawn.

Concerning the use of cannabis in India, Chopra writes:

In contrast to the other narcotic drugs, we found that the necessity for increase of dosage in order to produce the same effects subsequently was only rarely observed in those who took cannabis drugs habitually. The tolerance developed both in animals and man was generally slight, if any, and was in no way comparable to that tolerance developed to opiates. Its occurrence was observed only in those individuals who took excessive doses, after its prolonged use. Even then, it was hardly appreciable when cannabis was taken orally, but sometimes occurred when it was smoked ... Habitual use of bhang can be discontinued without much trouble, but withdrawal from ganja and charas habits, in our experience, is more difficult to achieve, and is sometimes accompanied by unpleasant symptoms, though they are negligible compared with those associated with withdrawal from opiates and even cocaine.

PHYSICAL AND MENTAL EFFECTS

Long-Lasting Effects

The Mayor's Committee compared the forty-eight users and twenty-four non-users from the standpoint of mental and physical deterioration resulting from long-term use of marihuana. They also conducted detailed quantitative measures on seventeen of those who had used it the longest (mean eight years, range two to sixteen; mean dose per day seven cigarettes, range two to eighteen). They concluded that the subjects 'had suffered no mental or physical deterioration as a result of their use of the drug'. Freedman and Rockmore also report that their sample of three hundred and ten, who had used marihuana an average of seven years, showed no mental or physical deterioration.[13]

13. Freedman, H. L. and M. J. Rockmore, 'Marihuana, Factor in Personality Evaluation and Army Maladjustment', *Journal of Clinical Psychopathology*, 7, and 8, 1946, pp. 765–82 and 221–36.

In India, the study of the mental, moral and physical effects of cannabis has had a long history, beginning with a seven-volume report issued by the Indian Hemp Drugs Commission in 1894. Their conclusions, as quoted by Walton, are as follows:

The evidence shows the moderate use of ganja or charas not to be appreciably harmful, while in the case of bhang drinking, the evidence shows the habit to be quite harmless ... The excessive use does cause injury ... tends to weaken the constitution and to render the consumer more susceptible to disease ... Moderate use of hemp drugs produces no injurious effects on the mind ... excessive use indicates and intensifies mental instability.

The commission continued, as quoted by Chopra: 'it [bhang] is the refreshing beverage of the people corresponding to beer in England and moderate indulgence in it is attended with less injurious consequences than similar consumption of alcohol in Europe.' Chopra writes, 'This view has been corroborated by our own experience in the field.'

Chopra provides numerous statistics on the effect of cannabis on health by dose size and mode of consumption. In the previously mentioned sample of 1,200 regular users, there was a distinct difference in the effects on health, as reported by the user, depending on whether bhang or ganja and charas were consumed. For bhang, 65 per cent reported no effect, 19 per cent minor impairment, 4 per cent marked impairment and 11 per cent slight improvement. For ganja and charas the comparable percentages were thirty-one, thirty-three, thirty-two, and four.[14] By dose level, 70 per cent of those using less than ten grains per day said there was no effect on health and 30 per cent reported improvement. By comparison, of those using more than ninety grains per day, 25 per cent claimed no effect, 31 per cent minor impairment, 44 per cent marked impairment and none claimed improvement of health. Forty per cent of the ganja and charas users reported sleep disturbance and insomnia as compared to 4 per cent of the bhang drinkers.

14. As described in the previous section the consumption of bhang was typically much lower and its effect less potent than ganja and charas.

Turning now to the relation between cannabis and psychosis, it is well established that transient psychotic reactions can be precipitated by using the drug, and, in susceptible individuals, this may occur even with moderate or occasional use. Out of a total of seventy-two persons used as experimental subjects the Mayor's Committee reports three cases of psychosis: one lasted four days, another six months, and one became psychotic two weeks after being returned to prison (duration not noted). The Committee concludes, 'that given the potential personality make-up and the right time and environment, marihuana may bring on a true psychotic state'.

Benabud especially stresses excessive use and environmental factors, pointing out that the rate of psychosis among the moderate-smoking country people is only one tenth that in the large cities.

The chronic cannabis psychosis reported by eastern writers has not been observed in this country. Most western authors, while recognizing the role of cannabis in precipitating acute transient psychoses, have questioned the causal role in chronic cases. Mayer-Gross writes: 'The chronic hashish psychoses described by earlier observers have proved to be cases of schizophrenia complicated by symptoms of cannabis intoxication.'[15] Allentuck states that 'a characteristic cannabis psychosis does not exist. Marihuana will not produce a psychosis *de novo* in a well-integrated stable person.'[16] And Murphy writes: 'The prevalence of *major* mental disorder among cannabis users appears to be little, if any, higher than that in the general population.' Since it is well established that cannabis use attracts the mentally unstable, Murphy raises the interesting question of 'whether the use of cannabis may not be protecting some individuals from a psychosis'.

15. Mayer-Gross, W., E. Slater and M. Roth, *Clinical Pyschiatry*, Cassell, London, 1954.
16. Allentuck, S., and K. M. Bowman, 'The Psychiatric Aspects of Marihuana Intoxication', *American Journal of Psychiatry*, 99, 1942, pp. 248–51.

CANNABIS AND CRIME

The Mayor's Committee found that many marihuana smokers were guilty of petty crimes, but there was no evidence that the practice was associated with major crimes. On the contrary 'professional' criminals considered marihuana smokers to be inferior and unreliable and would not associate with them. The Committee also investigated thirty-nine schools and found that marihuana was used by small numbers in certain schools, but that it was not a large-scale practice. Finally, they report that although marihuana smoking causes disinhibition, it does not alter the basic personality of the user or 'evoke responses which would be totally alien to him in his undrugged state'.

More recent assessments tend to agree with these findings. The Ad Hoc Panel on Drug Abuse at the 1962 White House Conference states, 'Although marihuana has long held the reputation of inciting individuals to commit sexual offences and other anti-social acts, evidence is inadequate to substantiate this.'[17] Maurer and Vogel write:

While there may be occasional violent psychopaths who have used marihuana, have committed crimes of violence, and who have, in court, explained their actions as uncontrollable violence resulting from the use of the drug, these are exceptions to the general run of marihuana users.[18]

In addition to impulsive acts performed under acute cannabis intoxication, there are frequent references in the literature to criminals using the drug to provide courage to commit violent acts. There has been no evidence offered to substantiate this claim; rather, Chopra writes as follows regarding premeditated crime:

In some cases these drugs not only do not lead to it, but actually act as deterrents. We have already observed that one of the important actions of these drugs is to quieten and stupefy the individual so that there is no tendency to violence, as is not infrequently found

17. *White House Conference on Narcotic and Drug Abuse*, U.S. Government Printing Office, Washington, 1963.

18. Maurer, D. W. and V. H. Vogel, *Narcotics and Narcotics Addiction*, Charles C. Thomas, Springfield, Illinois, 1962.

in cases of alcoholic intoxication. The result of continued and excessive use of these drugs in our experience in India is to make the individual timid rather than lead him to commit violent crimes.

It is interesting that a number of observers, particularly in countries other than the United States, consider alcohol to be a worse offender than cannabis in causing crime. For instance, an editorial in the *South African Medical Journal* states:

Dagga produces in the smoker drowsiness, euphoria and occasional psychotic episodes, but alcohol is guilty of even graver action. It is not certain to what extent dagga contributes to the commission of crime in this country. Alcohol does so in undeniable measure.[19]

In the United States, probably the most serious accusation made regarding marihuana smoking is that it often leads to the use of heroin.[18] The Mayor's Committee found no evidence of this, stating, 'The instances are extremely rare where the habit of marihuana smoking is associated with addiction to these other narcotics.' Nevertheless, it is difficult to see how the association with criminal pedlars, who often also sell heroin, can fail to influence some marihuana users to become addicted to heroin.

SUMMARY AND APPRAISAL

Cannabis is an hallucinogen whose effects are somewhat similar to, though much milder than, peyote and LSD. The confirmed user takes it daily or more frequently, and through experience and careful regulation of the dose is able to consistently limit the effects to euphoria and other desired qualities. Unlike peyote, there are typically no claims of benefit other than the immediate effects. Mild tolerance and physical dependence may develop when the more potent preparations are used to excess; however, they are virtually non-existent for occasional or moderate regular users. There are apparently no

19. Editorial, 'Dagga', *South African Medical Journal*, 25: 17, 1951, pp. 284–6.

deleterious physical effects resulting from moderate use, though excessive indulgence noted in some eastern countries contributes to a variety of ailments. The most serious hazard is the precipitation of transient psychoses. Unstable individuals may experience a psychotic episode from even a small amount, and although they typically recover within a few days, some psychoses triggered by cannabis reactions may last for several months. In eastern countries, where cannabis is taken in large amounts, some authors feel that it is directly or indirectly responsible for a sizeable portion of the intakes in psychiatric hospitals.

In this country cannabis is not used to excess by eastern standards; however, it does attract a disproportionate number of poorly adjusted and non-productive young persons in the lower socio-economic strata. The extent to which legal prohibition and social stigma prevent other groups from indulging is a matter of conjecture. In eastern countries cannabis is currently also largely restricted to the lower classes; however, moderate use is not illegal, socially condemned, nor necessarily considered indicative of personality defects. The reputation of cannabis for inciting major crimes is unwarranted and it probably has no more effect than alcohol in this respect.

Of those familiar with the use of marihuana in this country, there is general agreement that the legal penalties imposed for its use are much too severe. Laws controlling marihuana are similar or identical to those pertaining to the opiates, including the mandatory imposition of long prison sentences for certain offences. Many judges have complained that these laws have resulted in excessive sentences (five to ten years) for relatively minor offences with marihuana. The 1962 White House Conference made the following recommendation: 'It is the opinion of the Panel that the hazards of marihuana *per se* have been exaggerated and that long criminal sentences imposed on an occasional user or possessor are in poor social perspective.'

The cultural attitude toward narcotics is, of course, a very important determiner of legal and social measures adopted for their control. An interesting commentary on the extent to which these attitudes resist change and influence factual interpretation is afforded by the lively debate that followed the publishing of the Mayor's Committee Report on Marihuana in 1944. This was an extensive study conducted under the auspices of the New York Academy of Medicine at the request of Mayor La Guardia. Its findings tended to minimize the seriousness of the marihuana problem in New York and set off a series of attacks from those with opposing viewpoints. An American Medical Association editorial commented: 'Public officials will do well to disregard this unscientific uncritical study, and continue to regard marihuana as a menace wherever it is purveyed.'[20] And, as Taylor points out, 'We have done so ever since.'[21] Anslinger, the Commissioner of Narcotics, wrote, 'The Bureau immediately detected the superficiality and hollowness of its findings and denounced it.'[22] The authors expressed dismay that the report was attacked on the grounds that the findings represented a public danger, rather than on its scientific aspects.[23] Walton, a leading authority on cannabis, wrote:

The report in question came generally to the same conclusion that any other group of competent investigators might reach if they repeated the inquiry under the same conditions ... A scientific study should be expected to report merely what it finds, avoid propaganda and let the public do what it will with the results.[24]

Murphy raises the question of why cannabis is so regularly banned in countries where alcohol is permitted. He feels that one of the reasons is the positive value placed on action, and the hostility towards passivity:

20. Editorial, 'Marihuana Problems', *Journal of the American Medical Association*, 127, 1945, p. 1129.
21. Taylor, N., *Flight from Reality*, Duell, Sloan & Pearce, New York, 1949.
22. Anslinger, H. J. and W. G. Tompkins, *The Traffic in Narcotics*, Funk & Wagnalls, New York, 1953.
23. Bowman, K. M., 'Psychiatric Aspects of Marihuana Intoxication', *Journal of the American Medical Association*, 125, 1944, p. 376.
24. Walton, R. P., 'Marihuana Problems', *Journal of the American Medical Association*, 128, 1945, p. 383.

In Anglo-Saxon cultures inaction is looked down on and often feared, whereas over-activity, aided by alcohol or independent of alcohol, is considerably tolerated despite the social disturbance produced. It may be that we can ban cannabis simply because the people who use it, or would do so, carry little weight in social matters and are relatively easy to control; whereas the alcohol user often carries plenty of weight in social matters and is difficult to control, as the United States prohibition era showed. It has yet to be shown, however, that the one is more socially or personally disruptive than the other.

Marihuana and the 'O' Effect

S. H. Groff*

I have observed that besides a variation in the intensity of specific effects brought about by the use of marihuana grown in different parts of the world, there is also a variation in the *nature* of the effects it may arouse. The psychedelic effect and its relationship to consciousness expansion, and the parasympathetic effect on the central nervous system, have been quite thoroughly investigated and described, and its use in the healing arts in the form of an extract and a tincture has been listed in the Pharmacopeia of many countries. I have given the name 'O' effect to one specific property of some types of marihuana, because it seemed to be, at least semantically, a descriptive lowest common denominator for being understood when discussing this hypothesis with those having some experience in this area. To be sure, the 'O' is lent from the word opium, and

*Dr Groff is a psycho-physiologist who has had extensive experience with both psychedelic drugs and parachute jumping. He notes a similarity between the sensation felt in sky-diving during the period before the parachute opens, known as the 'free fall', and the 'high feeling' so frequently encountered in psychedelic drug sessions. It is interesting to compare this with a comment made by a member of the Royal Air Force that 'pilots flying at very high altitudes have reported hallucinations in which they seem to be outside the cabin looking at the shell of themselves on the inside.'

indeed a part of the meaning is meant to indicate that this is an undesirable effect. At the outset it should be made clear that it is not my intention to make any value judgement considering the use of opium for any means whatever, nor has the particular effect I am about to describe any relationship with yet another undesirable effect specific to opium, that of addiction. That marihuana does not have any addictive effect has been unequivocally authenticated through investigation, and need not be gone into further here. The specific effect I call the 'O' effect has often been described as that of being 'stoned out'. It is meant to describe a physical situation occurring concomitantly with other mind manifesting properties which the marihuana brings about. Contrary to what one would expect in that enlightened state, it seems almost impossible to get the body to respond to the desired normal motor function when this effect is present. I daresay that one being accustomed to a type of marihuana in which this effect is absent or negligible, when confronted with this new effect after having had experience with marihuana from some other part of the world, depending on his level of paranoia at the moment, may be thrust into a situation which creates an entirely negative experience for him. It has been reported for example that marihuana grown in certain regions of Morocco has either very little or no 'O' effect inherent to it, whereas the marihuana referred to as 'Congo Wheat' causes a rather high level of the 'O' effect. Further, it would seem that in the process of preparing hashish from marihuana, a greater level of the 'O' effect is always the result, since to my knowledge there is no hashish reported which does not have a noticeable 'O' effect resultant from its use. At this moment it is assumed by some that the active principle in marihuana is dependent on a group of substances called tetrahydrocannabinols and it would thus seem a rather simple task for the biochemist to test the quantity of these substances found in the various types of marihuana. However, I should like to point out that even after such an extensive research was done into the chemical presence of these substances one could always question whether it is truly these substances which are responsible for the ascribed effect, and problems as to the level of our biochemical powers of resolution at the moment will always remain subservient to subjective experimentation. This should be understood as an attempt to indicate a more complete and healthy attitude in one's approach to the problem, and shifts in emphasis are apparent as the story is retold or rewritten rather than misunderstood to imply a lessened faith in the value of biochemical research. Lastly, I should like to point out that it is of course possible that this effect that I have ascribed to marihuana may be nothing more than an individual's response to the marihuana, having nothing to do with the marihuana itself. There is no question in my mind that this is possible, and I am certain that if not the sole answer, it surely does play a role.

Two Letters, 1964

R. D. Laing and A. Esterson

The following two letters were written by English doctors after one of their colleagues was imprisoned for possession of marihuana. The letters were written to the editors of two medical journals who refused to print them because they 'did not wish to seem to take sides'.

1 June 1964

Dear Sir,

Last week in Glasgow several people, including a doctor, were sentenced to months of imprisonment after conviction on charges of being in possession of marihuana. Does not this case point urgently to the need for the medical profession to do what we can to dispel the mounting panic in the country, reflected in the Police and judiciary, at the effects of this drug that is not known to have any deleterious effects whatever?

As far as I know, marihuana has no addictive properties; it

has no harmful physiological effects; it induces no deterioration in the personality. The simplest short summary of its action is that it induces an enhanced sense of delight and serenity (see *Lancet* Editorial 9/11/63).

It is my impression that it is a useful therapeutic agent in people who feel mildly unreal and depersonalized, that is, people who would probably be diagnosed as ambulatory schizophrenics, with symptoms of depersonalization and derealization. I have never heard of a marihuana smoker who was an alcoholic.

There seems to me to be a strong case both to point out to doctors that it is possible for them to prescribe this drug with discrimination and, moreover, to think seriously about making it as available to the public as nicotine or alcohol. It seems to me that the bad effects of marihuana arise practically *entirely* through the need for young people to go underground if they wish to 'turn on'. One is reminded of the Prohibition period. Anyone who knows anything of this drug, knows how tragically ironic it is that the innocent delight it occasions should be associated in so many good people's minds with degeneracy and depravity.

I would be far happier if my own teenage children would, *without breaking the law*, smoke marihuana when they wished, rather than start on the road of so many of their elders to nicotine and ethyl alcohol addiction.

R. D. Laing, M.B., Ch.B., D.P.M.

2 June 1964

Dear Sir,

A wave of hysteria appears to have gripped the authorities and the popular press on the issue of marihuana. They seem to believe that this substance is dangerous and that members of the public must be protected from it. People who smoke it are being sent to prison as if they were dangerous criminals and last week in Glasgow a doctor was sentenced to six months' imprisonment for being in possession of a quantity.

In these circumstances should not the medical profession through its representatives try to stem the panic by placing the facts on marihuana before the public? Marihuana, far from being dangerous, appears to be completely harmless and under certain circumstances beneficial. It is non-addictive and unlike nicotine and ethyl alcohol it has no known deleterious physiological effects. Psychologically, it is known to enhance perception including self-perception and there is no scientifically respectable evidence to suggest that it causes any harm morally or mentally. On the contrary, there is evidence to suggest it may be useful in psychiatric conditions such as schizophrenia and states of depersonalization and derealization.

True, those who smoke it sometimes fall foul of the law but this is simply because smoking it is illegal. If the law was changed these people would not transgress, and since the law in this matter is based on a total misunderstanding of the effects of marihuana, is it not time that this change was made?

Yours sincerely,
A. Esterson, M.B., Ch.B., D.P.M.

Recent Trends in Cannabis Research

Julian Reeves, M.A., M.B.

There has been a curious accent on emotional stances in recent scientific research into Indian hemp. It has often seemed that the more strongly the researcher disapproved of any use of the drug by humans, the more readily opened were the purses of those who finance drug research: government agencies and industry.

The pharmaceutical industry in particular has an enormous commitment to selling and developing drugs unrelated to cannabis but for which the classical benefits of Indian hemp are claimed. Drugs to relax the mind and body and to relieve depression are market best-sellers. They help to pay for much of that expensively produced and totally useless advertising with which the pharmaceutical industry deluges the medical profession. The pharmaceutical industry, however, overtly ignores cannabis and its derivatives. The pleasure drug industries (alcoholic drinks and nicotine products) also have a great deal at stake.

In medical laboratories mice and rats have been getting a bellyful of the drug – administered in solution by hypodermic needle directly into the abdominal cavity. This practice seems impossible to correlate with the habits of human cannabis devotees, but the pretext is that intraperitoneal injection of drugs is routine for rat experiments. The results have been as bizarre as the mode of administration. At Oxford mice in the cages of Professor Paton have shown an inability to renew the structure of certain white blood cells in the usual way, which has been hastily interpreted as implying that the mice were suffering genetic damage of the total organism. Some animals have been so overwhelmed by the traumatic daily administration of the drug that they expired. Some, as reported to the American Chemical Association in October 1971, developed malignant growths of new tissue in their abdominal cavity, a form of cancer. This immediately suggests that malignant growths of the lung should be common among cannabis smokers. A sociological study using mass chest x-rays, as in tuberculosis detection, could easily be done. It could probably be done best in some country such as India, which has a part of its people ingesting cannabis from cradle to grave. However, it is medical doctrine that cancer of the lung is exceedingly rare except among heavy tobacco smokers living in cities. If this traditional view of lung cancer is correct, it would explain why the British Indian Hemp Report of 1894 did not note any incidence of lung cancer at that time among cannabis smokers. In fact their health was good.

On the other hand, human studies on volunteer subjects have yielded no dramatic results. The only news is but a confirmation of what was generally believed, i.e. that when men are high they behave in a preoccupied way with such things as motor cars to the extent of slowed reaction time in response to a need to brake or failing to notice road signs. The impairment of learned psycho-motor functions is however less than is caused by alcohol in the amounts commonly taken. One London practitioner is researching its use in muscular dystrophy, which he believes can sometimes be relieved by cannabis. And on the other hand commercial pharmacists have proven that in neither mice, rats, guinea pigs or monkeys does long-term ingestion of cannabis injure the animals in any way.

The medical uses for cannabis have not changed. Most prescriptions are for psychiatric indications, to ease nervous tension or for the relief of pain. No deaths have been recorded in the past decade from overdosage of medically prescribed cannabis. This safety record is far higher than that of any other drug which is prescribed for the same range of ailments. Without any expensive publicity from the manufacturers, more British doctors have taken to prescribing cannabis preparations in the past five years than did in the preceding decade.

Le Dane Report

The Non-Medical Use of Drugs (Canadian Government Commission)

OVERVIEW OF EFFECTS

153. *Physiological Effects.* The short-term physiological effects of cannabis are usually slight and apparently have little clinical significance. The following effects have been established in adequately controlled studies: increase in heart rate, swelling of the minor conjunctival blood vessels in the membranes around the eye, and minor unspecific changes in the electroencephalogram (EEG). Also commonly noted, but less well documented, are: a slight drying of the eyes and nasal passages, initially stimulated salivation followed by dryness of

the mouth, throat irritation and coughing during smoking, and increased urination. Less commonly, nausea, vomiting, diarrhoea or constipation are reported. These gastrointestinal disturbances rarely occur with smoked cannabis, although nausea is not uncommon when large quantities are taken orally. Changes in blood sugar level and blood pressure have been inconsistently reported. Appetite is usually stimulated. Contrary to popular belief, there is little evidence of pupil dilatation. In some individuals, incoordination, ataxia and tremors have been observed and chest pains, dizziness and fainting have occasionally been noted, usually at high doses. Physiological hangover effects have been described but are rare, even after considerable intoxication.

154. Cannabis has little acute physiological toxicity – sleep is the usual somatic consequence of over-dose. No deaths due directly to smoking or eating of cannabis have been documented and no reliable information exists regarding the lethal dose in humans. One fatality, however, was reportedly caused by distention of the bowel during a prolonged bout of gross overeating under the acute influence of cannabis.

155. There is little reliable information on the long-term effects of cannabis use. There are numerous reports from eastern countries of chronic ill-health among very heavy long-term users of hashish. Most commonly reported are minor respiratory and gastro-intestinal ailments. These studies rarely provide a control group of comparable non-users for a reference standard, and clinical findings are usually confounded with a variety of social, economic and cultural factors which are not easily untangled. Consequently, much important work remains to be done in this area. The British *Cannabis* report (1968) states:

Having reviewed all the material available to us, we find ourselves in agreement with the conclusion reached by the Indian Hemp Drugs Commission appointed by the Government of India (1893-4) and the New York Mayor's Committee on Marihuana (1944), that the long-term consumption of cannabis in *moderate* doses has no harmful effects.

. 156. Some observers have suggested that chronic smoking of cannabis might produce carcinogenic effects similar to those now attributed to the smoking of tobacco, although no evidence exists to support this view at this time. A meaningful comparison is difficult to make since the quantity of leaf consumed by the average cigarette smoker in North America is many times the amount of cannabis smoked by even heavy users. The present pattern of use by regular cannabis smokers in North America is more analogous to intermittent alcohol use (e.g., once or twice a week), than to the picture of chronic daily use presented by ordinary tobacco dependence. However, the deep inhalation technique usually used with cannabis might add respiratory complications.

157. Recently, there have been conflicting reports that large quantities of cannabis extract, injected into pregnant females of certain strains of rodents, may cause abnormalities in the offspring. These disparate results cannot be simply extrapolated to humans and at this time there is no scientific evidence that cannabis adversely affects human chromosomes or causes deformed children.

Part Four

Potentialities for Increasing Consciousness

Varieties of Consciousness

William James

One conclusion was forced upon my mind at that time, and my impression of its truth has ever since remained unshaken. It is that our normal waking consciousness, rational consciousness as we call it, is but one special type of consciousness, whilst all about it, parted from it by the flimsiest of screens, there lie potential forms of consciousness entirely different. We may go through life without suspecting their existence; but apply the requisite stimulus, and at a touch they are there in all their completeness, definite types of mentality which probably somewhere have their field of application. No account of the universe in its totality can be final which leaves these other forms of consciousness quite disregarded. How to regard them is the question – for they are so discontinuous with ordinary consciousness. Yet they may determine attitudes though they cannot furnish formulas, and open a region though they fail to give a map. At any rate, they forbid a premature closing of our accounts with reality.

Mysticism, Sacred and Profane

R. C. Zaehner

It is, of course, a well-known fact that certain drugs – and among them one may include alcohol – modify the normal human consciousness and produce what can literally be called ec-static states – states in which the human ego has the impression that it escapes from itself and 'stands outside' itself. Indian hemp and hashish have long been used in the East to produce precisely such a result.

A Psychedelic Experience: Fact or Fantasy

Alan Watts

What we know, positively and scientifically, about psychedelic chemicals is that they bring about certain alterations of sense perception, of emotional level and tone, of identity feeling, of the interpretation of sense data, and of the sensations of time and space. The nature of these alterations depends on three varieties: the chemical itself (type and dosage), the psycho-physiological state of the subject, and the social and aesthetic context of the experiment. Their physiological side effects are minimal, though there are conditions (e.g., disease of the liver) in which some of them may be harmful. They are not physiologically habit-forming in the same way as alcohol and tobacco, though some individuals may come to depend on them for other (i.e., 'neurotic') reasons. Their results are not easily predictable since they depend so largely upon such imponderables as the setting, and the attitudes and expectations of both the supervisor and the subject. The (enormous) scientific literature on the subject indicates that a majority of people have pleasant reactions, a largish minority have unpleasant but instructive and helpful reactions, while a very small minority have psychotic reactions lasting from hours to months. It has never been definitely established that they have led directly to a suicide. (I am referring specifically here to LSD-25, mescaline, the mushroom-derivative psilocybin, and the various forms of cannabis, such as hashish and marihuana.)

Psychometabolism

Sir Julian Huxley

Throughout evolution, the animal, with the aid of various bodily organs, utilizes the raw materials of its food, drink, and inspired air and transforms them into characteristic biochemical patterns which canalize and direct its physiological activities. This is metabolism. But with the aid of its brain, its organ of awareness or mind, it utilizes the raw materials of its subjective experience and transforms it into characteristic patterns of awareness which then canalize and help to direct its behaviour. This I venture to call psychometabolism.

During the latter stages of evolution, an increasingly efficient type of psychometabolism is superposed on and added to the universal physiological metabolism. Eventually, about 10 million years ago, purely biological evolution reached a limit, and the breakthrough to new advance was only brought about by the further elaboration of the psychometabolic apparatus of mind and brain. This gave rise to man: it endowed him with a second method of heredity based on the transmission of experience, and launched him on a new phase of evolution operating by cumulative tradition based on ideas and knowledge. Both novelties are of course superposed on the biological methods of transmission and evolution, which he also possesses.

In man, organizations of awareness become part of the evolutionary process by being incorporated in cultural tradition. Accordingly, in human evolution totally new kinds of organization are produced: organizations such as works of art, moral codes, scientific ideas, legal systems, and religions. We men are better able to evaluate, to comprehend, to grasp far more complex total patterns and situations than any other organism. We are capable of many things that no other animal is capable of:

conscious reflection, the idea of self, of death, and of the future in general; we have the capacity of framing conscious purposes which can then be translated into action, and of constructing values as norms for our activities. The result is that evolution in the psycho-social phase is primarily cultural and only to a minor extent genetic.

Of course all these new types of organization evolve like everything else. The science of comparative religion shows how religions have evolved and are still evolving. The history of science studies the evolution of scientific ideas and how they become operative in the psychosocial process.

Our mental or psychometabolic organizations fall into two main categories: those for dealing with the outer world and establishing a relation with external objects; and those for dealing with our inner world and relating our perceptions and concepts and emotional drives to each other and integrating them into a more or less harmonious whole. The ultimate aim is to deal with all kinds of conflict and to reduce mental friction, so as to get the maximum flow of what is often called mental energy . . .

A major job for all disciplines concerned with human affairs, whether biochemistry, psychology, psychiatry or social anthropology, is to investigate the extraordinary mechanisms underlying the organization and operation of awareness, so as to lay the foundation for and promote the realization of more meaningful and more effective possibilities in the psycho-social process of human evolution.

When we look at animal behaviour, it is clear that differences in possibilities of awareness between different species are primarily genetic. One species of bird prefers blue, another does not: the sign-stimulus which will release adaptive patterns of action in one species of bird, will not do so in another. There is obviously a genetic basis for the difference.

Equally obviously, there is a genetic basis for the difference between the genetically exceptional individual and the bulk of the species. All great advances in human history are due to the thought or action of a few exceptional individuals, though they take effect through the mass of people and in relation to the general social background. We have seen how, already in birds and mammals, the exceptional individual can be of some importance in the life of the species. In man, the exceptional individual can be of decisive importance.

Today, many workers in psychology and psychiatry and other behavioural and social sciences resist or even deny the idea that genetic factors are important for behaviour. I am sure that they are wrong. Of course environmental factors, including learning, are always operative, but so are genetic factors. To take an example, genetic differences in psychosomatic organization and somatotype are obviously correlated with differences in temperament, and these with different reactions to stress and proneness to different diseases.

Frequently, it is not so much complete genetic determination we have got to think about, but rather proneness to this or that reaction, a tendency to develop in this or that way. This comes out very clearly in regard to cancer: every different inbred strain of mice has a different degree of proneness for a different type of cancer – sometimes 40 per cent, sometimes 80 per cent, in a few cases 100 per cent. Professor Roger Williams of Texas has coined a new word, *propetology*, to denote genetic proneness. A science of propetology is badly needed.

The old-fashioned behaviourists simply denied any influence to genetic factors. For them everything was due to learning; and I am afraid that a number of ethologists and students of behaviour, especially in America, still stick to that point of view. They forget that even the *capacity* to learn, to learn at all, to learn at a definite time, to learn one kind of thing rather than another, to learn more or less quickly, must have some genetic basis.

One of the most curious discoveries of the past thirty or forty years has been that of the sensory morphisms, where a considerable proportion of the population has a sensory awareness different from that of the 'normal' majority. The best known cause is a taste-morphism. Phenylthiocarbamide (PTC) tastes very bitter to the majority of human beings, but a minority of about 25 per cent, varying somewhat in different ethnic groups, cannot taste it at all except in exceedingly high concentrations. As R. A. Fisher pointed out in his great book, *The Genetic Basis of Natural Selection*, in 1930, two sharply contrasted genetic characters like this cannot coexist indefinitely in a population unless there is a balance of biological advantage and disadvantage between them. Thus whenever we find such balanced polymorphisms, or *morphisms*, as they are more simply called, we know that there must be some selective balance involved. Quite recently it has been shown that PTC taste-morphism is correlated with thyroid function; here we begin to get some inkling of what advantage or disadvantage there may be.

Years ago, Fisher, Ford, and I tested all the captive chimpanzees in England for PTC sensitivity. We found, to our delight, that within the limits of statistical error they had the same proportion of non-tasters as human beings. People asked, 'How did you find out?' Actually it was quite simple; we offered them a sugar solution containing PTC. If they were non-tasters, they spat it in our faces: it was an all-or-nothing reaction. The fact that both chimpanzees and man react alike means that this balanced morphism must have been in existence in the higher primates for at least 10 million years.

There are a number of these sensory morphisms in man. There is a sex-linked morphism with regard to the smell of hydrogen cyanide, HCN; about 18 per cent of males are insensitive to it, which can be dangerous in a chemical works or laboratory. There is another smell-blindness with regard to the scent of Freesias. I personally am one of the considerable minority of human beings unable to smell Freesias; I can smell any other flower, but am absolutely insensitive to the particular smell of even the most fragrant Freesias. There are visual morphisms; the best known is red-green colour-blindness, which is also sex-linked. Another appears to be myopia. I remember years ago discussing with Professor H. J. Muller the puzzling fact of the considerable incidence of apparently genetic myopia in modern populations. However, he pointed out that during a considerable period of human history, from the time when people began doing fine, close work and up to the period when spectacles were invented, myopia would confer certain advantages. The short-sighted man would not only be employed on well-paid work, but would usually not be sent to war, so that there was less likelihood of his being killed. This would balance the obvious disadvantage of myopia in other aspects of life.

There are some very interesting biological problems concerning sensitivity to pain. Some human mutants are apparently insensitive to pain altogether and may incur terrible injuries because damaging agencies do not hurt them; but these are very rare. On the other hand, giraffes have mouth-cavities and tongues which appear to be surprisingly insensitive to pain. I always thought that they used their long beautiful tongues to strip the leaves off the extremely thorny acacia trees on which they often feed without getting pricked; but apparently this is not so. Recently in the London Zoo, giraffes have been tested with spiny hawthorn branches: they accept them and chew them just as readily as soft foliage. This surprising fact is worth further investigation.

At the other end of the psychometabolic scale from sensation, we have problems like schizophrenia. Apparently this too must involve a balanced morphism. First, in all countries and races there are about 1 per cent of schizophrenic people; secondly, the disease appears to have a strong genetic basis; and thirdly, as already mentioned, genetic theory makes it plain that a clearly disadvantageous genetic character like this cannot persist in this frequency in a population unless it is balanced by some compensating advantage. In this case it appears that the advantage is that schizophrenic individuals are considerably less sensitive than normal people to histamine, are much less prone to suffer from operative and wound shock, and do not suffer nearly so much from various allergies. Meanwhile, there are indications that some chemical substance, apparently something like adrenochrome or adrenolutin, is the genetically determined basis for schizophrenia, and in any case there is a chromatographically detectable so-called 'mauve-factor' in the urine of schizophrenics.

This biochemical abnormality presumably causes the abnormality of perception found in schizophrenics. The way the schizophrenic psychometabolizes his sensory experience and relates his sensations to build meaningful perceptions, is disordered. Accordingly he is subject to disorders of sensation and of all sorts of perception, including disorders of perception of time and space, and of association. Apparently, schizophrenic individuals show much less consistency in association tests than do normal people. The schizophrenic's world is neither consistently meaningful nor stable: this naturally puts him out of joint with his fellow human beings and makes communication with them difficult and frustrating, so that he retires much more into his own private world.

Hallucinogens like mescaline, lysergic acid, and psilocybin (from a Mexican fungus) appear to exert similar dislocating effects on perception, even in incredibly low doses. In addition, they can produce totally new types of experience: some of their effects can elicit something quite new from the human mind. They may have unpleasant effects if the subject is in a wrong psychological stage, and exceedingly pleasant and rewarding effects if he is in a right one. But in either case they may reveal possibilities of experience which the subject did not know existed at all. For this reason the term *psychedelic*, or mind-revealing, has been suggested for this type of psychotropic drug. In many ways their effect closely resembles a very brief but acute schizophrenia: perception is disordered in a way very like that seen in schizophrenic patients.

In psychedelic drugs we have a remarkable opportunity for interesting research. Nobody, so far as I know, has done any work on their effects on different types of psychologically normal people – people of high and low IQ, of different somatotypes, of different affective dispositions, on verbalizers and visualizers. This would be of extraordinary interest: we might find out not merely how to cure some defect, but how to promote creativity by enhancing the creative imagination.

Another problem is to discover whether psychedelics modify or enhance dreaming. The study of dreaming has received a great impetus since the recent discovery that dreaming is necessary for good mental health. If people are prevented from dreaming night after night, their mental health begins to suffer. Dreaming, it seems, provides a satisfactory way of psychometabolizing various facts and experiences that have proved resistant to the integrating efforts of our waking psychometabolic activity. Unconscious mechanisms take revenge and provide an outlet in dreams.

Early detection is another fact of the schizophrenia problem. Here too, study and research are obviously needed. Granted that there is a genetic proneness to schizophrenia, it should be possible in many cases to detect its symptoms in quite early stages of life. This could clearly best be done in the schools, so that it will be important to establish a close link between psychiatrists and school teachers. The teachers would pick out the children who are prone to schizophrenia; while the psychiatrists would then suggest appropriate methods of education and training to prevent the disease from developing.

Indeed, the subject of education in general clearly needs overhauling, in the light of the two views of the human organism that I have been advocating. Today, we have hardly begun to think of how to educate the organism as a whole – the mind-body, the joint psycho-physiological mechanism which we call the human child. We confine ourselves almost entirely to mental education through verbal means, with the crude physical education of games and physical training added as something quite separate. As my brother Aldous has stressed, we need non-verbal education as well, and education of the entire mind-body instead of 'mind' and 'body' separately.

It is not only in regard to schizophrenia that we are confronted with situations which demand immediate remedial measures, but later find ourselves impelled to adopt a preventive or a constructive attitude. Medical history is largely the story of people trying to cope with disease, then attempting to prevent disease from arising, and finally turning their knowledge to good account in the promotion of positive health. The same is true of the psychological approach. The psychiatrist starts with the mentally diseased person, tries to cure him, or at least to prevent his disease developing further, but in the course of this remedial process, he acquires knowledge which can be of extreme importance in building up a more fruitful normal personality. However, to achieve this, a new approach is needed. Psychiatry usually attempts to analyse the causes of the diseased condition and discover its origins. The very term *psychoanalysis* commits the Freudian practitioner to this approach. This is important, but is certainly not sufficient. All important biological phenomena are irreversible processes, whose end-results are biologically more significant than their origins. Accordingly, we must study the whole process, its end-results as well as its origins, its total pattern as well as its elements.

In psychology, pure and applied, medical and educational, our main aim should be to discover how to regulate the processes of psychometabolism so that they integrate experience in a more effective and less wasteful way and produce a more fruitful end-organization. For instance, I am sure that a study of the origin and strengthening of emotional bonds will repay a great deal of effort. Let me take John Bowlby's work as an example. He studied the development of children who had been deprived of maternal care (including care by a mother substitute) during a critical period of early life, and therefore were unable to form the primary affectional bond between infant and parent. Such children proved incapable of forming further emotional bonds and of developing a normal affectional and moral organization. This whole problem of building up affectional bonds, whether between members of a family or a social group, is fundamental for family life.

The overriding psychometabolic problem, of course, is how the developing human being can integrate his interior life, whether by reconciling emotional or intellectual conflict in a higher synthesis, or by reconciling diversity in a more embracing unity. Let me take the creative arts as an example. Thus the poet must reconcile diverse and even conflicting meanings in a single work of art, and, indeed, must employ multivalent or multi-significant words and phrases in the process. Good poems and paintings are among the highest products of man's psychometabolic activities. Milton's line, 'Then feed on thoughts that voluntary move harmonious numbers ...' beautifully expresses this psychometabolic concept of artistic creation, while Lowe's celebrated critical study, *The Road to Xanadu*, shows how Coleridge psychometabolized the raw materials of his personal experience, his reading and his conversations and discussions, and was able to integrate them into a single poem, 'Kubla Khan', with amazing emotional impact.

As an example of the emotional impact exercised by great art, let me recall a story of Bertrand Russell. When he was an undergraduate at Cambridge, he and a friend were going up his staircase in college and the friend quoted Blake's famous poem, 'Tiger, Tiger, Burning Bright'. Bertrand Russell had never heard or read this before, and was so overcome that he had to lean against the wall to prevent himself falling.

On the other hand, we all know that many poems and works of art fail sadly to achieve this desirable result. The way in which an operatively effective unitary pattern of intellectual, emotional and moral elements can be built up certainly deserves study, not merely in art, but also in morality, religion, and love.

Mysticism is another psychometabolic activity which needs much further research. A really scientific study of the great mystics of the past, of their modern successors, of yoga and other similar movements, undoubtedly would be of great value. The scientist need not, indeed must not, accept at their face value the claims of mysticism, for instance, of achieving union with God or the Absolute. But some mystics have certainly obtained results of great value and importance: they have been able to achieve an interior state of peace and strength which combines profound tranquillity and high psychological energy.

There is also the still much neglected subject of hypnotism

and hypnosis, with all its implications. One of the darker chapters in the history of science and medicine is the way in which the pioneer hypnotists were attacked and often hounded out of the medical profession. Even today, there is still clearly a great deal to be discovered in this strange and exciting subject.

The field of the psychiatrist and the psychologist today is nothing less than the comprehensive study of hypnosis, drugs, education, mysticism, and the subconscious, of mental disease and mental health, of the relation between normal and abnormal or supernormal experience. Backed by the concept of psychometabolism and the fact of the increasing importance of psychological organization of experience during evolution, they will be working for a better integration of all the psychological forces operating in man's life – emotional, imaginative, intellectual and moral – in such a way as to minimize conflict and maximize creativity. In so doing, they will be in harmony with the only desirable direction that our scientific vision indicates for the future evolution of man – a direction making for increased fulfilment of individual human beings and fuller achievement by human societies.

Culture and the Individual

Aldous Huxley

Between culture and the individual the relationship is, and always has been, strangely ambivalent. We are at once the beneficiaries of our culture and its victims. Without culture, and without that precondition of all culture, language, man would be no more than another species of baboon. It is to language and culture that we owe our humanity. And 'What a piece of work is a man!' says Hamlet: 'How noble in reason! how infinite in faculties! ... in action how like an angel! in apprehension, how like a god!' But, alas, in the intervals of being noble, rational and potentially infinite,

> man, proud man,
> Dressed in a little brief authority,
> Most ignorant of what he is most assured,
> His glassy essence, like an angry ape,
> Plays such fantastic tricks before high heaven
> As make the angels weep.

Genius and angry ape, player of fantastic tricks and god-like reasoner – in all these roles individuals are the products of a language and a culture. Working on the 12 or 13 billion neurons of a human brain, language and culture have given us law, science, ethics, philosophy; have made possible all the achievements, of talent and of sanctity. They have also given us fanaticism, superstition and dogmatic bumptiousness; nationalistic idolatry and mass murder in the name of God; rabble-rousing propaganda and organized lying. And, along with the salt of the earth, they have given us, generation after generation, countless millions of hypnotized conformists, the predestined victims of power-hungry rulers who are themselves the victims of all that is most senseless and inhuman in their cultural tradition.

Thanks to language and culture, human behaviour can be incomparably more intelligent, more original, creative and flexible than the behaviour of animals, whose brains are too small to accommodate the number of neurons necessary for the invention of language and the transmission of accumulated knowledge. But, thanks again to language and culture, human beings often behave with a stupidity, a lack of realism, a total inappropriateness, of which animals are incapable.

Trobriand Islander or Bostonian, Sicilian Catholic or Japanese Buddhist, each of us is born into some culture and passes his life within its confines. Between every human consciousness and the rest of the world stands an invisible fence, a network of traditional thinking-and-feeling patterns, of secondhand notions that have turned into axioms, of ancient slogans revered as divine revelations. What we see through the meshes of this net is never, of course, the unknowable 'thing in itself'. It is not even, in most cases, the thing as it impinges upon our senses and as our organism spontaneously reacts to it. What we ordinarily take in and respond to is a curious mixture of immediate experience with culturally conditioned symbol, of sense impressions with preconceived ideas about the nature of things. And by most people the symbolic elements in this cocktail of awareness are felt to be more important that the elements contributed by immediate experience. Inevitably so, for, to those who accept their culture totally and uncritically, words in the familiar language do not stand (however inadequately) for things. On the contrary, things stand for familiar words. Each unique event of their ongoing life is instantly and automatically classified as yet another concrete illustration of one of the verbalized, culture-hallowed abstractions drummed into their heads by childhood conditioning.

It goes without saying that many of the ideas handed down to us by the transmitters of culture are eminently sensible and realistic. (If they were not, the human species would now be extinct.) But, along with these useful concepts, every culture hands down a stock of unrealistic notions, some of which never made any sense, while others may once have possessed survival value, but have now, in the changed and changing circumstances of ongoing history, become completely irrelevant. Since human beings respond to symbols as promptly and unequivocally as they respond to the stimuli of unmediated experience, and since most of them naïvely believe that culture-hallowed words about things are as real as, or even realer than their perceptions of the things themselves, these outdated or intrinsically nonsensical notions do enormous harm. Thanks to the realistic ideas handed down by culture, mankind has survived and, in certain fields, progresses. But thanks to the pernicious nonsense drummed into every individual in the course of his acculturation, mankind, though surviving and progressing, has always been in trouble. History is the record, among other things, of the fantastic and generally fiendish tricks played upon itself by culture-maddened humanity. And the hideous game goes on.

What can, and what should, the individual do to improve

his ironically equivocal relationship with the culture in which he finds himself embedded? How can he continue to enjoy the benefits of culture without, at the same time, being stupefied or frenziedly intoxicated by its poisons? How can he become discriminating acculturated, rejecting what is silly or downright evil in his conditioning, and holding fast to that which makes for humane and intelligent behaviour?

A culture cannot be discriminately accepted, much less be modified, except by persons who have seen through it – by persons who have cut holes in the confining stockade of verbalized symbols and so are able to look at the world and, by reflection, at themselves in a new and relatively unprejudiced way. Such persons are not merely born; they must also be made. But how?

In the field of formal education, what the would-be hole cutter needs is knowledge. Knowledge of the past and present history of cultures in all their fantastic variety, and knowledge about the nature and limitations, the uses and abuses, of language. A man who knows that there have been many cultures, and that each culture claims to be the best and truest of all, will find it hard to take too seriously the boastings and dogmatizings of his own tradition. Similarly, a man who knows how symbols are related to experience, and who practises the kind of linguistic self-control taught by the exponents of *General Semantics*, is unlikely to take too seriously the absurd or dangerous nonsense that, within every culture, passes for philosophy, practical wisdom and political argument.

As a preparation for hole cutting, this kind of intellectual education is certainly valuable, but no less certainly insufficient. Training on the verbal level needs to be supplemented by training in wordless experiencing. We must learn how to be mentally silent, must cultivate the art of pure receptivity.

To be silently receptive – how childishly simple that seems! But in fact, as we very soon discover, how difficult! The universe in which men pass their lives is the creation of what Indian philosophy calls *Nama-Rupa*, Name and Form. Reality is a continuum, a fathomlessly mysterious and infinite Something, whose outward aspect is what we call Matter and whose inwardness is what we call Mind. Language is a device for taking the mystery out of Reality and making it amenable to human comprehension and manipulation. Acculturated man breaks up the continuum, attaches labels to a few of the fragments, projects the labels into the outside world and thus creates for himself an all-too-human universe of separate objects, each of which is merely the embodiment of a name, a particular illustration of some traditional abstraction. What we perceive takes on the pattern of the conceptual lattice through which it has been filtered. Pure receptivity is difficult because man's normal waking consciousness is always culturally conditioned. But normal waking consciousness, as William James pointed out many years ago, 'is but one type of consciousness, while all about it, parted from it by the filmiest of screens, there lie potential forms of consciousness entirely different. We may go through life without suspecting their existence; but apply the requisite stimulus, and at a touch they are there in all their completeness, definite types of mentality which probably somewhere have their field of application and adaptation. No account of the universe in its totality can be final which leaves these forms of consciousness disregarded.'

Like the culture by which it is conditioned, normal waking consciousness is at once our best friend and a most dangerous enemy. It helps us to survive and make progress; but at the same time it prevents us from actualizing some of our most valuable potentialities and, on occasion, gets us into all kinds of trouble. To become fully human, man, proud man, the player of fantastic tricks, must learn to get out of his own way; only then will his infinite faculties and angelic apprehension get a chance of coming to the surface. In Blake's words, we must 'cleanse the doors of perception'; for when the doors of perception are cleansed, 'everything appears to man as it is – infinite'. To normal waking consciousness things are the strictly finite and insulated embodiments of verbal labels. How can we break the habit of automatically imposing our prejudices and the memory of culture-hallowed words upon immediate experience? Answer: by the practice of pure receptivity and mental silence. These will cleanse the doors of perception and, in the process, make possible the emergence of other than normal forms of consciousness – aesthetic consciousness, visionary consciousness, mystical consciousness. Thanks to culture we are the heirs to vast accumulations of knowledge, to a priceless treasure of logic and scientific method, to thousands upon thousands of useful pieces of technological and organizational know-how. But the human mind-body possesses other sources of information, makes use of other types of reasoning, is gifted with an intrinsic wisdom that is independent of cultural conditioning.

Wordsworth writes that 'our meddling intellect [that part of the mind which uses language to take the mystery out of Reality] mis-shapes the beauteous forms of things: we murder to dissect.' Needless to say, we cannot get along without our meddling intellect. Verbalized conceptual thinking is indispensable. But even when they are used well, verbalized concepts mis-shape 'the beauteous forms of things'. And when (as happens so often) they are used badly, they mis-shape our lives by rationalizing ancient stupidities, by instigating mass murder, persecution and the playing of all the other fantastically ugly tricks that make the angels weep. Wise non-verbal passiveness is an antidote to unwise verbal activity and a necessary corrective to wise verbal activity. Verbalized concepts about experience need to be supplemented by direct, unmediated acquaintance with events as they present themselves to us.

It is the old story of the letter and the spirit. The letter is necessary, but must never be taken too seriously; for, divorced from the spirit, it cramps and finally kills. As for the spirit, it 'bloweth where it listeth' and, if we fail to consult the best cultural charts, we may be blown off our course and suffer shipwreck. At present most of us make the worst of both worlds. Ignoring the freely blowing winds of the spirit and relying on cultural maps which may be centuries out-of-date, we rush full speed ahead under the high-pressure steam of our own overweening self-confidence. The tickets we have sold ourselves assure us that our destination is some port in the Islands of the Blest. In fact it turns out, more often than not, to be Devil's Island.

Self-education on the non-verbal level is as old as civilization. 'Be still and know that I am God' – for the visionaries and mystics of every time and every place, this has been the first and greatest of the commandments. Poets listen to their Muse and in the same way the visionary and the mystic wait upon inspiration in a state of wise passiveness, of dynamic vacuity. In the western tradition this state is called 'the prayer of simple regard'. At the other end of the world it is described in terms that are psychological rather than theistic. In mental silence we 'look into our own Self-Nature', we 'hold fast to the Not-Thought which lies in thought', we 'become that which essentially we have always been'. By wise activity we can acquire useful analytical knowledge about the world, knowledge that can be communicated by means of verbal symbols. In the state of wise passiveness we make possible the emergence of forms of consciousness other than the utilitarian consciousness of normal waking life. Useful analytical knowledge about the world is replaced by some kind of biologically inessential but spiritually enlightening acquaintance with the world. For example, there can be direct aesthetic acquaintance with the world as beauty. Or there can be direct acquaintance with the intrinsic strangeness of existence, its wild implausibility. And finally there can be direct acquaintance with the world's unity. This immediate mystical experience of being at one with the fundamental Oneness that manifests itself in the infinite diversity of things and minds can never be adequately expressed in words. Like visionary experience, the experience of the mystic can be talked about only from the outside. Verbal symbols can never convey its inwardness.

It is through mental silence and the practice of wise passiveness that artists, visionaries and mystics have made themselves ready for the immediate experience of the world as beauty, as mystery and as unity. But silence and wise passiveness are not the only roads leading out of the all-too-human universe created by normal, culture-conditioned consciousness. In *Expostulation and Reply*, Wordsworth's bookish friend, Matthew, reproaches the poet because

> You look round on your Mother Earth,
> As if she for no purpose bore you;
> As if you were her first-born birth,
> And none had lived before you!

From the point of view of normal waking consciousness, this is sheer intellectual delinquency. But it is what the artist, the visionary and the mystic must do and, in fact, have always done. 'Look at a person, a landscape, any common object, as though you were seeing it for the first time.' This is one of the exercises in immediate, unverbalized awareness prescribed in the ancient texts of Tantric Buddhism. Artists, visionaries and mystics refuse to be enslaved to the culture-conditioned habits of feeling, thought and action which their society regards as right and natural. Whenever this seems desirable, they deliberately refrain from projecting upon reality those hallowed word patterns with which all human minds are so copiously stocked. They know as well as anyone else that culture and the language in which any given culture is rooted, are absolutely necessary and that, without them, the individual would not be human. But more vividly than the rest of mankind they also know that, to be *fully* human, the individual must learn to decondition himself, must be able to cut holes in the fence of verbalized symbols that hems him in.

In the exploration of the vast and mysterious world of human potentialities the great artists, visionaries and mystics have been trail-blazing pioneers. But where they have been, others can follow. Potentially, all of us are 'infinite in faculties and like gods in apprehension'. Modes of consciousness different from normal waking consciousness are within the reach of anyone who knows how to apply the necessary stimuli. The universe in which a human being lives can be transfigured into a new creation. We have only to cut a hole in the fence and look around us with what the philosopher, Plotinus, describes as 'that other kind of seeing, which everyone has but few make use of'.

Within our current systems of education, training on the non-verbal level is meagre in quantity and poor in quality. Moreover, its purpose, which is simply to help its recipients to be more 'like gods in apprehension' is neither clearly stated nor consistently pursued. We could and, most emphatically, we should do better in this very important field than we are doing now. The practical wisdom of earlier civilizations and the findings of adventurous spirits within our own tradition and in our own time are freely available. With their aid a curriculum and a methodology of non-verbal training could be worked out without much difficulty. Unhappily most persons in authority have a vested interest in the maintenance of cultural fences. They frown upon hole cutting as subversive and dismiss Plotinus' 'other kind of seeing' as a symptom of mental derangement. If an effective system of non-verbal education could be worked out, would the authorities allow it to be widely applied? It is an open question.

From the non-verbal world of culturally uncontaminated consciousness we pass to the sub-verbal world of physiology and biochemistry. A human being is a temperament and a product of cultural conditioning: he is also, and primarily, an extremely complex and delicate biochemical system, whose inwardness, as the system changes from one state of equilibrium to another, is changing consciousness. It is because each one of us is a biochemical system that (according to Housman)

> Malt does more than Milton can
> To justify God's ways to man.

Beer achieves its theological triumphs because in William James's words, 'Drunkenness is the great exciter of the *Yes* function in man.' And he adds that 'It is part of the deeper mystery and tragedy of life that whiffs and gleams of something that we immediately recognize as excellent should be vouchsafed to so many of us only in the fleeting earlier phases of what, in its totality, is so degrading a poisoning.' The tree is known by its fruits, and the fruits of too much reliance upon ethyl alcohol as an exciter of the *Yes* function are bitter indeed. No less bitter are the fruits of reliance upon such habit-forming sedatives, hallucinogens and mood elevators as opium and its derivatives, as cocaine (once so blithely recommended to his friends and patients by Dr Freud), as the barbiturates and amphetamine. But in recent years the pharmacologists have extracted or synthesized several compounds that powerfully affect the mind without doing any harm to the body, either at the time of ingestion or, through addiction, later on. Through these new psychedelics, the subject's normal waking consciousness may be modified in many different ways. It is as though, for each individual, his deeper self decides which kind of experience will be most advantageous. Having decided, it makes use of the drug's mind-changing powers to give the person what he needs. Thus, if it would be good for him to have deeply buried memories uncovered, deeply buried memories will duly be uncovered. In cases where this is of no great importance, something else will happen. Normal waking consciousness may be replaced by aesthetic consciousness, and the world will be perceived in all its unimaginable beauty, all the blazing intensity of its 'thereness'. And aesthetic consciousness may modulate into visionary consciousness. Thanks to yet another kind of seeing, the world will now reveal itself as not only unimaginably beautiful, but also fathomlessly mysterious – as a multitudinous abyss of possibility for ever actualizing itself into unprecedented forms. New insights into a new, transfigured world of givenness, new combinations of thought and fantasy – the stream of novelty pours through the world in a torrent, whose every drop is charged with meaning. There are the symbols whose meaning lies outside themselves in the given facts of visionary experience, and there are these given facts which signify only themselves. But 'only themselves' is also 'no less than the divine ground of all being'. 'Nothing but this' is at the same time 'the Suchness of all'. And now the aesthetic and the visionary consciousness deepen into mystical consciousness. The world is now seen as an infinite diversity that is yet a unity, and the beholder experiences himself as being at one with the infinite Oneness that manifests itself, totally present, at every point of space, at every instant in the flux of perpetual perishing and perpetual renewal. Our normal word-conditioned consciousness creates a universe of sharp distinctions, black and white, this and that, me and you and it. In the mystical consciousness of being at one with infinite Oneness, there is a reconciliation of opposites, a perception of the Not-Particular in particulars, a transcending of our ingrained subject-object relationships with things and persons; there is an immediate experience of our solidarity with all beings and a kind of organic conviction that in spite of the inscrutabilities of fate, in spite of our own dark stupidities and deliberate malevolence, yes, in spite of all that is so manifestly wrong with the world, it is yet, in some profound, paradoxical and entirely inexpressible way, All Right. For normal waking consciousness, the phrase, 'God is Love', is no more than a piece of wishful positive thinking. For the mystical consciousness, it is a self-evident truth.

Unprecedently rapid technological and demographic changes are steadily increasing the dangers by which we are surrounded, and at the same time are steadily diminishing the relevance of the traditional feeling-and-behaviour patterns imposed upon all individuals, rulers and ruled alike, by their culture. Always desirable, widespread training in the art of cutting holes in cultural fences is now the most urgent of necessities. Can such a training be speeded up and made more effective by a judicious use of the physically harmless psychedelics now available? On the basis of personal experience and the published evidence, I believe that it can. In my utopian fantasy, *Island*, I speculated in fictional terms about the ways in which a substance akin to psilocybin could be used to potentiate the non-verbal education of adolescents and to remind adults that the real world is very different from the mis-shapen universe they have created for themselves by means of their culture-conditioned prejudices. 'Having Fun with Fungi' –

that was how one waggish reviewer dismissed the matter. But which is better: to have Fun with Fungi or to have Idiocy with Ideology, to have Wars because of Words, to have Tomorrow's Misdeeds out of Yesterday's Miscreeds?

How should the psychedelics be administered? Under what circumstances, with what kind of preparation and follow-up? These are questions that must be answered empirically, by large-scale experiment. Man's collective mind has a high degree of viscosity and flows from one position to another with the reluctant deliberation of an ebbing tide of sludge. But in a world of explosive population increase, of headlong technological advance and of militant nationalism, the time at our disposal is strictly limited. We must discover, and discover very soon, new energy sources for overcoming our society's psychological inertia, better solvents for liquefying the sludgy stickiness of an anachronistic state of mind. On the verbal level an education in the nature and limitations, the uses and abuses of language; on the wordless level an education in mental silence and pure receptivity; and finally, through the use of harmless psychedelics, a course of chemically triggered conversion experiences or ecstasies – these, I believe, will provide all the sources of mental energy, all the solvents of conceptual sludge, that an individual requires. With their aid, he should be able to adapt himself selectively to his culture, rejecting its evils, stupidities and irrelevances, gratefully accepting all its treasures of accumulated knowledge, of rationality, human-heartedness and practical wisdom. If the number of such individuals is sufficiently great, if their quality is sufficiently high, they may be able to pass from discriminating acceptance of their culture to discriminating change and reform. Is this a hopefully utopian dream? Experiment can give us the answer, for the dream is pragmatic; the utopian hypotheses can be tested empirically. And in these oppressive times a little hope is surely no unwelcome visitant.

The Integration of Human Knowledge

Oliver L. Reiser

Professor Reiser is Chairman of the Department of Philosophy at the University of Pittsburgh, and is also Chairman of the International Committee for Scientific Humanism.

That man ... literally does stand mid-way between the supra-universes and the infra-universes, that he is in a sense at the crossroads of the universe, is indicated by calculations which show that while about 10^{27} atoms make a man's body, 10^{28} human bodies constitute enough material to build a star. Man lives his life in a middle-scale universe, suspended between two infinities, and he appears to possess characteristics derived from both domains.

... *evolution is not yet finished with the human organism, for still higher functions are in process of development.* Furthermore, we surmise that Humanity is a god in embryo, a developing being with those psychic powers of omniscience and omnipotence which man hitherto has assigned to his god. Such a theory of the source of man's extra-sensory powers would be in harmony with the view of E. Servadio that telepathic experience may be an original and archaic way of establishing understanding between individuals which, in the course of time, has been replaced by sign communication. Servadio does not believe that telepathic transference can be produced experimentally on a rational and conscious level. But this fact – if fact it be – that telepathy cannot be reproduced at the logical-rational level does not mean that it cannot be reproduced. According to our own three-level scheme of orientations, the coming superlogical level could reinstate a type of unity which would make it appear as a kind of regression to a more primitive mode of response, when in fact it is an adumbration of a coming unity. In that event, ESP and Psiphenomena generally are flickering and fitful anticipations of the integration of a giant organism in which humans function as neuroblasts of the world sensorium – cells in the social cortex which the electromagnetic society is beginning to proliferate.

If human organisms are embryonic cells in a super-organism which is still on its way, individual human beings, as the neuroblasts of the emerging organism, are also not finished products. New functions may emerge as embryogenesis continues, and Psi-phenomena may provide the experimental basis for such developments. The ESP faculties in those persons who possess it may be due to mutational changes in a few cells first, then more and more cells in successive generations, until the whole organ, the world sensorium, has perfected a new function in all individuals.

To explain ESP (telepathy and clairvoyance) one may suppose that the perceptive centres can respond to sensory and non-sensory stimuli. Therefore, vision in man is splitting into sensory and extra-sensory components. The evolutionary changes that are bringing this about would not appear in the size or weight of the brain but in the morphology of the neuron; accordingly the external appearance may bear no obvious relation to the chemical mutational changes within the neurons.

The Problem of Consciousness

Oliver L. Reiser

Beyond doubt the problem of establishing the missing connections between the phenomena of consciousness and the rest of our scientific knowledge is the most important unsolved problem of philosophy. This is the one phenomenon for which there is no existing physico-chemical model. Supposing – in an optimistic mood – that such a model does appear, will it come as a stroke of genius from one man – or will it come as a result of the gradual development of existing knowledge along established lines? At the moment we cannot say.

For the behaviourist, of course, there is no problem: he simply denies the existence of consciousness as a reality to be dealt with. But this is silly. I recall how one of my own teachers, Dr A. P. Weiss, a well-known behaviourist, once demanded of a philosopher (me) who used the term 'consciousness' – what do you mean by consciousness? The reply was: I mean by consciousness what you experience when you ask me that question: this silenced the behaviourist. One can define subjective terms – like 'redness', 'sweetness' etc. – only by denotative reference. In that manner, the term consciousness, for me, will refer to that complex of shifting patterns of present sensations, images, ideas and feelings, which all normal individuals experience. In the stream of time this is a fusion of past, present and future. In his classic treatise, *Principles of Psychology*, William James pictured the stream of consciousness as for ever flowing, never the same, with the stream as it flows leaving a record in the living brain.

Unfortunately the behaviourists (like B. F. Skinner) have had relatively slight interest in the human brain – it is the 'black box' into which one need not look too carefully in order to establish uniform and predictable connections (correlations) between stimuli and responses. But from the present viewpoint, the human brain is the master tissue of nature – the 'specific organ of civilization', as C. J. Herrick termed it. What goes on inside the skull of man is truly marvellous to consider, as Charles S. Sherrington has shown in his masterpiece, *Man On His Nature*. One of the more dramatic manifestations of the manner in which higher organizational factors may arise, in ways not directly related to sensory input or motor outgo, is provided by the delusional and hallucinatory phenomena induced by LSD (lysergic acid). Here, indeed, are 'intervening variables' with a vengeance.

Yoga

Ernest Wood

In the very extensive and varied yoga literature of India, both classical and modern, there is frequent reference to psychic powers, but not usually – somewhat to the surprise of the western inquirer – enthusiasm about them. They are regarded as coming by the way, and are not treated as something to be sought for or especially prized. Indeed, the highest authority of all, Patanjali, speaks of the arising of higher senses of hearing, touch, taste, and smell, but immediately adds: 'These powers of the spreading (or outgoing) mind are injurious to contemplation (samadhi).'

No objection to them is indicated otherwise than as temptations to linger by the wayside with these new enjoyments, and in fairness to the whole field of study Patanjali in about thirty aphorisms speaks of them and how they are produced. Some of these statements are somewhat obscure at our date, but Patanjali lists a variety of them as resulting from full meditation upon certain things. He also mentions that the powers arise also in other manners than by practice of yoga-meditation, listing them as sometimes occurring from birth, and sometimes produced by drugs, incantations (mantras), and austerities.

As examples of those produced by full meditation (i.e. concentration, meditation, and contemplation) may be mentioned: knowledge of past and future; understanding of the sounds made by all creatures; knowledge of past lives; knowing what others are thinking; prior knowledge of one's death; the attainment of various kinds of strength; perception of the small, the concealed, and the distant; knowledge of other inhabited regions; knowledge about the stars and their motions; knowledge of the interior of the body; control of hunger and thirst; steadiness; seeing the adepts in one's own interior light;

general intuition; understanding of the mind; entering the bodies of others; lightness and levitation; brightness; control of material elements; control of the senses; perfection of the body; quickness of the body, and the well-known set of eight powers beginning with smallness.

Patanjali does not give a list of the eight powers, but it appears frequently and widely in yoga literature. They are:

Minuteness (*anima*). To be as small as an atom, at will.

Expansion (*mahima*). To increase in size, at will.

Lightness (*laghima*). Neutralization of gravity, at will.

Reaching (*prapti*). To obtain anything or to reach any place, at will.

Acquirement (*prakamya*). To have the fulfilment of any wish, at will.

Lordship (*ishatwa*). Control of the energies of Nature, at will.

Self-control (*vashitwa*). Self-command and freedom from being influenced, at will.

Lordship (*ishatwa*). Control of the energies of Nature, at will.

These are interpreted in detail in various ways, subjective and objective, by various yogis, gurus, and writers.

Before leaving this topic, it seems desirable to point out that the raja-yogi is aiming at the experience of inward illumination beyond all sensation. He is aiming not to be governed by impulses of any kind from outside, however relatively superior. He aims at the mountain top (*kutastha*), not to 'rest' on any object (*alambana*.)

Prayer of the Heliotrope

Proclus

On earth one can see suns and moons in a terrestrial condition, and in the sky one can see all the different plants, stones, and animals living as spirits.

Treaty of the Vision of God

Nicolas de Cusa

This place which is surrounded by coinciding contradictions is no other than the wall of paradise, at the door of which the highest spirit of reason stands on guard, who one must force in order to enter.

Song of Enlightenment

Yoka Daishi

Hini the herb grows on the Himalays where no other grasses are found,
And the cows feeding on it give the purest milk, and this I always enjoy.

A Modern Myth

C. G. Jung

... I feel myself compelled, as once before when events were brewing of fateful consequence for Europe, to sound a note of warning. I know that, just as before, my voice is much too weak to reach the ear of the multitude. It is not presumption that drives me, but my conscience as a psychiatrist that bids me fulfil my duty and prepare those few who will hear me for coming events which are in accord with the end of an era. As we know from ancient Egyptian history, they are symptoms of psychic changes that always appear at the end of one Platonic month and at the beginning of another. They are, it seems, changes in the constellation of psychic dominants, of the archetypes, or 'gods' as they used to be called, which bring about, or accompany, long-lasting transformations of the collective psyche. This transformation started within the historical tradition and left traces behind it, first in the transition from the age of Taurus to that of Aries, and then from Aries to Pisces, whose beginning coincides with the rise of Christianity. We are now nearing that great change which may be expected when the spring-point enters Aquarius. It would be frivolous of me to conceal from the reader that reflections such as these are not only exceedingly unpopular but come perilously close to those turbid fantasies which becloud the minds of world-improvers and other interpreters of 'signs and portents'. But I must take this risk, even if it means putting my hard-won reputation for truthfulness, trustworthiness, and scientific judgement in jeopardy. I can assure my readers that I do not do this with a light heart. I am, to be quite frank, concerned for all those who are caught unprepared by the events in question and disconcerted by their incomprehensible nature. Since, so far as I know, no one has yet felt moved to examine and set forth the possible psychic consequences of this foreseeable change, I deem it my duty to do what I can in this respect. I undertake this thankless task in the expectation that my chisel will make no impression on the hard stone it meets.

Utopian Speculations

Henry Miller

This paragraph was quoted in Normal O. Brown's Life against Death *and he comments on Miller's text as follows: Utopian speculations, such as these of Henry Miller, must come back into fashion. They are a way of affirming faith in the possi-*

bility of solving problems that seem at the moment insoluble. Today even the survival of humanity is a utopian hope.

The cultural era is past. The new civilization, which may take centuries or a few thousand years to usher in, will not be *another* civilization – it will be the open stretch of realization which all the past civilizations have pointed to. The city, which was the birth-place of civilization, such as we know it to be, will exist no more. There will be nuclei of course, but they will be mobile and fluid. The peoples of the earth will no longer be shut off from one another within states but will flow freely over the surface of the earth and intermingle. There will be no fixed constellations of human aggregates. Governments will give way to management, using the word in a broad sense. The politician will become as superannuated as the dodo bird. The machine will never be dominated, as some imagine; it will be scrapped, eventually, but not before men have understood the nature of the mystery which binds them to their creation. The worship, investigation and subjugation of the machine will give way to the larger one of power – and of possession. Man will be forced to realize that power must be kept open, fluid and free. His aim will be not to possess power but to radiate it.

Ecstasy

Julius de Boer

A spontaneous mental devotion or even exaltation that might reasonably be called an 'ecstasy' within the physiological sphere can raise a personality type along affective, volitive, and cognitive steps to heights nearing the optimum of mental qualities. Such a normal ecstasy may take a poetic, or a religious, and certainly also a philosophical direction, without losing touch with scientific reality. It has been suggested that philosophy can, or must, rise to the level of science, but the reverse seems, relatively speaking, more rational: science must become philosophy on a scientific foundation. The desirable unity (synthesis) should comprise an optimum of categories embracing both science and philosophy, which might be called wisdom. It is to be hoped that we can look behind the words that we use to define our concepts, which sometimes seem mere word-play, and that we shall not lose sight of the reality of knowing and understanding, even though we have no other or better means than words, or similar symbols, to attain or approach what we may call our highest goal. A world-wide *significant science*, serving as the highest terminological authority, would be, if not absolutely necessary, at least highly desirable.

Cannabis and Opiates

William Burroughs

It is unfortunate that cannabis (the Latin term for preparations made from the hemp plant, such as marihuana and hashish), which is certainly the safest of the hallucinogen drugs, should be subject to the heaviest legal sanctions. Unquestionably this drug is very useful to the artist, activating trains of association that would otherwise be inaccessible, and I owe many of the scenes in *Naked Lunch* directly to the use of cannabis. Opiates, on the other hand, since they act to diminish awareness of surroundings and bodily processes, can only be a hindrance to the artist. Cannabis serves as a guide to psychic areas which can then be re-entered without it. I have now discontinued the use of cannabis for some years and find that I am able to achieve the same results by non-chemical means: flicker, music through head phones, cutups and foldins of my texts, and especially by training myself to think in association blocks instead of words, that is, cannabis, like all the hallucinogens, can be discontinued once the artist has familiarized himself with the areas opened up by the drug. Cannabis some-times causes anxiety in large doses, and this anxiety is prompt-ly relieved by apomorphine.

It would seem to me that cannabis and the other hallucino-gens provide a key to the creative process, and that a system-atic study of these drugs would open the way to non-chemical methods of expanding consciousness.

The Politics of Consciousness Expansion

Timothy Leary and Richard Alpert

Timothy Leary was recently sentenced to thirty years impris-onment and a fine of $30,000 for being found in possession of three ounces of marihuana when crossing the border from Mexico into Texas (see also Part Five).

EXPANSION-CONTRACTION. The tension between the flow-ing process and the fixed structure.

Inorganic processes: The expanding gaseous cloud whirls into temporary patterned structures. The structures always changing, hurtling towards eventual entropy.

Organic processes: Watery, electro-biochemical globules cluster into cells. Cells cluster into temporary hardened forms (vegetative or animal), themselves always changing, eventually returning to the entropic.

Social processes: The free expansive vision is moulded into the institutional. Hardly has the institutional mortar set before there is a new cortical upheaval, an explosive, often ecstatic or prophetic revelation. The prophet is promptly jailed. A hundred years later his followers are jailing the next vision-ary.

One is led naïvely to exclaim: will man never learn the lesson of cyclical process?

Naïve question, which fails to appreciate the necessary

tension of the expansion-contraction play. Membrane contracts. Life force bursts membrane. Establishment controls vision. Vision bursts establishment.

The expansion process in physics and biology is described in evolutionary terms.

The expansion process in human affairs is defined in terms of the word 'freedom'.

We measure social evolution in terms of increased freedom – external or internal. Freedom to step out of the tribal game and move to construct a new social form. Freedom to move in space. Freedom to experience. Freedom to explore.

The administration always recognizes intuitively the next evolutionary step that will leave it behind. To cast this drama in terms of saints and pharisees is entertaining, but outmoded.

The drama is genetic. Neurophysiological.

Where, then, will the next evolutionary step occur? Within the human cortex. We *know* that science has produced methods for dramatically altering and expanding human awareness and potentialities. The uncharted realm lies behind your own forehead. Internal geography. Internal politics. Internal control. Internal freedom.

The nervous system can be changed, integrated, recircuited, expanded in its function. These possibilities naturally threaten every branch of the Establishment. The dangers of external change appear to frighten us less than the peril of internal change.

There are obvious avenues toward this next stage of human evolution.

Biochemical methods of increasing cortical efficiency. 'Biochemicals' in the human body, in plants, and in drugs. There exist in nature hundreds of botanical species with psychedelic ('mind-opening') powers. There exists around the indole circle a wide variety of psychedelic compounds. Cortical vitamins.

The existence of these substances has been known for thousands of years, but has been maintained as a well-guarded secret. The sanctity of botanical supply. Now, the mind-opening substances (e.g., mescaline, LSD, psilocybin) are available for the first time in limitless mass-produced quantities. What a threat! What a challenge!

The danger, of course, is not physical. A recent editorial in the *Medical Tribune* clearly recognizes the physiological safety of consciousness-expanding drugs. Nor is the danger psychological. In studies reported by Ditman, McGlothlin, Leary, Savage, up to 90 per cent of subjects taking these drugs in supportive environments testify enthusiastically.

The danger is not physical or psychological, but social-political, for the effect of consciousness-expanding drugs will be to transform our concepts of human nature, of human potentialities, of existence. Man is about to make use of that fabulous electrical network he carries around in his skull. Present social establishments had better be prepared for the change. Our favourite concepts are standing in the way of a floodtide, two billion years building up. The verbal dam is collapsing.

In totalitarian states, the use and control of instruments for external freedom – the automobile, the private aeroplane – are reserved for the government bureaucracy and the professional élite. Even in democracies, the traditional means for expanding or contracting consciousness (internal freedom) such as the printing press, the radio transmitter, the motion picture, are restricted by law and remain under government control.

Now consider consciousness-expanding drugs. No language. No trained operators. Lots of reactionaries whose monopoly is threatened. A few people who do see an inevitable development of a new language, a transfiguration of every one of our social forms. And these few, of course, the ones who have taken the internal voyage.

It is possible that in twenty years our psychological and experiential language (pitifully small in English) will have multiplied to cover realms of experience and forms of thinking now unknown. In twenty years, every social institution will have been transformed by the new insights provided by consciousness-expanding experiences. Many new social institutions will have developed to handle the expressions of the potentiated nervous system.

The political issue involves control: 'automobile' means that the free citizen moves *his* own car in external space. Internal automobile. Auto-administration. The freedom and control of one's experimental machinery. Licensing will be necessary. You must be trained to operate. You must demonstrate your proficiency to handle consciousness-expanding drugs without danger to yourself or the public. The Fifth Freedom – the freedom to expand your own consciousness – cannot be denied without due cause.

The open cortex produces an ecstatic state. The nervous system operating free of learned abstraction is a completely adequate, completely efficient, ecstatic organ. To deny this is to rank man's learned tribal concepts above two billion years' endowment. An irreverent act. Trust your inherent machinery. Be entertained by the social game you play. Remember, man's natural state is ecstatic wonder, ecstatic intuition, ecstatic accurate movement. Don't settle for less.

The Process

Brion Gysin

When they blackened my face, darkness swirled down like the beating of drums. As they put the flails in my hands and began to play our music, I fell to the ground. When Hamid fell, Bou Jeloud jumped into him. Even now, I'm afraid. Bou Jeloud is the Father of Fear: he is, also, the Father of Flocks. The Good Shepherd works for him. When the goats, gently grazing, brusquely frisk and skitter away, he is counting his herd. When you shiver like someone just walked on your grave, that's him! That's Pan, the Father of Skins. Did you almost jump out of your skin, just then, Hassan Merikani? I've still got you under my skin.

How did you like it up there? I know it got under your skin – and I don't mean the fleas. We let you sleep late, so breakfast was goat cheese and honey on fresh golden platters of bread from my sister's mud-oven out in the yard where our dinner, the rooster, was crowing to his last morning sun. My uncles, the Master Musicians, were lolling about in their big woollen jellabas and white turbans, sipping mint tea, their kif-pipes and their flutes. They never work in their lives so they loll about easy. They cop a tithe of one tenth of the crops in the lush valley below. It's always been so. They're musicians and play for the king. Every sultan who ever lived in his palace in Fez, signed a *dahir* or order-in-council, giving us the full power of our right to play to the king in the morning to wake him and, on Fridays, to pipe him down from his throne to his knees in the mosque. We have privileges, rights.

Late in August, each Master Musician slips away up to the borders of Rif country, in the blue mountains miles up, over, beyond and above our own Little Hills. High above those kif meadows of Ketama, where I've never been, hangs the ruin of an old fortified monastery from which, so they say, the Old Man of the Mountain once ruled the world. His adepts were called the Assassins because of the hashish they smoke – Hashishins were monks who ran naked in August, ran naked and mad through the meadows of kif. When they fell in their cells like a stone, the Old Man scraped off their skins with a knife because their shaved bodies were covered with gum from the kif flowers. *That* gum is hashish. They spread out the gum on great marble slabs where they pressed it and cut it in cubes which the Master sent out all over the world to Marseilles and to Hollywood, even. That trade is finished, now, too.

Now, we just run into the valley to snatch up a bundle of grass to take home. We have privileges, rights but, yes, we're afraid of that valley and glad in our hearts that the castle above is a ruin and the Old Man is not there any more; for, they say, he could point a long skinny finger like *that*, at any one adept of his standing sentry up there on the tower and that adept would leap, would throw himself down to smash on the rocks in the valley below because he knew that his moment had come. We don't like to be told. *Hamdullah!* we still have plenty of kif.

There is so much kif smoked in my village you can see it rise over the hedges of prickly pear and the thatched roofs of our houses. You can see the kif smoke rising blue, like a veil for the winds to catch up and drop back on this village of mine like a blessing. We're invisible, here in our hills. The music picks up like a current turned on and the kids are all out in the leafy green lanes, bawling:

> Ha! Bou Jeloud!
> Bou Jeloud the Piper met Aissha Amoka!
> Ha! Bou Jeloud!

My uncles, the Master Musicians, know all the music but our women know the words to tease Bou Jeloud. When night falls, they sit with their drums in some place apart from the men and they sing over the fire:

> O Brother Bou Jeloud, come up in our hills
> As God is our guide, you can have all the girls
> Allah, allalai i lalli
> Allah, alla lai wai wa!
>
> O Brother Bou Jeloud, don't hide in the melons
> Eyes blacker than pips, false eyebrows like felons
> O Brother Bou Jeloud; good-bye, good-bye
> Your rotten straw hat cocked over one eye.

Women tease Bou Jeloud just to make him run after them. That's all women want. Bou Jeloud wants Aissha Amoka; that means Crazy Aissha. He's crazy for Aissha. She drifts around after dark, cool and casual, near springs and running water with a silvery-blue face in the moonlight where she pulls back her veils like a wanton to show you her twinkling tits. Her face and her breasts are a beautiful blue, all starry with sparkling lights. She coos at you in the husky voice of a dove: 'Young man, can you tell me the time?' If you answer her one single word you are lost. From that day forever, you are her slave! Her slave!

The Teachings of Don Juan

Carlos Castenada

As in the case of Sitting Bull no matter what the mixture that went into the pipe may have contained, the experience is certainly relevant to the scheme of this anthology.

Sunday, 7 February 1965

My second attempt with the smoke took place about midday on Sunday 31 January. I woke up the following day in the early evening. I had the sensation of possessing an unusual power to recollect whatever don Juan had said to me during the experience. His words were imprinted on my mind. I kept on hearing them with extraordinary clarity and persistence. During this attempt another fact became obvious to me: my entire body had become numb soon after I began to swallow the fine powder, which got into my mouth every time I sucked the pipe. Thus I not only inhaled the smoke, but also ingested the mixture.

I tried to narrate my experience to don Juan; he said I had done nothing important. I mentioned that I could remember everything that had happened, but he did not want to hear about it. Every memory was precise and unmistakable. The smoking procedure had been the same as in the previous attempt. It was almost as if the two experiences were perfectly juxtaposable, and I could start my recollection from the time the first experience ended. I clearly remembered that from the time I fell to the ground on my side I was completely devoid of feeling or thought. Yet my clarity was not impaired in any way. I remember thinking my last thought at about the time the room became a vertical plane: 'I must have clunked my head on the floor, yet I don't feel any pain.'

From that point on I could only see and hear. I could repeat every word don Juan had said. I followed each one of his directions. They seemed clear, logical, and easy. He said that my body was disappearing and only my head was going to remain, and in such a condition the only way to stay awake and move around was by becoming a crow. He commanded me to make an effort to wink, adding that whenever I was capable of winking I would be ready to proceed. Then he told me that my body had vanished completely and all I had was my head; he said the head never disappears because the head is what turns into a crow.

He ordered me to wink. He must have repeated this command, and all his other commands countless times, because I could remember all of them with extraordinary clarity. I must have winked, because he said I was ready and ordered me to straighten up my head and put it on my chin. He said that in the chin were the crow's legs. He commanded me to feel the legs and observe that they were coming out slowly. He then said that I was not solid yet, that I had to grow a tail, and that the tail would come out of my neck. He ordered me to extend the tail like a fan, and to feel how it swept the floor.

Then he talked about the crow's wings, and said they would come out of my cheekbones. He said it was hard and painful. He commanded me to unfold them. He said they had to be extremely long, as long as I could stretch them, otherwise I would not be able to fly. He told me the wings were coming out and were long and beautiful, and that I had to flap them until they were real wings.

He talked about the top of my head next and said it was still very large and heavy, and its bulk would prevent my flying. He told me that the way to reduce its size was by winking; with every wink my head would become smaller. He ordered me to wink until the top weight was gone and I could jump freely. Then he told me I had reduced my head to the size of a crow, and that I had to walk around and hop until I had lost my stiffness.

There was one last thing I had to change, he said, before I could fly. It was the most difficult change, and to accomplish it I had to be docile and do exactly as he told me. I had to learn to see like a crow. He said that my mouth and nose were going to grow between my eyes until I had a strong beak. He said that crows see straight to the side, and commanded me to turn my head and look at him with one eye. He said that if I wanted to change and look with the other eye I had to shake my beak down, and that that movement would make me look through the other eye. He ordered me to shift from one eye to the other. And then he said I was ready to fly, and that the only way to fly was to have him toss me into the air.

I had no difficulty whatsoever eliciting the corresponding sensation to each one of his commands. I had the perception of growing bird's legs, which were weak and wobbly at first. I felt a tail coming out of the back of my neck and wings out of my cheekbones. The wings were folded deeply. I felt them coming out by degrees. The process was hard but not painful. Then I winked my head down to the size of a crow. But the most astonishing effect was accomplished with my eyes. My bird's sight!

When don Juan directed me to grow a beak, I had an annoying sensation of lack of air. Then something bulged out and created a block in front of me. But it was not until don Juan directed me to see laterally that my eyes actually were capable of having a full view to the side. I could wink one eye at a time and shift the focusing from one eye to the other. But the sight of the room and all the things in it was not like an ordinary sight. Yet it was impossible to tell in what way it was different. Perhaps it was lopsided, or perhaps things were out of focus. Don Juan became very big and glowy. Something about him was comforting and safe. Then the images blurred; they lost their outlines, and became sharp abstract patterns that flickered for a while.

Sunday, 28 March 1965

On Thursday 18 March I smoked again the hallucinogenic mixture. The initial procedure was different in small details.

I had to refill the pipe bowl once. After I had finished the first batch, don Juan directed me to clean the bowl, but he poured the mixture into the bowl himself because I lacked muscular coordination. It took a great deal of effort to move my arms. There was enough mixture in my bag for one refill. Don Juan looked at the bag and said this was my last attempt with the smoke until the next year because I had used up all my provisions.

He turned the little bag inside out and shook the dust into the dish that held the charcoals. It burned with an orange glow, as if he had placed a sheet of transparent material over the charcoals. The sheet burst into flame, and then it cracked into an intricate pattern of lines. Something zigzagged inside the lines at high speed. Don Juan told me to look at the movement in the lines. I saw something that looked like a small marble rolling back and forth in the glowing area. He leaned over, put his hand into the glow, picked out the marble, and placed it in the pipe bowl. He ordered me to take a puff. I had a clear impression that he had put the small ball into the pipe so that I would inhale it. In a moment the room lost its horizontal position. I felt a profound numbness, a sensation of heaviness.

When I awakened, I was lying on my back at the bottom of a shallow irrigation ditch, immersed in water up to my chin. Someone was holding my head up. It was don Juan. The first thought I had was that the water in the channel had an unusual quality; it was cold and heavy. It slapped lightly against me, and my thoughts cleared with every movement it made. At first the water had a bright green halo, or fluorescence, which soon dissolved, leaving only a stream of ordinary water.

I asked don Juan about the time of day. He said it was early morning. After a while I was completely awake, and got out of the water.

'You must tell me all you saw,' don Juan said when we got to his house. He also said he had been trying to 'bring me back' for three days, and had had a very difficult time doing it. I made numerous attempts to describe what I had seen, but I could not concentrate. Later on, during the early evening, I felt I was ready to talk with don Juan, and I began to tell him what I remembered from the time I had fallen on my side, but he did not want to hear about it. He said the only interesting part was what I saw and did after he 'tossed me into the air and I flew away'.

All I could remember was a series of dreamlike images or scenes. They had no sequential order. I had the impression that each one of them was like an isolated bubble, floating into focus and then moving away. They were not, however, merely scenes to look at. I was inside them. I took part in them. When I tried to recollect them at first, I had the sensation that they were vague, diffused flashes, but as I thought about them I realized that each one of them was extremely clear although totally unrelated to ordinary seeing – hence, the sensation of vagueness. The images were few and simple.

As soon as don Juan mentioned that he had 'tossed me into the air' I had a faint recollection of an absolutely clear scene in which I was looking straight at him from some distance away. I was looking at his face only. It was monumental in size. It was flat and had an intense glow. His hair was yellowish, and it moved. Each part of his face moved by itself, projecting a sort of amber light.

The next image was one in which don Juan had actually tossed me up, or hurled me, in a straight onward direction. I remember I 'extended my wings and flew'. I felt alone, cutting through the air, painfully moving straight ahead. It was more like walking than like flying. It tired my body. There was no feeling of flowing free, no exuberance.

Then I remembered an instant in which I was motionless, looking at a mass of sharp, dark edges set in an area that had a dull, painful light; next I saw a field with an infinite variety of lights. The lights moved and flickered and changed their luminosity. They were almost like colours. Their intensity dazzled me.

At another moment, an object was almost against my eye. It was a thick, pointed object; it had a definite pinkish glow. I

felt a sudden tremor somewhere in my body and saw a multitude of similar pink forms coming towards me. They all moved
on me. I jumped away.

The last scene I remembered was three silvery birds. They
radiated a shiny, metallic light, almost like stainless steel, but
intense and moving and alive. I liked them. We flew together.

Don Juan did not make any comments on my recounting.

Tuesday, 23 March 1965

The following conversation took place the next day, after the
recounting of my experience.

Don Juan said: 'It does not take much to become a crow.
You did it and now you will always be one.'

'What happened after I became a crow, don Juan? Did I fly
for three days?'

'No, you came back at nightfall as I had told you to.'

'But how did I come back?'

'You were very tired and went to sleep. That is all.'

'I mean did I fly back?'

'I have already told you. You obeyed me and came back to
the house. But don't concern yourself with that matter. It is of
no importance.'

'What is important, then?'

'In your whole trip there was only one thing of great value
– the silvery birds!'

'What was so special about them? They were just birds.'

'Not just birds – they were crows.'

'Were they white crows, don Juan?'

'The black feathers of a crow are really silvery. The crows
shine so intensely that they are not bothered by other birds.'

'Why did their feathers look silvery?'

'Because you were seeing as a crow sees. A bird that looks
dark to us looks white to a crow. The white pigeons, for instance, are pink or bluish to a crow; seagulls are yellow. Now,
try to remember how you joined them.'

I thought about it, but the birds were a dim, disassociated

image which had no continuity. I told him I could remember only that I felt I had flown with them. He asked me whether I had joined them in the air or on the ground, but I could not possibly answer that. He became almost angry with me. He demanded that I think about it. He said: 'All this will not mean a damn; it will be only a mad dream unless you remember correctly.' I strained myself to recollect, but I could not.

Saturday, 3 April 1965

Today I thought of another image in my 'dream' about the silvery birds. I remembered seeing a dark mass with myriads of pinholes. In fact, the mass was a dark cluster of little holes. I don't know why I thought it was soft. As I was looking at it, three birds flew straight at me. One of them made a noise; then all three of them were next to me on the ground.

I described the image to don Juan. He asked me from what direction the birds had come. I said I couldn't possibly determine that. He became quite impatient and accused me of being inflexible in my thinking. He said I could very well remember if I tried to, and that I was afraid to let myself become less rigid. He said that I was thinking in terms of men and crows, and that I was neither a man nor a crow at the time that I wanted to recollect.

He asked me to remember what the crow had said to me. I tried to think about it, but my mind played on scores of other things instead. I couldn't concentrate.

Sunday, 4 April 1965

I took a long hike today. It got quite dark before I reached don Juan's house. I was thinking about the crows when suddenly a very strange 'thought' crossed my mind. It was more like an impression or a feeling than a thought. The bird that had made the noise said they were coming from the north and were going south, and when we met again they would be coming the same way.

I told don Juan what I had thought up, or maybe remembered. He said, 'Don't think about whether you remembered it or made it up. Such thoughts fit men only. They do not fit crows, especially those you saw, for they are the emissaries of your fate. You are already a crow. You will never change that. From now on the crows will tell you with their flight about every turn of your fate. In which direction did you fly with them?'

'I couldn't know that, don Juan!'

'If you think properly you will remember. Sit on the floor and tell me the position in which you were when the birds flew to you. Close your eyes and make a line on the floor.'

I followed his suggestion and determined the point.

'Don't open your eyes yet!' He proceeded, 'In which direction did you all fly in relation to that point?'

I made another mark on the ground.

Taking these points of orientation as a reference, don Juan interpreted the different patterns of flight the crows would observe to foretell my personal future or fate. He set up the four points of the compass as the axis of the crows' flight.

I asked him whether the crows always followed the cardinal points to tell a man's fate. He said that the orientation was mine alone; whatever the crows did in my first meeting with them was of crucial importance. He insisted on my recalling every detail, for the message and the pattern of the 'emissaries' were an individual, personalized matter.

There was one more thing he insisted I should remember, and that was the time of day when the emissaries left me. He asked me to think of the difference in the light around me between the time when I 'began to fly' and the time when the silvery birds 'flew with me'. When I first had the sensation of painful flight, it was dark. But when I saw the birds, everything was reddish – light red, or perhaps orange.

He said: 'That means it was late in the day; the sun was not down yet. When it is completely dark a crow is blind with whiteness and not with darkness, the way we are at night. This indication of the time places your last emissaries at the end of the day. They will call you, and as they fly above your head, they will become silvery white; you will see them shining against the sky, and it will mean your time is up. It will mean you are going to die and become a crow yourself.'

'What if I see them during the morning?'

'You won't see them in the morning!'

'But crows fly all day.'

'Not your emissaries, you fool!'

'How about *your* emissaries, don Juan?'

'Mine will come in the morning. There will also be three of them. My benefactor told me that one could shout them back to black if one does not want to die. But now I know it can't be done. My benefactor was given to shouting, and to all the clatter and violence of the devil's weed. I know the smoke is different because he has no passion. He is fair. When your silvery emissaries come for you, there is no need to shout at them. Just fly with them as you have already done. After they have collected you they will reverse directions, and there will be four of them flying away.'

Saturday, 10 April 1965

I had been experiencing brief flashes of disassociation, or shallow states of non-ordinary reality.

One element from the hallucinogenic experience with the mushrooms kept recurring in my thoughts: the soft, dark mass of pinholes. I continued to visualize it as a grease or an oil bubble which began to draw me to its centre. It was almost as if the centre would open up and swallow me, and for very brief moments I experienced something resembling a state of non-ordinary reality. As a result I suffered moments of profound agitation, anxiety, and discomfort, and I wilfully strove to end the experiences as soon as they began.

Today I discussed this condition with don Juan. I asked for advice. He seemed to be unconcerned and told me to disregard the experiences because they were meaningless, or rather valueless. He said the only experiences worth my effort and concern would be those in which I saw a crow; any other kind of 'vision' would be merely the product of my fears. He reminded me again that in order to partake of the smoke it was necessary to lead a strong, quiet life. Personally I seemed to have reached a dangerous threshold. I told him I felt I could not go on; there was something truly frightening about the mushrooms.

In going over the images I recalled from my hallucinogenic experience, I had come to the unavoidable conclusion that I had seen the world in a way that was structurally different from ordinary vision. In other states of non-ordinary reality I had undergone, the forms and the patterns I had visualized were always within the confines of my visual conception of the world. But the sensation of seeing under the influence of the hallucinogenic smoke mixture was not the same. Everything I saw was in front of me in a direct line of vision; nothing was above or below that line of vision.

Every image had an irritating flatness, and yet, disconcertingly, a profound depth. Perhaps it would be more accurate to say that the images were a conglomerate of unbelievably sharp details set inside fields of different light; the light in the fields moved, creating an effect of rotation.

After probing and exerting myself to remember, I was forced to make a series of analogies or similes in order to 'understand' what I had 'seen'. Don Juan's face, for instance, looked as if he had been submerged in water. The water seemed to move in a continuous flow over his face and hair. It so magnified them that I could see every pore in his skin or every hair on his head whenever I focused my vision. On the other hand, I saw masses of matter that were flat and full of edges, but did not move because there was no fluctuation in the light that came from them.

I asked don Juan what were the things that I had seen. He said that because this was the first time I was seeing as a crow the images were not clear or important, and that later on with practice I would be able to recognize everything.

I brought up the issue of the difference I had detected in the movement of light. 'Things that are alive', he said, 'move inside, and a crow can easily see when something is dead, or about to die, because the movement has stopped or is slowing down to a stop. A crow can also tell when something is moving too fast, and by the same token a crow can tell when something is moving just right.'

'What does it mean when something is moving too fast, or just right?'

'It means a crow can actually tell what to avoid and what to seek. When something is moving too fast inside, it means it is about to explode violently, or to leap forward, and a crow will avoid it. When it moves inside just right, it is a pleasing sight and a crow will seek it.'

'Do rocks move inside?'

'No, not rocks or dead animals or dead trees. But they are beautiful to look at. That is why crows hang around dead bodies. They like to look at them. No light moves inside them.'

'But when the flesh rots, doesn't it change or move?'

'Yes, but that is a different movement. What a crow sees then is millions of things moving inside the flesh with a light of their own, and that is what a crow likes to see. It is truly an unforgettable sight.'

'Have you seen it yourself, don Juan?'

'Anybody who learns to become a crow can see it. You will see it yourself.'

At this point I asked don Juan the unavoidable question.

'Did I really become a crow? I mean would anyone seeing me have thought I was an ordinary crow?'

'No. You can't think that way when dealing with the power of the allies. Such questions make no sense, and yet to become a crow is the simplest of all matters. It is almost like frolicking; it has little usefulness. As I have already told you, the smoke is not for those who seek power. It is only for those who crave to see. I learned to become a crow because these birds are the most effective of all. No other birds bother them, except perhaps larger, hungry eagles, but crows fly in groups and can defend themselves. Men don't bother crows either, and that is an important point. Any man can distinguish a large eagle, especially an unusual eagle, or any other large, unusual bird, but who cares about a crow? A crow is safe. It is ideal in size and nature. It can go safely into any place without attracting attention. On the other hand, it is possible to become a lion or a bear, but that is rather dangerous. Such a creature is too large; it takes too much energy to become one. One can also become a cricket, or a lizard, or even an ant, but that is even more dangerous, because large animals prey on small creatures.'

I argued that what he was saying meant that one really changed into a crow, or a cricket, or anything else. But he insisted I was misunderstanding.

'It takes a very long time to learn to be a proper crow,' he said. 'But you did not change, nor did you stop being a man. There is something else.'

'Can you tell me what the something else is, don Juan?'

'Perhaps now you know it yourself. Maybe if you were not so afraid of becoming mad, or of losing your body, you would understand this marvellous secret. But perhaps you must wait until you lose your fear to understand what I mean.'

Part Five
The Scene Today and the Law

The Holy Barbarians

Lawrence Lipton

The euphoria that the beats who use marihuana are seeking is not the wholly passive, sedative, pacifying experience that the users of commercial tranquillizers want. On the contrary, they are looking for a greater sense of aliveness, a heightened sense of awareness. Of all the euphoric, hypnotic and hallucinogenic drugs, marihuana is the mildest and also the most conductive to social usage. The joint is passed around the pad and shared, not for reasons of economy but as a *social ritual*. Once the group is high, the magic circle is complete. Confidences are exchanged, personal problems are discussed – with a frankness that is difficult to achieve under normal circumstances – music is listened to with rapt concentration, poetry is read aloud and its images, visual and acoustical, communicated with maximum effect. The Eros is felt in the magic circle of marihuana with far greater force, as a unifying principle in human relationships, than at any other time except, perhaps, in the mutual metaphysical orgasm. The magic circle is, in fact, a symbol of and a preparation for the metaphysical orgasm. While marihuana does not give the user the sense of timelessness to the same degree that peyote does, or LSD or other drugs, it does so sufficiently to impart a sense of *presence*, a here-and-nowness that gives the user a heightened sense of awareness and immediacy.

Memoirs of a Kif Smoker

Michael Pickering

The following article was written by a sixteen-year-old English boy and appeared in his local parish magazine.

When you first arrive at Tangier in Morocco, you recoil with horror when you are approached by young men trying to sell you marihuana or hashish or whatever you like to call it (in Morocco it is universally called 'kif'). You have thoughts of glassy-eyed junkies wasting away in dens full of drug addicts. After a few days or a few weeks (or never at all with some people) you begin to get a different impression – you find that most of the people you know smoke or have smoked it, and that those who have are not one jot different from those who have never touched it. So, urged on by your friends and trying to cover up your anxiety, you taste a little.

At first it is horrible: you feel weak and tired and depressed, with none of the light and joy they'd told you to expect. But you are given more reassuring words – it's only because of your scarcely repressed fears that cause your subconscious to try and reject the effect. Keep on trying and it will come. It does after one or two times, with effects that are impossible to describe accurately and which give some of the most wonderful experiences of your life.

Kif itself is a plant that grows or can grow all over the world – even in England, though the product I am told is not very good. The Rif mountains in the north of Morocco grow some of the best. The leaves of the plant are finely chopped and sorted (a very skilled process) and often a little tobacco added. It is smoked in tiny clay bowls at the end of long wooden pipes, which are sometimes beautifully carved or decorated, each filling gives only three or four drags – the ash being neatly blown out before the pipe is refilled.

The effects, usually coming on after two or three or four pipefuls, are different for each person, but several general characteristics are usually common to everybody. First of all, you suddenly notice as if for the first time in your life, how fantastically beautiful everything in the world is – even little things you hardly thought worth looking at before ... all colours become incredibly bright and intense, and sounds and touches full of beauty. When I first got high on kif, I was in a filthy youth hostel in Casablanca – but lying on a table was a small alcohol heater someone was using for cooking; it was dark and the heater was shooting out a long bright blue flame. Suddenly this flame was to me the most beautiful object in the world – the only thing worth looking at – it was full of exquisite wisps of orange and red – it was swirling round and round in the air, always emitting a lovely hissing noise that filled the whole room. It became for me all sorts of things – a flaming torch sweeping through the sky or a gurgling river of fire leaping from the table.

One example of thousands. But there is much more than just the heightening of the senses. You begin to think think think. More profoundly and more interestingly than ever before. You have fantastic ideas thrown up by your imagination which knows no bounds or restraints. And you feel an intense physical exhilaration – that makes you want to leap around. Everything in the world suddenly becomes true and real – you can see deep into people's minds by just looking at their eyes – you can tell everything about them, their thoughts, characters, dreams and secrets. You can see what people are really like – their 'image' is shattered – and so is yours – you start behaving as you really are. Politeness for the sake of politeness is impossible, or if tried, it is completely unconvincing. You become obsessed with the beauty of everything around you – a small noise made with your mouth is wonderful – you repeat it over and over again. To any observer you appear crazy – but this is nothing to you – you are in your own lovely world creating thoughts and visions and sounds and sights – creating whatever you like – doing whatever you like – you have woken up at last and start seeing the world as it really is for the first time – the kif has drawn the veil from your eyes and there is only life and growth and creation.

All very well. What happens afterwards? Answer, nothing. When the effect wears off, you are as you were before – but with a difference – in many ways you still see the world as it was when you were high – the flame is just as beautiful an object as before. Your whole life is enriched, your imagination deeper, and your mind is more active. There is not the slightest chance of getting hooked (addicted) to kif, unlike opium or heroin, which are different altogether; there are no bad effects no headaches or hangovers, no depression or 'let-down' feeling. Moroccans who have smoked it for sixty years or more have no ill effects.

It is strange to realize that kif and 'drugs' like it are regarded as the height of evil and corruption in European countries. Strange also that here it is alcohol (highly respectable in western countries) that has this same association of sin and wickedness (it being illegal for a native of a Moslem country to drink). But nobody can claim that alcohol (and tobacco), unlike kif, are not addict-forming or without harmful effects.

Two Statements

Judge John M. Murtagh

Judge Murtagh is Administrative Judge of the City of New York's Criminal Court.

1959: 'Our drug laws are immoral in principle and ineffectual in operation.'
25 April 1966: 'If there is a success in fighting the problem of narcotics addiction, it will be due to the scientists. We of the law are asses, and our approach is at best an utter disgrace.

Basically, it is a public health matter. Punishment should be limited to deviant conduct which harms the rest of us. An enforcement law corrupts more than it corrects.'

The Case of Timothy Leary

New York Daily News Report

Laredo, Texas, 11 March (UPI) – Dr Timothy Leary, 45, former Harvard professor nationally known for experiments with such hallucinogenic drugs as LSD and Peyote, was convicted today on two marihuana charges and sentenced to a maximum of thirty years in federal prison. His eighteen-year-old daughter, Susan, was ordered sent to a federal reformatory.

Federal Judge Ben C. Connally also fined Leary $30,000. Susan drew an indeterminate term. Defence attorneys said they would appeal.

Leary was found guilty of charges of transporting marihuana and failing to pay tax on it.

Connally gave Leary and his daughter ten days to wind up their affairs. They plan to return to their Millbrook, N.Y. home immediately. At the end of ten days, both must submit to psychiatric examination before Connally determines final sentence.

SEIZED AT BORDER

Leary, Susan, his son John, sixteen, and two companions were arrested at the Mexican border 22 December. Susan was found guilty of failing to pay tax on marihuana and John was not charged. A woman customs inspector made Miss Leary undress and found three ounces of marihuana in a silver snuffbox. Leary said the marihuana was his.

Before the case went to the jury, Connally dismissed a charge of smuggling marihuana against Leary. He dismissed charges of smuggling and unlawful transportation of marihuana against Miss Leary.

Leary had freely admitted using marihuana and said it was less dangerous than alcohol. He was convicted of unlawful transportation, for which he was sentenced to twenty years in prison and fined $20,000, and of failure to pay tax on marihuana, for which he was sentenced to ten years and fined $10,000.

DROP SMUGGLING COUNT

Connally said he dismissed the smuggling count because Leary, by his own admission, had the marihuana when he left New York.

In earlier interviews, Leary had denied being dismissed as a Harvard professor for his drug experiments. He said he was fired in an argument over salary.

(Leary had been operating a foundation in Millbrook in connection with his experiments in drugs. 11 March 1966.)

Sympathizers throughout the United States and in fact all over the world have recently formed a Timothy Leary Defence Fund. The following statements by eminent authorities and officials are being used by them to show the current legal penalties for the use of marihuana in the States are excessive.

'It is the opinion of the panel that the hazards of marihuana *per se* have been exaggerated and that long criminal sentences imposed on an occasional user or possessor of the drug are in poor social perspective.' *White House Conference on Narcotics and Drug Abuse,* 1962.)

'Dr S. J. Holmes, Director of the Narcotic Addiction Unit of the Alcoholism and Drug Addiction Research Foundation in Toronto, believes it is "fantastic and ridiculous" that a person caught with one marihuana cigarette can be sent to prison. "The situation is a disgrace to our civilization and merits much consideration." (*Toronto Globe and Mail,* 17 February 1966.)

'The continued linking of marihuana with opiates and cocaine results in excessively harsh penalties at both federal and state levels.' (Sub-committee on Narcotics of the Public Health Committee, N.Y. County Medical Society. Donald B. Louria, M.D., Chairman, March, 1966.)

'The penalty provisions applicable to marihuana users under state and federal law are about the same as those applied to heroin users. These penalties are entirely disproportionate to the seriousness of the offending behaviour and lead to gross injustice and undesirable social consequences ... The moderate or occasional marihuana user is not a significant social menace.' (Alfred R. Lindesmith, Ph.D., Professor of Sociology, Indiana University in *The Addict and the Law*, 1965.)

'Physicians and social scientists have defaulted leadership and responsibility in dealing with the pleasure-giving drugs, and law-enforcement agencies and legislatures have far exceeded their legitimate areas of concern.' (Joel Fort, M.D., Director, Special Problems Centre, San Francisco, former Consultant to World Health Organization, in *Utopiates*, ed. R. Blum, 1965.)

'The laws are now turning half the people on our campuses and a good portion of our leading citizens into criminals and law breakers. It is like Prohibition when the laws had nothing to do with the practices and beliefs of the people.' (Rev. Howard R. Moody of Judson Memorial Church, *Village Voice*, 31 March 1966.)

Abuse of American Law

Henry Smith Williams

The following statement was made in 1938 only a year after legislation to control the use of marihuana was introduced in the USA.

A Marihuana Tax bill was introduced and presently enacted as Federal law. And the foundation was thus laid for a racket that should quite eclipse even the billion-dollar illicit drug industry that the Harrison Act (as misinterpreted) developed and fostered. For the new drug has qualities that put it in a class by itself.

For example: marihuana, despite its high-sounding name, is merely a product of the familiar hemp plant – an agricultural product to which (according to statements made before the Congressional committee) upward of 10,000 acres of land in the United States are devoted. Leaves and flowers of any of these plants supply material for the marihuana cigarettes which we are asked to believe are a menace to American youth today.

But that is only the beginning. The hemp plant is not only cultivated extensively, but it grows wild in countless fields, neglected gardens, fence corners, and back yards ... But with the aid of newspaper propaganda already started, an interest will be created in the alleged allurements of marihuana smoking; and the army of inspectors sent out to explore the millions of fields on which the weed may grow need only apply, with slight modifications, the methods learned in the conduct of the narcotics racket, in order to develop a marihuana industry that should eclipse the billion-dollar illicit narcotics racket of today.

Racketeers who developed a billion-dollar illicit drug industry, using opium that had to be smuggled into the country, should have no difficulty at all in developing a five-billion dollar racket with marihuana – provided only that the press can be induced to stimulate curiosity by giving the drug publicity.

Already a good beginning has been made. A recent magazine article conveyed the impression that marihuana is rampant as a chief promoter of sex crimes; it being noted in particular that several hideous crimes committed in Los Angeles were instigated by use of this drug.

The Law in Colorado

Colorado Daily News Report

Boulder District Judge William E. Buck Monday declared the state law governing narcotics unconstitutional and dismissed charges against twelve defendants involved in February's crackdown on marihuana in the city.

The action came at a seven-hour hearing on the case, during which defence attorneys Jim R. Carrigan and Robert Ryan argued for dismissal on grounds that marihuana is not a narcotic, is not addicting, does not cause physical damage and thus is not covered by state narcotics laws.

Colorado statute 48 6-1 was ruled unconstitutional by Buck on two grounds.

That marihuana exhibits characteristics different from a narcotic as defined by law, and

That the State Board of Health has been given the power to define a narcotic. Buck ruled this an unconstitutional delegation of legislative power.

Charges were dismissed against (*names omitted for obvious reasons*).

The twelve were arrested last February on charges ranging from possession of the plant, to use and sale.

Captain Joseph Moomow, head of the Denver police laboratories, and University Pharmacologist Dr Harold C. Heim testified for the defence in the case.

Stanley F. Johnson, Boulder deputy district attorney, said, 'We defended the statute as best we could. There are two or three avenues left open for us to follow. Actually, we just have not yet decided which one to follow.' He said there is a possibility of asking the state legislature to do something about the statute, and added, 'It may be carried to the supreme court.'

Johnson said he would argue the case on the basis of the statute as it exists.

The argument of the defence attorneys were that marihuana was placed in an unreasonable classification with heroin and morphine: cruel and unusual punishment for marihuana smokers, paralleling those of heroin and morphine; delegation of legislative power to the Board of Health, and the fact that marihuana is not an addictive drug.

Moomow, in his testimony for the defence, said, 'Dr Heim and I agreed on all of the material physiological and psychological effects. Marihuana has no addictive powers, it does not have the habit-forming characteristics even tobacco may have.'

Speaking of the law itself Moomow said, 'There are a number of categories for drugs. To put all drugs in one law is foolish. There is a distinction between marihuana and other drugs.'

Moomow said however he does feel that marihuana should be illegal. 'There is no excuse for its existence or use,' he said, 'but it just should not be classified with the other drugs.'

The defence's second major witness, Heim, added that ... 'marihuana is not addicting, there is no recorded instance where marihuana has been fatal, as barbiturates and heroin can be. Based on pharmaceutical evidence, the body doesn't respond to it the same way it does to morphine or heroin. It is not in the same league, and that was the point I was trying to make.

'I do not feel it is a safe drug to go on smoking. It should be curtailed, but it just is in a different league than the others,' Heim said.

According to Moomow, the law was set up by the state health board, and was patterned after a recommended law of the Federal Narcotics Bureau.

Tom Andrews, federal narcotics bureau chief in Denver, said, 'The Federal Narcotics Act of 1956 covers the possession, acquisition, transfer and sale of narcotics. There is no federal law against illegal use.' Federal authorities could not prosecute for use, according to Andrews, but he said they could, if the federal attorney desires, prosecute on the charges of possession and sale.

'We'll wait and see what happens,' Andrews said. 'If we

have to tighten our belts, spit on our hands, and start over again, we will.'

Both Andrews and Moomow stressed the connections between crime and marihuana. 'Denver police are active against illegal use,' Andrews said, 'we consider it a disorderly factor.'

The question now pending, according to Johnson, is whether carrying the case to a state court constitutes double jeopardy. 'We're studying the thing fully,' Johnson said.

The ramifications of Boulder District Judge William E. Buck's decision Monday that Colorado's narcotics statutes are unconstitutional are momentous, according to a Boulder lawyer.

The barrister, who requested his name be withheld, said the ruling in effect left Boulder County with no narcotics laws. He added, however, that he felt Judge Buck's decision was correct and fair.

The Defence attorneys, he said, based their argument on four points.

The unrealistic classification of marihuana with such drugs as heroin and morphine.

The cruel and unusual punishment for the sale of marihuana to persons under twenty-five years of age. (The statute provided the death penalty for this.)

The delegation of legislative power to the state board of health in that the board could determine the definition of a narcotic.

The irrebuttable presumption of fact, i.e., that heroin, morphine and marihuana are addictive drugs.

Another lawyer, who also wished to remain unnamed, said the defence was not contending that the use, possession and sale of marihuana should not be an offence.

He said the penalties provided by the current statute, especially the death sentence, were completely out of proportion to the offence.

——, one of the defendants, said, 'I didn't expect this motion to be granted. I was ecstatic. I'm glad it's over. Buck showed extreme courage.'

——, another defendant, said, 'I knew they were going to argue the motion, but I never thought it would be accepted. We were already tried by some newspapers before we were put on trial in court. Judge Buck made a good decision.'

—— had entered a plea of guilty which was dismissed when the charge was ruled unconstitutional. He said, 'I was surprised. Even my lawyer didn't think it would go through. I feel we were given some unfair publicity during this whole thing. Buck was a good judge. He realized the law was incorrect. He was not just being a good guy.'

——, also a defendant, said, 'I was stunned by it all. It's nice to know that twelve nice people are not going to jail.' In reference to the publicity given the case, she said, 'What I saw really disgusted me.'

'I knew the lawyers were going to make this motion,' said ——, 'but I was surprised at the way it should have come out.'

Professor Albert R. Menard Jr, of the Fleming Law School, said, 'The ruling has a reasonable possibility of standing since it was reached after full argument.' (21 April 1964.)

Nigeria Whispers

Akin Davies

In May 1966, a British tourist and an American were both sentenced in Lagos to fifteen years' imprisonment, on charges of growing and smoking Indian hemp. The following article by a Nigerian journalist will help to explain why.

There is a growing trend in the more economically advanced countries to indulge at leisure in the exploration of the personality. At a certain stage of development, there is less need to produce and more time to spend consuming. This is healthy. If used properly, marihuana could be helpful at this stage of development. However, countries which are only beginning to develop a more complex economic structure must channel all their energies into creating a new system. This means that they must sacrifice more of their pleasures.

People who smoke hemp seem on the whole to be less aggressive than people who drink alcohol. Hemp smoking may have a positive value for certain social functions. In my country, Nigeria, and in other parts of Africa the main trouble with it seems to be its abuse by terrorist organizations of the type made famous by the Assassins of ancient Persia. The system works something like this. An unscrupulous politician decides to build a private army. He goes around the country and finds unemployed young men who are not too intelligent and close to starvation. He sees to it that every day they each get food, pocket money, and a supply of marihuana (a luxury for a poor man). What they must do in return is to carry out his orders: beat up, kill, or kidnap political opponents, perhaps plunder or burn a house now and then. They are usually called the 'party stalwarts'.

Recently there was rioting in western Nigeria which went on for three months. The army and the police failed to quell the rioting. Gangs of 'party stalwarts' armed with guns and locally manufactured flame-throwers which sprayed victims with burning petrol are reported to have killed 567 people. The Government, as most Governments do, tried to minimize the casualties and gave an official figure of 153. The Government neither replied to the demands of the opposition nor applied emergency measures to cope with the situation. It was this aloofness, plus the attempt to minimize casualties, which was the signal for desperate action. The army took over. The news was received with joy by Nigerian circles abroad, and the change was popular at home also.

One of the first acts of the Military Government was to issue a decree making it punishable by death to grow marihuana, and by up to twenty years of prison for merely being in possession of it. This seems extremely excessive, but must be considered as a reaction to the misdeeds of the gangs of 'party stalwarts'. It is to be hoped that the law can be modified when a way is found to prevent politicians from forming such private armies. In the meantime, we Nigerians have to stop getting high for a while and develop our country.

Notes from Tartaros

Neal Phillips

Neal Phillips, an American teacher of English, is at present serving a four and a half year sentence in the Greek prison of Tartaros for being in possession of three kilos of Indian hemp.

ANTON THE CONNECTION finally drove his colour poem in here. I know now he is high enough to survive bomb blast and fallout.

What a jolt your opening into a dialogue of deliverance gave to my twisted system. I seem to be chopping cotton fields with an iron handled hoe and could believe it was true except that a hoe with an iron handle can't happen since old Abe Lincoln cut our chains but the handle IS iron so it must be me who is not here. But where? I seem to be this unstable (a pure act of will) gentleman who is the acknowledged leader of the fools and one-armed beggars but has a steaming head and a very bad look in his eye who STILL has not been flushed although they pulled the handle hard. On the way down I found there's a bottom to despair. As for the rest, if this is bottom (and it must be close because it's at the far edge of human conception) then WOW! I've arrived and learned to live here, which gives rise to fright rather than comfort. But the case is not finally closed. They must be given every possible reason for giving me a full pardon. Life seems no longer real. I am consumed now by this constant vision of a man like me stumbling away through the snapping fields of flowers one afternoon ... I went to Hydra to rent a house and do some writing. Fuzz followed me for three days, found no evidence of selling. They busted me. They spoke very poor English, I no Greek at all. I asked for Consulate and they refused. I asked that they write questions in English and they both couldn't and wouldn't. I asked that I write answers in English and they refused. They twisted my story into pure nonsense. Had a Court of Inquiry five bloody days later, had lawyer appointed by police as they didn't allow me to call Consulate until too late to obtain my own lawyer. The lawyer spoke about 200 words of English and was working for the police besides. The court interpreter spoke no more English than the lawyer. They merely read off papers prepared by the police – again in Greek – handcuffed me, and pushed me into an outdoor cement compound where I lived with 120 half-kicked junkies through a long winter on the far side of sense. Went to court and was convicted before I started. As they had absolutely no evidence of selling, they convicted me as 'a member of an international gang' solely on the basis of my own testimony to the police. Wow! There is nothing lower than narcotics fuzz, Anton, they are worse than terminal cancer. So now we must say from everywhere and repeatedly that a grotesque mistake has been made. I mean, can that be called a pre-trial procedure? After all, how long would the Greek people take it if the police who questioned them knew only 200 words of Greek and wrote down the answers in Chinese? Is there any difference? Does that procedure not leave an endless margin for malice and misunderstanding? Under what set of principles do we accept a procedure which puts such unlimited power in the hands of the police? And if we do not accept it in principle, then how can we accept it in fact? Also: they gave me four and a half years, and while it is within the wide limits of the law it happens to be a stiff penalty. I've seen several hundred hashish cases here, and the biggest holder of all (sixty-seven kilos) who was in addition convicted of selling (I was not) got three years. Endless examples of bigger 'narcotics crimes' here with sentences down to six months. According to my lawyer, there is no hope. Especially since my crime is narcotics, as there has NEVER been a pardon issued for a narcotics case . . .

Cannot write much except letters here and run the risk of having them translated which would strike a mortal blow to my pardon possibilities, but the imagery here is overpowering and so darkly beautiful that it can never be erased. A hundred kilos of galloping horrors in a one kilo bag. I've fallen through the crust of the earth and am walking through Tartaros on my face. Very slow, very painful, very impressive. Reduced to simple instinct I win with ease, but the victory tastes like last year's herring. In the next cell sixteen murderers masturbate in close harmony, all still looking for the regret which precedes guilt which must come before deliverance. Dimitraki the Blank-Faced Beggar Boy spreads his cheeks several times nightly on the next cot to receive the sperm of hatred. His reward is but promise of cigarettes that will never be delivered. Promises are in fact all he really wants, because when he never receives them it proves to him what he always thought about a world that never delivers, has never delivered, and never will deliver, being but sliding panels that change shape and colour and pitch and texture and back out of reach before his needy hand. Dimitraki. One comes to hope that his ship will never come in, for now he knows a constant disappointment, but at least he can predict it and prefers it to confusion. But Greek junkies win all the prizes, Anton. They are beneath contempt here, beaten and brutalized by the police and nobody cares, live in the worst prison on the least food, get the worst medical attention. They have one defence: to become so despicable that not even a fuzz will slap them down.

'Gimme a cigarette,' says the guard. 'You can't talk to me like that!' shrieks Junkie, as he whips out the top of a sardine can and slashes his forearm twenty times and blood spurts everywhere. Fuzz turns green and phones for ambulance. Junkie chases him to phone and wipes blood all over his uniform while he speaks. 'You're sub-human!' says Fuzz in agony. 'Once more and I'll cut my throat right before your eyes,' says Junkie. 'Stop! You win!' says Fuzz in despair. 'OK, I win,' says Junkie and speeds away to a warm bed for a day or two. I once saw a junkie get so mad at the ruling of the fuzz-scorekeeper at a volleyball game that he slashed his abdomen open, pulled his entire stomach out in his hands, and tried to hand the bloody mess to the guard. 'That's what you wanted? Then don't be afraid to take it!' No end to it, so extreme is the self-mortification. They commit these acts not in the name of humility but in the name of pride, for they choose to drop themselves below the lowest level the fuzz can feature for them in order to maintain the freedom of at least controlling their own fate. Partly illusion, partly courage of truth, but at least we know now that even though absolute humility and absolute indifference become almost indistinguishable at times, and that the two of them turn to pride when they become the final refusal to be judged by all standards social and finally human, then at least my friends are proud of their distinctive vision and willing to chase it through the swamps until it wins ...

A man came in today having just received a two-year sentence for importing, possessing, and selling ninety kilos. I got four and a half years for importing and possessing three kilos, and I was not convicted of selling. They really hated me ...

The American Embassy of Athens has done absolutely nothing to help me. I must put the thumb on those people, they are offering zero and I am in terrible trouble without even a tiny bit of aid from them, like acknowledging my existence as a human being or something.

The Queen is having a baby, so they're cancelling five years off every sentence EXCEPT NARCOTICS. Do you see what I've run up against? Narcotics, hell! If everybody were high here they wouldn't even need a court, or a Queen either. The page runs out, sun comes up. I must go out and break rocks for five hours now before they'll give me a handful of olives and black bread for lunch. Always bread and olives. Another five hours in the afternoon. They are punishing me, but when I groan I groan for them and not one time for me. It is all an intermediate point on the way to beginning ...

The rock slide was started by a homicidal nut two hours

before schedule and caught me half-prepared, was too far underneath the overhang. Got out with a little Jehovah's Witness (he won't carry a rifle so they gave him twenty years) under my arm but went underneath at the last instant and my left hand was mangled. Stared at it for hours under morphine. Handsomely pulverized. Ghoulishly gnarled. Hurts but as expected just melts into other greater pains and is indistinguishable.

My lawyer writes that the American Embassy is showing no interest in the case whatsoever. The Greek government must be made to feel that the Teahead Troopers are after them. Hit them from here, hit them from there, from the other side, it looks as if their *tourist identity* is threatened, and that is the source of their heartbeat. Hoeing cotton now like Miles's grandfather, but mine's got snakes and scorpions in it. One-handed. Pressed a scorpion between the pages of Sartre's *St Genet*. Plans to flee later jell now. Cold criminal wit. Know every police mind in existence and every step from here to there. Don't want to do it as November is a bad month to bleed, but if pardon is denied ... Zinc dawn emerges. Better the lonely night. Sleep is a distant memory, so is wakefulness. Keys rattle in the concrete rampart. They're coming.

There is a young (twenty-four) New Zealand schoolteacher in here with me, busted selling two kilos to narcotics fuzz (they trapped him) in Athens. He got O N E Y E A R. Anyway he has done four months and cannot hold out any longer, has lost thirteen kilos, has long vacant spells, howls at night, so his Embassy is sending doctors up and trying to get him out early. He's been fucked about a hundred times, just overpowered and balled, also beaten here and there, was forcibly given an overdose of heroin and nearly died, etc. None of that in New Zealand jails, he says. Sorry as hell for him but can't help. End scene: his mother will shriek with terror when he finally walks out.

Marihuana and Alcohol

Anthony Storr

In Britain today increasing anxiety over the use of drugs by young people is prevalent among parents, school-teachers, dons and Government officials. Some of their anxiety is justified; but much of it is based upon ignorance and fear, fanned by emotional articles in the daily press which makes extravagant statements, such as 'drug addiction is a venereal disease of the soul'. The fact is that we know relatively little about addiction, and until we know more from the sober results of controlled research, any new legislation will be premature and may defeat its own object . . .

Indian hemp, marihuana or hashish has been known and used for centuries, especially in Muslim countries where alcohol is forbidden. Although a few people may become dependent upon its use, marihuana is not a drug of addiction and is, medically speaking, far less harmful than cigarettes or alcohol. Yet the possession of marihuana is, in this country [Great Britain], illegal and in 1964 a Glasgow doctor was sent to prison for having it . . . The idea that the use of marihuana necessarily leads to addiction to other drugs springs from the fact that it is illegal and has thus become associated with black market activities . . .

Marihuana is currently popular at Oxford and other universities. It is generally smoked in the company of others and its chief effect seems to be an enhanced appreciation of music and colour together with a feeling of relaxation and peace. A mystical experience of being at one with the universe is common, which is why the drug has been highly valued in eastern religions. Unlike alcohol, marihuana does not lead to aggressive behaviour, nor is it aphrodisiac. There is no hang-over, nor so far as is known, any deleterious effect. As with other drugs, there may be some danger that people turn to it as an habitual escape from life's problems. Its supposed pleasures have at times been rather tediously over-sold.

The Oxford Scene and the Law

Stephen Abrams

THE PROBLEM OF CANNABIS

The use of cannabis (marihuana and hashish) is increasing, and the rate of increase is accelerating. It is obvious that the police are no longer able to control the situation, though the possession of cannabis carries a penalty, in this country, of up to ten years in prison. The most enlightened approach to the problem would seem to lie in the enactment of a campaign of public information to warn young people of the dangers of smoking cannabis. This is what the Home Secretary proposes to do. But there are two reasons to believe that this campaign is likely to fail. Sensational mass publicity concerning the effects and availability of cannabis is probably the leading cause of the increase in illicit traffic. To have any chance of success a publicity campaign would have to be able to point to documentary evidence of the dangers of cannabis, and such evidence is apparently lacking. If people are informed of the pleasures of cannabis and not convinced of its dangers, the result will be disastrous for the purpose of law enforcement.

Dr Joel Fort, a consultant on drug addiction to the World Health Organization, Lecturer in Criminology at the University of California, and former staff member of the US hospital for drug addicts in Lexington, Kentucky, has stated bluntly that 'cannabis is a valuable pleasure-giving drug, probably much safer than alcohol'.[1] This view is shared by *Guy's Hospital Gazette*, where it has been argued that 'the available

1. Fort, Joel, 'Social and Legal Response to Pleasure Giving Drugs', in Blum, Richard (ed.), *Utopiates*, Atherton Press, New York, 1964.

evidence shows that marihuana is not a drug of addiction and has no known harmful effects ... (the problem of marihuana has been) created by an ill-informed society rather than the drug itself'.[2] The *Lancet*, having considered the evidence, has recently called for discussion of the possibility of repealing the laws prohibiting cannabis.[3] Unless statements such as these can be effectively answered and then suppressed, the Law will seem to be an ass, and civil disobedience will result, culminating in a protest movement along the lines of CND.

At present it is not known for certain whether cannabis is dangerous. But this does not justify the view that it is perfectly safe and should be made freely available to everyone. It is an established principle of pharmacology that a drug should not be made generally available until its safety has been established by means of controlled clinical trials. Here lies the great difficulty in the present situation. For various reasons it has not been possible to obtain the scientific information that is necessary to make a fair assessment of the social and medical problem of cannabis. There are few experimenters who would be prepared to risk working in such a controversial field. Furthermore, the drug has been removed from the Pharmacopoeia, and is virtually unavailable for research purposes. To be in possession of cannabis or to import it, one must hold a licence issued by the Home Secretary. Given such a licence, one would find that international controls make the purchase of cannabis difficult. For such reasons, the average number of scientific papers published annually on the subject of cannabis has recently been about four or five, and these have been mainly chemical studies. Those who have a legitimate right and a scientific reason to possess cannabis find that they cannot obtain it, but their students have no difficulty in purchasing it for the purpose of 'getting stoned'. One could, of course, take the risk of performing research with illegally bought supplies; and I am informed by the editor of one of the British Psychological Society journals that his fellow editors would probably

2. 'Drugs and Prejudice', *Guy's Hospital Gazette*, 79, 1965.
3. 'Pop "Pot"', *Lancet*, 1963, II, 989 f.

consider publishing research on cannabis on its scientific merit and without reference to the source of supply. But in such a case the investigator would risk prosecution and dismissal from his job. It is to be hoped that the Home Office will recognize that the present situation is intolerable, and that they will make cannabis seized at the customs available to legitimate research workers.

The best that can be done at the moment to shed some light on the problem of cannabis is to report on the casual observations that one has been able to make concerning the actual conditions of its use. To be meaningful, such observations should be confined to a normal and respectable community of cannabis smokers. That is, the group under observation should be, as far as possible, representative of the country as a whole in all respects other than its use of cannabis in preference to alcohol. The closest approximation to such a group is the sub-culture of cannabis users within a university community. The members of a university may not be strictly representative of the country as a whole, but they assume a special importance as future leaders of the country. The use of cannabis is widespread within the universities, and if this drug is damaging the minds of future members of parliament, captains of industry, scientists and teachers, drastic action is obviously called for. I live in Oxford where there are several hundred undergraduates and an increasing number of Dons on the 'pot scene'. The observations I have been able to make are probably biased in various ways, and I accept that their validity may be called into question. But I am obliged to report what I have seen and the conclusions I have drawn in the hope that they may, in a modest way, assist in the determination of public policy and the planning of properly controlled experimental research.

THE OXFORD SCENE

Undergraduates introduced the large-scale use of cannabis to Oxford in the autumn of 1963, about the time that pop music, pop art and pop culture became a country-wide intellectual fad. The standards set by the leading pop groups are not merely sartorial. This is an open secret, as should be obvious from the names of some of the groups, and the titles and words of many of their songs. Jazz is marihuana music, and has been ever since it began in New Orleans. Before 1963, there had been a small and very private 'scene' composed of people who had been introduced to cannabis in North Africa or America. At the end of the Long Vac a young poet brought fifteen kilos of 'kif' from Morocco in a sleeping bag. CND was then in its death agony, and the undergraduates who had deserted it found a new and refreshingly different cause to support in 'pot'.

It is well to refer to 'pot-smoking' as a social cause, because it is an important part of the reaction that is now setting in against excessive materialism in our society. The 'tea-head', as he is called, does not merely proclaim his cause as a defensive reaction. The feeling seems to be that it was wrong to blame the Bomb, America, Russia and the Police for one's sense of frustration and inadequacy. A much more mature attitude upon which some hold the survival of society may depend is to recognize that one tends to project the worst part of one's character on to some external 'threat' which conveniently accepts the blame for the mess that lies inside. The attitude of undergraduates has become increasingly introverted. In part this has led to experiments with drugs – and in part it has been the result of these experiments. The view of the 'tea-heads' and of their hero, the American folk-rock singer Bob Dylan, is that CND and other social causes were a great hoax. They seem to believe that any excessive involvement in politics constitutes playing the other fellow's game and an acceptance of his rules.

It is very difficult to estimate the number of members of the University who make use of cannabis. At one time I kept a list which grew to 257 names before I decided that it would be prudent to destroy the list in fairness to my informants. I am continuously surprised by meeting someone for the first time at a party, a university society or a coffee house and learning that he smokes cannabis and does so with a group whose existence had previously been unknown to me. Without any claim to accuracy I should think that there are at least 500 junior members of the University who smoke cannabis when it is available. In addition, the drug is now being used by a few dozen of the younger Dons, though it has not yet been smoked in the Senior Common Rooms. Some of these Dons were undergraduates when cannabis was introduced to Oxford, but others have been 'turned on' by their students. Some of the older and more eminent Dons have also experimented with cannabis. Most of these Dons are people who have taken LSD, mescaline or other hallucinogens and regard cannabis as a comparatively innocuous drug to be taken out of curiosity or to find out whether it is safe for one's students.

If I were to say that the cannabis users tend to be the more 'switched-on' members of the university, I should be speaking redundantly. The smokers seem to be a fairly representative cross-section of junior members. They tend to be more adventurous and more extroverted than the average, but there are many exceptions. Surprisingly, the majority seem to have attended public schools, but all social classes and races appear to be represented in roughly the same proportion as within the university generally. The academic record of the smokers is difficult to judge, but it does not seem to be unsatisfactory, and I doubt that there are grounds for serious concern. The self-aggrandizing politicians from the Union and the athletes are two groups which are notably absent. On the other hand there are among the cannabis smokers a certain number of malcontents and weak or disturbed individuals of the kind who would be expected to join whatever protest movement was most popular at the moment.

It is interesting that many undergraduates seem to be congenitally unable to experience the effects of cannabis, however many times they try. Were this not so the proportion of smokers within the University would be considerably higher than it is. To my knowledge, no serious research has yet been done on susceptibility to cannabis, but I have reached the opinion that self-acceptance and relaxation, two of the principal rewards, must be present in some degree for the drug to produce its effects. It would therefore appear that 'tea-heads' must be fairly well-balanced individuals, at least to begin with.

I have been able to interview a large number of individuals, at Oxford and elsewhere, who have been smoking cannabis for periods of up to nineteen years and I have been unable to find any obvious physical or mental deterioration associated with its use over a long period. These persons have satisfied me that they have been able to discontinue the use of the drug at will or when required by external circumstances and that they have not experienced withdrawal symptoms except of the most trivial kind. Several state that they found it much more difficult to give up cigarettes. I cannot therefore regard such persons as addicts to cannabis. I would compare them with people who have used alcohol for periods of up to nineteen years. On this topic I should add that there is no evidence that the dosage of cannabis increases over time, and it is not evident that the frequency of smoking increases once the individual has established his pattern of cannabis use. Furthermore, the great majority only smoke when they have easy access to cannabis. Thus they usually discontinue smoking during the vacs and when they 'go down'.

It has often been asserted that drug use of any kind is a form of escapism and should be strongly discouraged on that ground alone. To this one student has replied: 'Of course, anyone who rejects the Protestant Ethic or some other related set of social obligations, such as Marxism, can expect to be branded as an escapist for refusing to do someone else's dirty work.' But I have gained the impression that cannabis is a poor escape route. Alcohol may blot out reality, but cannabis tends to magnify it. If one 'turns on' when one is feeling bad, cannabis usually has the effect of making one feel miserable. The sort of person who wants to escape from reality may turn to heroin or they may turn to the Church, but they are unlikely to continue to smoke cannabis. On the other hand, if intelligently used, cannabis can provide the necessary relief that will enable a person to ride out a difficult period in his life. It is evidently a much safer agent for such purposes than barbiturates and amphetamines, both of which are dangerous drugs leading to addiction, mental illness and, for several thousand people each year, death.

Another criticism that is frequently made is that cannabis leads to violence and crime. Professor G. Joachimoglu has stated that 'the French word *assassin* for murderer is derived from hashish, because at the crisis, when these people are excited and experiencing the full effect of the hashish, they act criminally'.[4] I find this extremely difficult to believe. During the so-called 'crisis' the most violent activity that is likely to occur is uninhibited dancing. I have observed hundreds of persons under the influence of cannabis and have never seen a single act of violence committed. I have known many people who have been arrested for possession of cannabis, but I know of no instance where a person has been arrested, in Oxford at least, for disorderly behaviour under the influence of cannabis. Furthermore, I have had the opportunity of observing the same persons under the influence of both cannabis and alcohol and seen that the latter drug sometimes gives rise to viciousness of many kinds whereas the former leads to a sense of peace. Indeed one of the possible dangers of cannabis is that it may reduce aggressiveness to below the level that is socially acceptable.

Much has been made of the supposed aphrodisiacal quality of cannabis. Shaw once argued that the great majority of sexual encounters take place out of boredom because the individuals concerned cannot think of anything else to do. Under the influence of cannabis, when most things are pleasant, there is always something else to do and sex is unlikely to take place unless it is uppermost in the minds of both individuals.

Under the influence of cannabis, people tend to behave as if they had regressed to that time in one's life when innocence makes all things seem possible. It is this naïve enthusiasm,

4. Joachimoglu, G., remark in discussion, in Wolstenholme, G. E. W. and Julie Knight, (eds.) *Hashish: Its Chemistry and Pharmacology*, J. & A. Churchill, London, 1965, p. 14.

more than anything else, which is the attraction of cannabis. It is a world in which pretentiousness is automatically and kindly deflated and prejudice ceases to exist. The pleasures of cannabis are innocent and simple.

The price of cannabis in Oxford tends to be about eight or nine pounds an ounce for hashish, which is more frequently used, and a pound or so less for marihuana. This works out at about the price of a pint of bitter for the evening's entertainment. Whatever the profits may be in retailing other drugs, the margin in selling cannabis is very slim, and no one in Oxford makes a living at it. 'Pushers' tend to be smokers who want to make a pound or two a week and get their smokes for free. They stay in business for a few months until they become well known and then quietly retire. The smokers take turns acting as pushers. Those who never push to make a profit are usually willing to sell small quantities of cannabis at cost to friends who have temporarily exhausted their supplies, in return for similar favours in future. One point which is clear, and indeed admitted by the authorities, is that in this country there is no organized criminal conspiracy behind the sale of cannabis. Sometimes the drug is smuggled into the country on a one shot basis by students. The major supplies are brought into the ports by merchant seamen acting for themselves and are sold to anyone who is waiting around the docks. Smaller quantities are sometimes sent through the post.

One tends to be introduced to cannabis at Oxford in a casual way. Cigarettes are frequently and openly passed around at parties and small informal social gatherings. No one is urged to smoke, and it is rare to be overtly asked to join in. One tends to observe the behaviour of friends under the influence of cannabis and to contrast this with one's own reactions under alcohol. An impressive point is that the cannabis smokers do not become ill or wake up with a hangover the next morning. One takes the odd puff until finally one night one becomes properly stoned. One then tends to be 'turned on' by friends and eventually introduced to the pusher of the day.

Cannabis is usually smoked in a small group in congenial

surroundings in rooms in college or in digs. The atmosphere is rather like that of a sherry party. A gramophone is the most essential prop. As the drug begins to take effect, within a few minutes, there is usually an increase in physical activity, accompanied by great mirth. One may feel a compulsion to dance. Sensory experience of all kinds is enhanced and there is an air of conviviality. The usual 'high' is an innocuous evening spent listening to music, dancing, talking and eating. One may also venture out to a party, a colour film, or even to a pub, and during the day it is pleasant to punt on the river or visit the Ashmolean art gallery. Many persons find they are able to do intellectual or artistic work under the influence of cannabis; and I know of a case of one young man successfully sitting an examination for a fellowship when he was 'high'.

The usual textbook account of cannabis intoxication suggests that hallucinations frequently occur and that the user falls into a stupor at the end of the cannabis experience. Neither observation is confirmed in Oxford. I have been told of just one case of an hallucination, by a girl who claims to have seen a castle at the end of Little Clarendon Street. What does happen is that spatial dimensions are distorted, and the surroundings take on a warm glow. The only reason that smokers often fall asleep is that the drug is usually taken at night. If it is taken during the day the effect wears off within about three hours. It is unusual to smoke every day. The average seems to be once or twice a week.

My observations tend to confirm the opinion of those authorities who find cannabis to be a relatively innocuous habit and probably less dangerous than alcohol. I find it hard to think of cannabis as a social menace. Yet a contradictory view is held by the legal authorities, and it must be based on evidence of some kind. There is more than prejudice to it. I think the answer is that the effects of cannabis have been confused with the people who make use of it. This can also be seen in connection with the great variability in the effects of alcohol. Both drugs create states of increased suggestibility, and the nature of the experience depends on personal and social factors. The society of Oxford is probably a highly favourable environment for the use of cannabis, bringing out what is best in the experience. But it is not necessary to accept that in other environments cannabis produces harmful effects. Its use by criminals may be an example. It is true that some criminals smoke cannabis, but that is probably due to the fact that they have special access to illicit channels of supply. I should expect that the use of cannabis would have the effect of reducing the crime rate. This, of course, is an untested hypothesis.

One glaring inconsistency is that in the Middle East hospitals are filled with so-called hashish addicts whereas there is no evidence of mental deterioration among cannabis smokers in the West. However, in the Middle East cannabis is often mixed with opium; the opium content may be as high as 50 per cent. In addition, in Egypt and other countries cannabis is often taken together with datura seeds which are known to produce progressive and fairly rapid mental deterioration. It may be that the addiction is to opium and that the major ill-effects are produced by datura. Malnutrition may be another factor.

It is important that the use of cannabis in this country be under governmental control. But there is, as Professor Macdonald of Manchester University remarked recently, 'there is a big feeling in this country that prohibiting a drug is not really the way to solve the problem'.[5]

Cannabis: The Wootton Report

General Conclusion and Recommendations

67. The evidence before us shows that:
An increasing number of people, mainly young, in all classes of society are experimenting with this drug, and substantial numbers use it regularly for social pleasure.

5. Macdonald, A. D., Chairman's concluding remarks, in Wolstenholme, G. E. W. and Julie Knight, (eds.) *Hashish: Its Chemistry and Pharmacology*, London, J. & A. Churchill, 1965, p. 93.

There is no evidence that this activity is causing violent crime or aggressive anti-social behaviour, or is producing in otherwise normal people conditions of dependence or psychosis, requiring medical treatment.

The experience of many other countries is that once it is established cannabis-smoking tends to spread. In some parts of western society where interest in mood-altering drugs is growing, there are indications that it may become a functional equivalent of alcohol.

In spite of the threat of severe penalties and considerable effort at enforcement the use of cannabis in the United Kingdom does not appear to be diminishing. There is a body of opinion that criticizes the present legislative treatment of cannabis on the grounds that it exaggerates the dangers of the drug, and needlessly interferes with civil liberty.

68. The controversy that has arisen in the United Kingdom about the proper evaluation of cannabis in the list of psychoactive drugs, should be resolved as quickly as possible, so that both the law and its enforcement as well as programmes of health education, may be relevant to what is known about the dangers of cannabis-smoking in this country, and may receive full public support. What are those dangers?

69. There are still a number of imponderables. The substance most commonly used in the United Kingdom is the concentrated form of resin, more potent than the leaf products used widely in America and in Asia. The active principles of this substance have not yet been fully identified; the immediate effects of the burning process are not yet understood; and the long-term physical and mental effects, if any, of chronic use have not been scientifically tested. There is at present no routine method of detecting the drug in body fluids in the user.

70. Notwithstanding the limits of present knowledge, it is clear that cannabis is a potent drug, having as wide a capacity as alcohol to alter mood, judgement and functional ability. In that sense, we agree with the conclusion[1] recently published in

1. The *Journal of the American Medical Association*, vol. 204, no. 13, 24 June 1968.

the USA by the council on Mental Health, the Committee on Alcoholism and Drug Dependence of the National Research Council, and the National Academy of Science that cannabis is a 'dangerous' drug. But we think it also clear that, in terms of *physical* harmfulness, cannabis is very much less dangerous than the opiates, amphetamines and barbiturates, and also less dangerous than alcohol. The implications of its mental effects are much less clear. Psychosis or psychological dependence, it is true, do not seem to be frequent consequences of cannabis-smoking. But the subjectivity of the mental effects of cannabis makes it particularly difficult to measure the total effect of cannabis experience on any individual, or to assess what changes even a moderate and seemingly responsible habit might bring in the smoker's relationships with family and friends, study or work. We think that too little is known about the patterns of use to predict that in western society it will produce social influences similar to those of alcohol. It was significant that even those of our witnesses who saw least danger in the drug were concerned to discourage juveniles from using it.

71. We conclude, therefore that in the interests of public health it is necessary to maintain restrictions on the availability and use of this drug. For the purpose of enforcing these restrictions there is no alternative to the criminal law and its penalties. As we have already stressed however (paragraph 15) it is difficult to draw a hard and fast line between actions that are purely self-regarding and those that involve wider social consequences. It is particularly difficult to do so when the matter at issue is the use of a drug with wide appeal as a relaxant, and the possibly deleterious effects of which – at least in the United Kingdom – are still unknown. Smoking cannabis may be an act of simple enjoyment, a demonstration of self-neglect or an indication of social irresponsibility. Distinctions such as these cannot be written into the law, but can and should be recognized by the courts in their consideration of cannabis offences and offenders. The measures that we now suggest are intended to meet the needs of the immediate situation as we see

it. They should be kept under review in the light of experience and research.

Legalization

72. Some of our witnesses argued that possession of cannabis should be legalized at once. Most of us felt that the uncertainties just mentioned ruled this out in the near future: legalization could not be reversed if the cost of 'accepting' cannabis were later found to be higher than expected; and even if cannabis were ultimately found to be no more, or even less, harmful than alcohol, there would still be room for debate whether it would be in the interests of public health to extend the range of socially acceptable drugs. Those of us who did not wish to rule out the possibility of eventual legalization agreed that this could not be introduced before an exhaustive study of the problems of transition and of necessary safeguards had been made. Safeguards against adulteration would have to be investigated and standards of inspection would have to be agreed; sources of supply would have to be considered; importation from countries where the supply was still illegal would present a particularly difficult problem; it might be necessary to devise a licensing system for manufacturing synthetics; much thought would have to be given to the mode of distribution; an attempt would have to be made to define permitted limits of intoxication and methods of detection; and special measures to protect minors would have to be incorporated into any such new law. It was clear therefore to all of us that the legalization of cannabis would involve difficult and complex problems most of which have not been given much thought even by those who favour legalization. Nevertheless we do not entirely discount the possibility that properly organized research may one day produce information which could justify further consideration of the practical problems of legalization.

Research

73. It will be clear from this Report that there is still a great deal that we do not know about cannabis. Precise description of the chemical structure and behavioural effects of its active constituents has not yet proceeded far. Chemical research on the synthesis of the active principles of cannabis and some of their derivatives has only recently begun to yield results. Accurate scientific knowledge is lacking of the personality of those who habitually use cannabis, of the significance of the circumstances in which it is used, and of the psychological, physiological and social consequences of its long-term use. No detailed information is available about the extent of cannabis use by immigrants and the effects of this on United Kingdom social conditions. No data exist on which to form reliable estimates of prevalence or to make meaningful projections of the possible growth of cannabis-taking, still less to gauge the social consequences of any such growth. The social consequences of the advent of synthetics may be important, but little scientific information has so far been assembled to guide us. Further study of all these things will be difficult and time-consuming. In a matter as complex and continuously changing as that of cannabis use in our society it is not reasonable to suppose that research alone will provide sure answers to all the problems. We were glad therefore to learn of the setting up, by the Medical Research Council, of three working parties specially to study problems of drug dependence, and of the formation of the new Institute for the Study of Drug Dependence. We have no doubt that these developments will lead to a much needed enlargement of inquiry into the cannabis problem and we most strongly urge that every encouragement, both academic and financial, be given to suitable projects.

74. It is not within our competence to make detailed recommendations as to the kind of investigation that should be undertaken; but we think it useful to indicate the general areas in which research might be most immediately helpful. Information is needed about the pharmacological effects of natural

cannabis, in its different forms, both on man and on experimental animals. The effects of synthetic derivatives should be studied as a matter of urgency. There is a pressing need for chemical tests, both qualitative and quantitative, to detect the presence of cannabis and its metabolites in the body fluids of users. Clinical reports of ill-effects, both immediate and long-term, following cannabis use are still haphazard and ill-documented. There is a need methodically to investigate possible cases of cannabis psychosis and, in particular, to study the concomitant effect of other drugs and of the abuse of alcohol in these cases. The possible therapeutic use of cannabis and its synthetic derivatives also deserves further investigation. There is also an immediate need for sociological studies to establish the prevalence of usage, and to define more closely the different social groups, and the personality patterns, of consumers of cannabis as well as the effects of the drug-use upon their social efficiency. More information is urgently needed on the incidence of cannabis-taking by adolescents, and the extent to which this is made up of the transient use of the drug at parties and weekends and of sustained regular use. It would be helpful to see if there are differentiating characteristics between users who take only cannabis, users who take other drugs besides cannabis, and people who used to take cannabis but have now given up all drug-use.

75. The present legal position is unhelpful to research. Cannabis may be obtained for research if the Home Office gives authority, but, as the law stands, any research requiring it to be smoked by human beings is illegal except on Crown premises. There is considerable uncertainty as to whether hospital or university premises are exempt. These legal uncertainties have made it virtually impossible to undertake this kind of research. However, merely to remove the restriction on premises would be insufficient to allow the relevant research to be carried out. As social factors are so important in the use of cannabis qualified workers should be free to study these phenomena by observation and laboratory and social experiments without the risk of prosecution.

The need for changes in the law relating to cannabis

76. The maximum penalties for any offence relating to cannabis are, on summary conviction, a fine not exceeding £250 or imprisonment for not more than twelve months or both, and, on conviction on indictment, a fine not exceeding £1,000 or imprisonment for not more than ten years or both. These penalties are common to all drugs prohibited or controlled under the Dangerous Drugs Act 1965, including heroin. Originally introduced in the Dangerous Drugs Act of 1920 (to deal with traffic in opiates) and increased by the Dangerous Drugs and Poisons (Amendment) Act 1923, they were applied to offences relating to Indian hemp by the Dangerous Drugs Act 1925 and have since remained virtually unchanged.

77. Article 36 of the Single Convention obliges Parties to penalize intentional offences of possession (and trafficking) but not of use. The selection of penalties is left for domestic law to determine. The Dangerous Drugs Act 1965 imposes the same penalties for unlawful possession as for unlawful supply. A high maximum penalty for possession has been justified in the past by the argument that it must allow for due punishment of the trafficker, who is more likely to be found in possession than in the act of supply.

78. While maximum penalties for dangerous drugs offences have stood unaltered, the general law on the treatment of offenders has been changed considerably. More alternatives to custodial treatment have been developed, and great flexibility introduced into sentencing. Scientific studies have increased understanding of the origins of anti-social behaviour and of the relative effectiveness of deterrent and other approaches. In common with offenders against other laws the drugs offender has no doubt benefited by these developments. At the same time it seems to us that the penalties for cannabis offences have gone unreviewed for too long. Now that experience here (and overseas) has shown misuse of drugs to be a complex and rapidly changing social problem, it seems to us essential that the law should progressively be recast to give greater flexibility of

control over individual drugs, and of adjustment of the relevant penalties in accordance with the dangers presented by a specific drug or form of drug-taking.

79. The tables in the Appendix on pages 360–71 give analyses of:

A.   penalties inflicted for cannabis offences under the Dangerous Drugs Act 1965 in the years 1964-6 and for offences under the Drugs (Prevention of Misuse) Act 1964 in the years 1965 and 1966;

B.   penalties inflicted in 1967 for cannabis offences, other Dangerous Drugs Act offences, and offences under the Drugs (Prevention of Misuse) Act;

C.   cannabis prosecutions and disposals in 1967 related to age groups and weights of the drug.

80. These tables show some notable features about the cases dealt with by courts in 1967. Over two thirds of all cannabis offenders (and nearly all found guilty of possessing more than 1 kg.) did not have a record of non-drug offences. Nine out of ten of all cannabis offences were for possessing less than thirty grams. About a quarter of all cannabis offenders were sent to prison (or borstal, detention centre, or approved school); only about 13 per cent were made subject to a probation order; and about 17 per cent of first offenders were sent to prison. There was notably greater emphasis on fines and imprisonment for possession of cannabis than of other dangerous drugs, but less use of probation and conditional discharge for possession of cannabis than for possession either of other dangerous drugs or of amphetamines and other 1964 Act drugs. Average fines for possession offences in 1967 were £36 in the case of cannabis: £39 in the case of other dangerous drugs: and £28 10s. 0d. in the case of 1964 Act drugs.

81. We believe that the association of cannabis in legislation with heroin and the other opiates is entirely inappropriate and that new and quite separate legislation to deal specially and separately with cannabis and its synthetic derivatives should be introduced as soon as possible. We are also convinced that

the present penalties for possession and supply are altogether too high.

82. Several of our witnesses also drew attention to the principle of absolute liability on which drugs legislation had been constructed, and to the effect of various High Court judgements that *mens rea* does not have to be proved before a person can be convicted of an offence of possession. They argued that in the circumstances it was not surprising that defendants made allegations of 'planting' by unknown persons or the police, or that some sections of the public should feel disinclined to bring evidence of offences to the notice of the authorities. It was outside the scope of our inquiry to examine these matters in general. We were glad to note, however, that following the judgement of the House of Lords in the case of *Warner v. Commissioner of Police for the Metropolis*, the Home Secretary undertook to examine, in conjunction with the Law Commission, the whole question of absolute liability in relation to drug offences. So far as cannabis is concerned, we have found nothing to justify making possession without knowledge an offence to which the law provides no defence, but we think that the form which defences might take is best left to be determined by the Home Secretary's review.

83. From our study of the statistics and other evidence about the supply of cannabis in the United Kingdom we have come to the conclusions that the traditional view of the supplier as a large-scale criminal is an over-simplification, and that having a heavy maximum penalty for possession to allow for punishment of the large-scale trafficker exaggerates the criminality of drug-taking itself. It seems clear that in cannabis 'society' there is a regular give and take of the drug and that many users are in a position to supply it, and do supply it, in very small quantities without real criminal intent. None of our witnesses felt that 'amateur' activities of this kind should be described as trafficking or singled out for particularly severe penalties. On the other hand, the margin between casual supply and purposeful profiteering is not so wide that a trafficker needs to be in regular possession of very large amounts to find

his operations worth while. The courts today face considerable difficulty in penetrating the ambiguity of 'possession', particularly since the norms of moderate drug-taking are not widely known. There is therefore a real risk, when the range of penalties is so extensive, that the courts may treat drug-takers with more, and drug-traffickers with less, severity than they deserve.

84. We considered the practicability of reducing this risk by distinguishing more clearly in the law between possession intended for use and possession intended for supply. One approach, which we understand has been tried in some countries overseas, would be to provide a specific offence of possession with intent to supply, attracting higher penalties than the offence of simple possession and with an onus on the defendant, after the prosecution had shown him to be knowingly in possession of a prohibited drug, to prove, on the balance of probabilities, that he did not intend to supply it to another person. It may be that such a provision would be valuable in clarifying the true nature of offences of possession, but it cannot be fully considered apart from the broad balance of obligations on prosecution and defence. We therefore recommend that the possibilities should be further examined in the Home Secretary's review of the question of strict liability. Subject to this, however, we think that a test of intent could produce further uncertainty in the law which it is our wish to remove.

85. Another course might be to devise a formula based on the amount of the drug found in a person's possession for determining the penalty to be imposed. Thus a person having, say, thirty grams or less of cannabis leaf or resin in his possession without authority at the time of his arrest would be liable only to a small fine; unauthorized possession of larger amounts would attract a higher penalty. Such a formula, however, would present serious difficulties for enforcement because of the practical requirements for determining the amount, type and purity of any drug found with sufficient exactitude to sustain proceedings for unauthorized possession of more than

the specified amount; for establishing, when synthetic alternatives become available, comparable norms attracting a fine only; and for dealing with the problems of adulteration and identification. The introduction of a quantitative formula might also have an effect on trafficking. The limitation of risk to a small fine might not only lead small-scale traffickers to conduct their operations on a wider scale and more openly, it might also encourage professional criminals to become involved in this activity: once a large consignment had been imported and concealed a well-organized distribution of small amounts could be carried on with virtual impunity. We have concluded that these difficulties make it impracticable to introduce a quantitative formula into cannabis offences at this time.

86. After the fullest consideration we have come back to the view that the only practical way to legislate for the situation over the next few years, is to retain the principle of a single offence namely unlawful possession, sale or supply of cannabis or its derivatives. This offence should carry a low range of penalties on summary conviction but a substantially higher range on indictment. If such legislation were brought in we would anticipate that the police would proceed on indictment only in those cases in which they believed that there was organized large-scale trafficking. Offences involving simple possession and small-scale trafficking would, we hope, be dealt with summarily.[2]

87. In considering the scale of penalties our main aim, having regard to our view of the known effects of cannabis, is to remove for practical purposes, the prospect of imprisonment for possession of a small amount and to demonstrate that taking the drug in moderation is a relatively minor offence. Thus we would hope that juvenile experiments in taking cannabis

2. In England and Wales offences are dealt with summarily at a magistrates' court, the verdict being decided by the magistrate. Trial on indictment takes place at a court of assize or quarter sessions where the verdict is decided by a jury.

In Scotland offences are dealt with both summarily and on indictment at a Sheriff Court. Trial on indictment may also take place in the High Court.

would be recognized for what they are, and not treated as antisocial acts or evidence of unsatisfactory moral character. On the other hand, we would expect repeated convictions for possession of cannabis – in the same way as convictions for drunkenness – to carry certain social implications and penalties, e.g. in certain kinds of employment where evidence of a drug habit might be thought to be a disqualification. In our view the cannabis-taker who is open to reason is more likely to be deterred by considerations of this kind than by a scale of penalties.

88. On summary conviction we think that the fine should be limited to £100. In many ways we would have preferred to have suggested no alternative prison sentence. It has, however, been represented to us that in United Kingdom law, hybrid offences, such as we are suggesting, normally carry some prison sentence on summary conviction, and that this gives the judiciary useful discretion in dealing suitably with difficult individual cases. In this instance we can foresee situations where a person, repeatedly engaging in small-scale trafficking, but nevertheless trafficking of a blatantly commercial nature, would not be deterred by modest fines, whereas a short prison sentence without the panoply of proceedings by indictment would be appropriate. We recommend therefore that on summary conviction there be a maximum alternative penalty of four months' imprisonment. In choosing this period we have been influenced by the fact that a four-month sentence on summary conviction is one which allows the defendant an option of going for trial by jury ... a not inconsiderable civil liberty. It is relevant to add that under section 39 of the Criminal Justice Act 1967 a court which imposed a sentence of not more than six months' imprisonment for a cannabis offence, would be obliged to suspend that sentence except in certain conditions, of which the most important are that the offender has already served a sentence of borstal training or imprisonment, or is already on probation or under conditional discharge.

89. It is socially undesirable for an organized criminal underworld to be able to make large profits from any illicit activity. Therefore we recommend that on indictment the offence should be punishable by an unlimited fine or a sentence of imprisonment not exceeding two years or both. The maximum penalty for smuggling cannabis imposed by the Customs and Excise Act 1952 (as amended by the Dangerous Drugs Act 1967) should be reduced from ten to two years. The existing provision under the Dangerous Drugs Act 1965 whereby proceedings or indictment are subject to the fiat of the Director of Public Prosecutions should be retained. In our view, however, such proceedings should normally only be appropriate in dealing with the large-scale trafficker.

90. It is our explicit opinion that any legislation directed towards a complex and changing problem like the use of cannabis cannot be regarded as final. For the foreseeable future, however, our objective is clear: to bring about a situation in which it is extremely unlikely that anyone will go to prison for an offence involving only possession for personal use or for supply on a very limited scale. We recommend that over the next three years the Advisory Committee should keep that objective under review and be ready to propose further measures if the objective is not being realized.

Use of premises for cannabis smoking or dealing

91. Section 5 of the Dangerous Drugs Act 1965 makes it an offence for an occupier to 'permit' premises to be used for smoking or dealing in cannabis or cannabis resin and for any person to be concerned in the management of premises used for any such purpose. The object of this provision, which was first enacted in the Dangerous Drugs Act 1964 (on the model of a long-standing provision about opium-smoking, now to be found in section 8 of the 1965 Act), was to discourage communal smoking and trafficking in cannabis in premises of public resort by placing the onus on the occupiers or managers to

ensure that such premises were not used for these purposes. The precise effect of the law is now the subject of an appeal to the House of Lords. In considering the present provisions we have assumed that the question of the appropriateness of strict liability in the offence will be examined in the Home Secretary's general review (paragraph 82).

92. In favour of the provision it was represented to us that if landlords or occupiers could not be held responsible, smoking parties would tend to increase, and drug-traffickers would be likely to use them to introduce smokers to other types of drugs. This would expose many young people to serious dangers outside the purview of routine checks by the police. In these circumstances it was urged that there should be a special obligation on those in charge of premises to prevent such activities. In the case of public premises, we were told that those having illicit possession of drugs found it easy to evade arrest by simply throwing the drugs on the floor. Unless those in charge of premises had a special obligation to prevent the use of, or traffic in, drugs, their tolerance of these activities, it was said, could make for a considerable increase in the misuse of drugs.

93. The 'pot party' is the natural focus for public disquiet about cannabis – and for the myths about the drug. If it were clear that intoxication, aggressive behaviour, sexual excesses, multiple drug use and crime were the predictable results of social smoking of cannabis, there would be a strong case for special steps to protect young people and for trying to enlist the help of these in charge of private premises. But, as is shown by the comparison we have drawn above between cannabis and other drugs, there is no evidence that taking cannabis in any special way stimulates behaviour of this kind. If cannabis is taken at a 'wild party' it is not because it supplies the spark to what would otherwise not catch fire.

94. Whatever may be the justification for the provisions of section 8 of the Dangerous Drugs Act 1965 in regard to the smoking of opium (see paragraph 91) we are convinced that there is no sufficient justification, in the harmfulness of can-

nabis, for placing occupiers and landlords of private premises under any special obligation to prevent cannabis-smoking, and there is even less justification for doing so in respect of cannabis-dealing (since this is not distinctively different from dealing in any other kinds of drug). We therefore recommend that section 5 should be repealed in relation to premises to which the public has no access.

95. We think that occupiers and managers of premises open to the public are in a different position. Society expects those who undertake to provide services and entertainment for the public to conduct their premises in a proper way, and it is not unreasonable to place on them a duty to prevent open use of, or trafficking in, drugs. Even here, however, it is evident that the duty may be more onerous in some directions than in others. It is easy enough to detect the odour of burning cannabis, but much more difficult to confirm that an exchange of tablets between two customers is a breach of the law. We think that a reasonable course would be to redefine the scope of section 5 so as to apply it only to premises open to the public, to exclude the reference to dealing in the drug, and to remove the absolute nature of the liability on managers.

96. We are aware that there are some types of premises which are, strictly, not open to the public, but are not private premises in the conventional sense. The Private Places of Entertainment (Licensing) Act 1967 provides, on adoption by a local authority, for a measure of supervision over certain types of club. Although this Act may not cover all the kinds of premises which, reasonably, should be subject to the obligation we have proposed for public premises, we are satisfied that the main sectors about which we know the police to be most concerned are covered by our proposals.

Powers of arrest and search

97. In paragraph 81 we have recommended the separation of cannabis from the opiates in drugs legislation and in para-

graph 88 and 89 we have proposed a reduction in penalties. Depending on the form and context in which legislative effect were given to these changes, consequential adjustments would have to be made in the present provisions which govern police powers of arrest and search in relation to cannabis offences. The present position is that under Section 2 of the Criminal Law Act 1967 the police have power to *arrest without warrant* any person who has committed or attempted to commit, or whom they have reasonable grounds to suspect to have committed or attempted to commit an 'arrestable offence'. Such an offence is one which is punishable with a sentence of at least five years' imprisonment. In England and Wales this power may be exercised in respect of offences against the Dangerous Drugs Act 1965 (i.e. including cannabis offences) which, on conviction, carry a possible penalty of up to ten years' imprisonment. The Criminal Law Act does not apply to Scotland and Northern Ireland and in those countries the police powers of arrest without warrant for cannabis offences derive from section 15 of the Dangerous Drugs Act 1965, as amended by section 6 of the Dangerous Drugs Act 1967. Under these provisions the police have power to arrest without warrant any person who either has, or who is suspected of having, committed or attempted to commit a dangerous drugs offence, only if they have reasonable grounds for believing that that person will abscond unless arrested, or whose name and address are unknown to the police and cannot be ascertained by them, or in whose case the police are not satisfied that the name and address given to them are true. As regards powers of *search* section 6 of the Dangerous Drugs Act 1967 introduced – for drugs scheduled under the Dangerous Drugs Act 1965 *and* the Drugs (Prevention of Misuse) Act 1964 – new powers enabling the police to search persons and vehicles on suspicion. If the penalties for cannabis offences are reduced as we propose and if cannabis were excluded from the Dangerous Drugs Act 1965 the case for retaining these police-powers would have to be reopened. This question of police powers cannot be realistically considered in relation to cannabis alone and it has been outside our task to examine the general issues. In the course of our inquiry, however, we have been made strongly aware both of concern about the effect of the exercise of these powers upon the relationship between the police and the public, and of the difficulties faced by enforcement authorities in recent years for which these wide powers of arrest and search have been thought to be essential. Because these features have contributed to so much of the current 'protest' against the existing law we recommend that as a matter of urgency the Advisory Committee should begin a general review of police powers of arrest and search in relation to all drug offences with a view to advising the Secretary of State on any changes that may appear appropriate, particularly as regards cannabis. In the meantime, however, changes in cannabis legislation should go forward without any specific recommendation about arrest and search. This omission will not have any immediate practical consequences in that the powers referred to will stand for the other drugs; search on suspicion is normally for drugs in a general sense rather than for cannabis specifically.

Control of synthetic cannabinols

98. Neither the Single Convention on Narcotic Drugs 1961 nor the Dangerous Drugs Act 1965 applies to synthetic cannabinols. Preliminary reports have suggested that some substances in this group are more potent than the natural product. So far no manufacturer of such substances for non-scientific or non-medical purposes has come to notice, but such a development may be expected as soon as the necessary technical processes have been evolved. Without further amendment the powers available in the Pharmacy and Poisons Act 1933 and the Drugs (Prevention of Misuse) Act 1964 would permit controls to be applied to manufacture, distribution and sale and to limit authorized possession. We think that these powers should be sufficient, but we recommend that the position should be kept under review.

99. At present cannabis can be prescribed by doctors in the form of extract of cannabis and alcoholic tincture of cannabis. Until very recently the demand for these preparations has been virtually negligible. In recent months however, there has been a striking increase in the amounts prescribed. Our inquiries, supported by what we were told by our witnesses, indicate that there are a number of doctors who are beginning to experiment with the use of cannabis in the treatment of disturbed adolescents, heroin and amphetamine dependence and even alcoholism. Whilst we do not expect cannabis prescription will ever become standard medication in the treatment of these conditions, it is quite likely that the amount dispensed on medical prescriptions will continue to increase and that this process may be accelerated when synthetic cannabis derivatives, properly standardized, become available. We see no objection to this and believe that any new legislation should be such as to permit its continuance. We think, however, that when cannabis or its derivatives are prescribed, records of the kind that can be inspected by H.M. Inspectors of Drugs should be available. This will enable the prescribing trend over the next few years to be kept under methodical review.

EDUCATION

100. The law alone cannot dispose of the problem of cannabis. However wise the law and whatever it says there will be those who will use cannabis and some who will suffer by it. Education too has a part to play. By 'education' we do not mean formal propaganda (the need for which it has been outside our terms of reference to consider); a proper understanding of the significance of cannabis in our society at this time cannot be given simply by description of the effects of the drug and the relevant law. Rather do we mean the general process of questioning, observations, argument and assessment by which society commonly forms balanced attitudes to community

problems and dangers. We hope that this report will contribute to an understanding both of the facts (and uncertainties) about cannabis and of the wider issues surrounding the problem of its control.

101. The following is a summary of our recommendations:

(1) We recommend that in the interest of public health, it is necessary for the time being to maintain restrictions on the availability of cannabis (paragraphs 70 and 71).

(2) Every encouragement, both academic and financial, should be given to suitable projects for inquiry into the cannabis problem (paragraph 73). Suggestions about areas in which research is required are made in paragraph 74.

(3) The law should progressively be recast to give Parliament greater flexibility of control over individual drugs (paragraph 78).

(4) The association in legislation of cannabis with heroin and the other opiates is inappropriate and new legislation to deal specially and separately with cannabis and its synthetic derivatives should be introduced as soon as possible (paragraph 81).

(5) Unlawful possession of cannabis without knowledge should not be an offence for which the law provides no defence (paragraph 82). The practicability of distinguishing between possession intended for use and possession intended for supply should be examined (paragraph 84).

(6) Possession of a small amount of cannabis should not normally be regarded as a serious crime to be punished by imprisonment (paragraphs 87 and 90).

(7) The offence of unlawful possession, sale or supply of cannabis should be punishable on summary conviction with a fine not exceeding £100, or imprisonment for a term not exceeding four months, or both such fine and imprisonment. On conviction on indictment the penalty should be an unlimited fine, or imprisonment for a

term not exceeding two years or both such fine and imprisonment (paragraphs 86, 88 and 89).

(8) The existing law which inhibits research requiring the smoking of cannabis (section 5, Dangerous Drugs Act 1965) should be amended to allow qualified workers to study its use both by observation and by laboratory and social experiments (paragraph 75).

(9) Section 5 of the Dangerous Drugs Act 1965 (permitting premises to be used for smoking cannabis, etc.) should be redefined in scope so as to apply only to premises open to the public, to exclude the reference to dealing in cannabis and cannabis resin, and to remove the absolute nature of the liability on managers (paragraphs 94 and 95).

(10) The Advisory Committee should undertake, as a matter of urgency, a review of police powers of arrest and search in relation to drug offences generally with a view to advising the Secretary of State on any changes that may be appropriate in the law, particularly as regards cannabis (paragraph 97).

(11) The development of the manufacture of synthetic cannabinols should be kept under review and, if necessary, control should be imposed under powers provided by the Pharmacy and Poisons Act 1933 and the Drugs (Prevention of Misuse) Act 1964 (paragraph 98).

(12) Preparations of cannabis and its derivatives should continue to be available on prescription for purposes of medical treatment and research. Provision should be made in legislation for records to be maintained so that the position can be kept under review (paragraph 99).

102. We wish to express our most cordial appreciation of the help that we have had from our secretaries, Dr E. G. Lucas and Mr D. G. Turner. Their skill in clarifying issues and their patience in feeding our seemingly insatiable appetite for drafts and redrafts far surpassed anything that we had a right to expect. We would also like to extend our thanks to those other officials of the Home Office, Ministry of Health and Scottish

Home and Health Department who assisted us with valuable information and advice.

WOOTTON OF ABINGER
Chairman

K. J. P. BARRACLOUGH
THOMAS H. BEWLEY
P. E. BRODIE*
P. H. CONNELL
J. D. P. GRAHAM
C. R. B. JOYCE
AUBREY LEWIS
NICOLAS MALLESON
H. W. PALMER
TIMOTHY RAISON
MICHAEL SCHOFIELD*

E. G. LUCAS
D. G. TURNER
Joint Secretaries
4 October 1968

Marihuana: Is It Time for a Change in Our Laws?

Newsweek, *7 September 1970*

... There are, by now, precious few American communities of any size that cannot offer such stories of their own: tales of pot puffed in unexpected places, of the offspring of prominent people – and sometimes even the notables themselves who have tried marihuana. With the possible exception of speeding on the highways, pot smoking is almost certainly the most widely committed crime in the United States today. Dr Stanley F. Yolles, former director of the National Institute of Mental Health, has estimated that the number of Americans who have

* Subject to reservations.

tried it at least once may be as high as 20 million. The Pentagon says that about 30 per cent of the US troops in Vietnam smoke it, and most observers consider this estimate conservative. In several large universities where surveys have been taken, the proportion of under-graduate users tops 50 per cent and is rising. Only in the days of Prohibition have so many Americans tasted a forbidden fruit so frequently and with so little remorse.

And now, as in the days of Prohibition, debate is welling up over a law that some suspect may be more damaging than the behaviour it is designed to prohibit. Questions never raised while marihuana was the monopoly of ghetto blacks and jazz musicians are being voiced now that the drug has spread to the middle class. 'When the kids who used it came from socially deprived backgrounds,' notes Inspector Joseph Rinken of the San Francisco narcotics squad, 'nobody gave a damn. But now it's my kids and your kids and everybody's kids.' Even Kennedy kids – Robert F. Kennedy Jr and his cousin Robert Shriver 3rd, both sixteen, got into trouble over marihuana just last month. And so some of the hard questions are finally being posed.

Is marihuana all that harmful? The conventional wisdom is challenged these days not only by spaced-out hippies and middle-aged mystics of the Timothy Leary stripe, but also by some responsible scientists who have studied the drug. The medical establishment and the government continue to say that it is dangerous, but now for the first time they are pressing forward with research to try to establish the facts.

Even assuming the drug is dangerous, do the current punishments fit the crime? If there is any area of broad agreement in the raging controversy over marihuana, it is on this point – almost all authorities believe that the penalties prescribed by law have been too harsh. The cultivation, possession or sale of grass is illegal under the laws of all fifty states and the Federal government, and some of the statutes carry fairly Draconian punishments. In Virginia only last year, for example, a twenty-year-old youth was sentenced to twenty years imprisonment for possession of six pounds of marihuana (he was later paroled), and in Michigan radical leader John Sinclair was given nine-to-ten years after handing two joints, free, to an undercover narcotics agent. The Nixon Administration, which came into office pledged to take a hard line on all drug offences, has done a turnabout on marihuana: it is now sponsoring Federal legislation that would reduce possession of pot, for first offenders, from a felony to a misdemeanour with a maximum sentence of one year. A number of states have already done the same or seem about to – and even where the legal penalties are still heavy, many courts tend to let first offenders off with probation.

Finally, and fundamentally, are any criminal penalties for pot smoking either justified or wise? The thought alone is enough to offend most policemen, many parents and some doctors, but a few venturesome voices have recently risen to argue that marihuana be made legal. The August issue of a New England medical journal called the *Massachusetts Physician* recommended editorially that grass be placed under the same controls as alcohol. And a forty-one-year-old Stanford University law professor (and former Justice Department prosecutor) named John Kaplan has just published a book entitled *Marijuana: The New Prohibition,* in which he contends that if there are any benefits of pot laws – and he can discern few – they are far outweighed by the damage they have done to American society. The current approach, Kaplan argues, ties up police and courts in a hopeless enforcement effort, turns a large segment of the younger generation at least technically into criminals, breeds disrespect for the law, spreads suspicion between parents and children, encourages disbelief of warnings about the dangers of harder drugs and forces marihuana smokers into contact with underground drug pedlars who frequently tempt them with far more hazardous wares.

The Gentle Moves to Legal Pot

Sunday Times (Spectrum)

American lawyers in New York this month were told at a conference on the defence of drug cases that marihuana could be legalized in the US in three years. At the same time the chief of the New York narcotics squad told me that the laws on marihuana should be changed. So what are the current odds on legalization?

The conference heard the great white hope of the pro-pot lobby Dr Norman Zinberg, psychiatry professor at Harvard Medical School, predicting that pot would be off the statute books in three to five years because there were no hard medical facts saying that it was harmful.

And Prof. John Kaplan of Stanford University Law School, whose book *Marijuana: The New Prohibition* is the pot lobbyist's bible, forecast lawful marihuana in seven years by a simple erosion of the existing law. The first state to legalize it would be New York, they thought.

And on the face of it the predictions of the academics are not unreasonable. The narcotics officer, deputy-chief inspector John McCahey told me that the serious epidemic of heroin and pills had put pot in the shade. 'For the present it is a violation of the law, but no one's going to jump up and down if they find it,' he said. 'It's got to be re-evaluated.'

The facts are that 75 per cent of the yearly rate of 13,000 convictions for selling drugs in New York City concern heroin, 18 per cent pills and only 7 per cent pot. While inspector McCahey could not say that his squad turned a blind eye to pot users he admitted that if someone rang up and told him there were 50 kids on the beach smoking their heads off he could not spare any of his 700 men for the job. Even if they found one smoker, the time involved in finding out where the drug came from was better spent uncovering a heroin pusher.

But the same is not true, of course, for the mid-states where pot may still be a distant rumour or in California where it is *the* problem. In Britain, too, where drugs convictions totalled 6,095 last year more than two thirds were concerned with cannabis.

In the meantime there are gross inconsistences in the execution of other countries' pot laws. In the US a man can be given 33 years for the possession of one marihuana cigarette in Texas and get off with a small fine in New York.

One of the most liberal attitudes to pot is found in Denmark. Last year the public prosecutor advised police and lower courts to be lenient on individual users and since then they have, as a rule, been let off with a warning (they would probably get a £10 fine and a suspended sentence in London).

And in Holland, of course, Amsterdam's municipality runs a youth club, The Paradiso, where soft drugs are openly taken. Outside the club first-time cannabis offenders may get off with one week on probation and a small fine. The latest betting is that either Holland or Denmark will be the first countries to legalize pot.

Unfortunately it is unlikely to happen in Britain where less than a dozen lawyers regularly defend drugs cases. But a London solicitor, Bernard Simons, who was the only British lawyer at the New York conference, says this is exactly why such teach-ins are necessary. 'The unfortunate result of the almost total ignorance of drug law practice among some magistrates, prosecutors and defenders is that sentences are often imposed in the provinces which are totally out of keeping with London standards,' he said.

PETER PRINGLE

Letter to *International Times*

October 1968

Dear IT,

I just read IT of Sept. 6 in which you published a letter of Robert Pontin in Erzincan prison. Soon I'll be a year in a Turkish prison. I got sentenced to 30 years. I appealed to the Supreme Court in Ankara but no results. Same sentence, 30 years. For what? That's what I'm asking myself so often. I carried 2 kilos of shit for my own use with me from Pakistan. Got busted in Istanbul because some German told Interpol and received a reward. They gave me 15 years for smuggling, 15 years for selling. No proof at all for selling, but they beat you with a wooden stick on your feet, hands, etc., here till you admit what they want you to say. The scene in Turkey is very bad at the moment. Lots of people get busted. In the last few weeks they have deported about 75 beats.

I also know that there are many others sentenced to two-and-a-half years, several to eight years four months, and two like me to 30 years – one still has to be sentenced. For what? Are we murderers? They treat us like this, we get beaten up by guards, get one bread and a soup a day. Consulates are not helping very much in Turkey. What can we do? How many years do we have to rot in a Turk prison? – no amnesties. Isn't there anybody who can help? Once more a warning to all beats, etc., who come back from the East. One day they might be so unlucky to get busted, like me. I am coming to Turkey for more than 4 years, been East three times, and I didn't know that sentences like this were possible.

Not nice to experience it this way. HELP!!!!

I heard once something about an organization called 'Release'. Could you write me back about it and inform me a bit. I'm trying to keep cool, and stoned, which is pretty difficult at times being the only foreigner between 400 Turks.

It's already Monday today, shitty rainy day, cold and windy. Just an hour ago I received a note from Ankara on which was written the date when I'll be free again. No chance to escape those 30 years. I've got them, that's a fact. The dossiers are closed, as a formality they send you the note. My freedom is far away, the date on the paper was 1998, March 10th, 6 o'clock a.m.

It is maybe interesting to know that I got busted together with my chick. After we had been in prison 2 months and I had taken the guilt on me her parents got her out, on 30,000 liras expenses. I wasn't that lucky. I've not got the bread. For my parents I'm as good as dead.

> Hans Van Der Aar,
> Pasakapi Ceza-Evi,
> Uskudar, Istanbul,
> Turkey.

Hell among the Turkish Delights

International Times, No. 50

Article 5 Declaration of Human Rights: No one shall be subjected to torture or to cruel, inhuman or degrading punishment.

This is the situation:

There are forty-six Europeans and Americans known to us in Turkish jails serving sentences for narcotics offences, mainly hash. Five of them are British. Sentences range from two-and-a-half to 30 years. Article 1 one of the Turkish Drug Laws states: '403.1. Whoever manufactures, imports or exports narcotics or attempts to perpetrate such offences without possessing a licence shall be punished by heavy imprisonment for not less than 10 years. 403.2. If the narcotic indicated in the foregoing paragraph is either heroin, hashish, cocaine or morphine, the perpetrator shall be punished by life imprisonment.' Para. 5 (111) states: 'In case of a commission of the crime by those organizing or governing or participating, the punishments ... shall be doubled. Under conditions described in the 2nd paragraph, the perpetrators shall be sentenced to death.'

PRISON CONDITIONS

a) *Cells*: Sometimes more than thirty prisoners to a cell. Bedding must be purchased by the prisoner.

b) *Clothing*: Nothing is provided by the prison authorities. Prisoner X (English) 'he has been given an eiderdown by the Consul'. Prisoner Y (English) 'he will shortly be receiving a pair of shoes from the Consul'. – William Whitlock, Parliamentary Under-Secretary of State, Foreign Office.

c) *Air*: 'The air stinks' Prisoner Y.

d) *Diet*: A daily piece of bread and a bowl of soup. Prisoners can survive if they are able to pay for further nourishment. 'If I have to live on what the Turkish Government gives us, I'll be dead in a few years.' – Prisoner Z (German).

e) *Medical*: Prisoner Z – sent to mental hospital for reasons undiscovered by the prisoner. '450 people, 150 beds, the rest sleeping on the floor, people without clothes ...' One British inmate, according to Prisoner Y, had to wait 2 months before an operation for swallowing a fish hook and when he went to hospital he was chained to the bed. 'The Director General of jails in Turkey went on to stress that British prisoners were given preferential treatment in Turkish jails and I have every reason to believe this is so' – William Whitlock, Parliamentary Under-Secretary of State. 7.1.69. Prisoner Y reports that invalids lie on the floors all day, insufficient beds.

WHAT HAS BEEN DONE

I. Col. James Allason, Tory MP for Hemel Hempstead, wrote to ask the Foreign Office what they are doing to ensure reasonable conditions of imprisonment and what representation they have made about the excessive length of sentences (15.11.68). William Whitlock, Parliamentary Under-Secretary of State, replied, 'We have given very close consideration to the pros and cons of protesting about the length of sentences and the conditions in prison ... We have concluded that the Turkish authorities would in all probability regard any such move as interference in their internal affairs.'

2. As a result of articles published in the *Guardian, Sunday Times* and the *New American,* London based correspondents of Turkish newspapers have sent to Turkey extracts from these articles which, according to reliable sources, have received major publicity and caused an uproar in Turkey. 'You may however like to know that the Director General of Jails in Turkey has already protested to the Consul about what was considered to be misleading publicity here.' – William Whitlock. 7.1.69.

3. Col. Allason tells the *Guardian* that he is 'disappointed by the Parliamentary Under-Secretary of State's letter'. He will continue the campaign.

4. *The Times,* who have kept out of the controversy altogether, print a report from their Turkish correspondent (20.1.69) 'Indignation expressed outside Turkey at harsh sentences imposed on narcotics offenders and at grim prison conditions is being met by Turkish indignation at an invasion of drug seeking young travellers.' (The reference to Turkish 'indignation' conflicts with reports arriving in Britain about Turkish reactions.) 'Prison conditions by western standards are dismal.' *The Times*, 20.1.69.

5. Following lobbying by Harvey Matusow and me, an ITN camera crew attempts to get permission to go to Turkey and film several prisoners. Application is referred to Turkey through the Turkish Embassy in London. Application is refused.

6. Najat Somnez, Turkish press attaché in London, lunches with Matusow and me and explains how shocked Turkey is about these slurs on her prison system and national integrity.

WHAT MUST BE DONE

46 PRISONERS MUST BE RESCUED. Their treatment conditions are cruel and inhuman, and the best parts of their lives are being wasted mainly because Turkey wants to improve her image and attract rich American tourists. The Turkish penal code, which allows exchange of prisoners (English drug offenders exchanged for Turks serving sentences in Britain) is impracticable, according to William Whitlock, who appears to disparage the 'excessive publicity' about European prisoners in his letter to Col. Allason.

WHAT YOU CAN DO

It's down to the people now. YOU have to protest, each one of you. Tell your friends to avoid Turkey. Don't go yourself. If you must, forget about drugs, it's not worth the risk. If you want to visit prisoners or write to them, contact me thru BIT for details. Write to your MP. Write to William Whitlock. Write or phone the Turkish Embassy, ask what is being done. We need your support and your activity. Involvement starts HERE and NOW. Don't wait for the next person to do something because the next person is waiting for you. Establish whether or not you feel strongly about these poor cats in Turkish jails. The next step is to translate feelings into Energy. The place is HERE. The time is NOW. YOU supply the ACTION.

*

We cannot print the names of prisoners X, Y & Z because reports from Turkey indicate that they are being penalized for activities on their behalf in England. We can tell you that they are all in on hash charges and that the sum total of their sentences is 48 years. Our grateful thanks on behalf of all prisoners in Turkey and people immediately involved in this campaign, to Nicholas de Jongh of the *Guardian* and Col. James Allason, MP., for their energetic support.

JANE DE MENDELSSOHN

The Release Report
Caroline Coon and Rufus Harris

Case 4

19.7.67
Mike, 19 years, unemployed
Simon, aged 17, unemployed
Steve, 25 years, unemployed
David, 22 years, unemployed
Peter, 20 years, unemployed
Jane, 29 years, journalist
Ann, 18 years, employed
Mike – Possession cannabis and LSD, allowing premises to be used
Simon – Possession cannabis and LSD
Steve – Possession 1 lb. cannabis, obstruction
David – Possession 1 lb. cannabis, obstruction
Peter – Possession tablets
Jane – Possession cannabis
Anne – Possession LSD
West London Court, September 1967
Inner London Session, 20–22 December 1967
Legal representation. Legal Aid.

Results

Mike and Simon, borstal. Anne two years' probation. Jane nine months, reduced to absolute discharge on appeal. Steve, David and Peter did not answer bail and probably left the country.

Previous convictions

Mike – previous larceny
Simon – previous larceny and drugs
Steve – none
David – none
Peter – none
Roger – previous drugs
Jane and Anne – none.

Remarks

The police broke down the door of the flat and found several people there. While the raid was in progress David and Steve came to the gate of the house. They were pushed down the steps by a policeman who informed them that because they were now on the premises they could be searched. Steve was later charged with being in possession of one pound of cannabis and David was later also charged with possession of the substance that had been found on Steve. Of the thirteen people taken to the police station only six were charged.

In court it was said that most of the LSD and cannabis in the flat belonged to an Indian who had been staying there. By the time the case came to Sessions this Indian had been arrested elsewhere and convicted on a drugs charge and had left the country. Mike and Simon pleaded not guilty. The premises were in their name but they claimed to have no knowledge of what was there. However, they were found guilty and sentenced to borstal, and the judge said that had they been old enough he would have sent them to prison for a very long time. While on bail, Mike had again been arrested for another drugs offence and been given a small fine. Steve, David and Peter did not surrender to bail and were thought to have left the country.

Ann pleaded guilty to the small quantity of LSD she had been charged with and called her father as a character witness.

When arrested she had only been in London two weeks, having come down to find a job, as her family were emigrating to Australia. However, because of the case they decided to remain in the country until it was over. Jane pleaded guilty to possessing a small quantity of cannabis. She was a journalist investigating the drug world for a newspaper and was able to call witnesses to substantiate this defence. Her Counsel, believing that he had an easy case, thought it unnecessary to call the witnesses, but Jane was sentenced to nine months' imprisonment. Up to this time she had used a lawyer that she had found for herself, but after her sentence she asked Release to help her find another solicitor to handle her appeal. The judge heard the appeal eight weeks later and taking into account that this was her first offence, and that the cannabis was purchased in the course of searching for material for a newspaper article, reduced the sentence, which he described as 'wholly wrong', to an absolute discharge.

Appendix

Tables A, B and C from *Cannabis: The Wootton Report*
General Conclusion and Recommendations (see pages 325–45)

Table A   Penalties Inflicted under the Drugs (Prevention of Misuse) Act 1964

	Discharge		Recognizances	Hospital Order	Fit Person Order	Detention Centre	Borstal or Approved School	Probation Orders			Fines		
	Absolute	Con-ditional						Months 12 or less	13–24	25–36	Under £10	£10-£25	£26-£50
1965[1]	10	131	1	8	1	48	29	67	105	26	119	255	54
									198			439	
1966	69	129	11	25	1	48	54	59	131	36	107	268	73
									226			474	

£51-£100	£101-£200	£201-£500	£501-£1000	Prison Sentences						Total Penalties	Total Persons Convicted
				Under 3 Mths	3–6 Mths	7–12 Mths	13 Mths -2 yrs.	Over 2–5 yrs.	Over 5 yrs.		
5	6	–	–	46	94	3	9	–	–	1017	958[2]
				152							
17	7	2	–	49	217	11	16	–	–	1330	1216[2]
				293							

Table A   Part Two
Penalties Inflicted under the Dangerous Drugs Act 1965 (Cannabis Only)

	Discharge		Recognizances	Hospital Order	Fit Person Order	Detention Centre	Borstal or Approved School	Probation Orders					
	Absolute	Con-ditiona						Months 12 or less	13–24	25–36	Under £10	£10–£25	£26–£50
1964[3]	5	34	–	7	–	15	4	13	43	10	26	124	62
									66				
1965[3]	3	41	2	3	–	19	9	21	58	13	37	198	69
									92				
1966[3]	12	99	–	2	1	42	35	31	108	32	85	300	166
									171				

NOTES:
1 The Drugs (Prevention of Misuse) Act came into effect on 31 October 1964 and the few prosecutions between then and 31 December 1964 have for convenience been included in the figures for 1965.
2 The discrepancy between total penalties and total persons convicted arises because where a person was convicted on more than one charge each fine and/or prison sentence inflicted is presented. Where concurrent prison sentences were inflicted, the highest sentence only is presented, but all consecutive prison sentences are included.
3 The numbers of persons convicted under the Dangerous Drugs Act for the three years were as follows: (see table at foot of opposite page)

Fines				Prison Sentences						Total Penalties	Total Persons Convicted
£51-£100	£101-£200	£201-£500	£501-£1000	Under 3 Mths	3–6 Mths	7–12 Mths	13 Mths -2 yrs.	Over 2–5 yrs.	Over 5 yrs.		
15	6	3	–	44	147	51	20	18	1	648	532[2]
\{ 236 \}				\{ 281 \}							
36	4	3	–	50	125	33	6	14	–	744	620[2]
\{ 347 \}				\{ 228 \}							
46	10	5	1	41	156	59	13	17	–	1261	1109[2]
\{ 613 \}				\{ 286 \}							

Year	Cannabis	Opium	Manufactured drugs	Total
1964	532	14	78	624
1965	620	13	111	744
1966	1109	36	208	1353

Table B   Analysis of Proceedings by Category of Offence 1967

	Unlawful Possession			Premises Offences			Unlawful Import			Unlawful Supply			Unlawful Procuring		
	a	b	c	a	b	c	a	b	c	a	b	c	a	b	c
No. of charges brought*	2507	456	2170	139	6	2	38	9	4	30	33	1	4	22	–
Charge withdrawn or dismissed	312	45	176	20	1	1	1	–	–	4	1	–			
Hospital or Guardianship order	2	–	2												
No. of convictions	2193	411	1992	119	5	1	37	9	4	26	32	1	4	22	–
Absolute discharge	11	4	17							1	–	–			
Recognizances	1	2	2												
Conditional discharge	169	46	211	11	–	–	1	–	–	1	–	–	–	2	–
Hospital Order (S.60., Mental Health Act, 1959)	6	1	1												
Probation Order	309	109	395	9	–	–				2	10	–	3	10	–
Fit Person Order	–	–	1												
Fine	1114	89	801	66	2	–	15	4	1	12	7	1	–	2	–
Attendance Centre	1	6	1												
Remand Home	–	–	–												
Detention Centre	39	16	97							3	1	–			
Approved School	6	–	8												
Police Cells	1	–	–												
Imprisonment w/o fine	465	102	301	28	3	1	16	3	2	6	8	–	1	5	–
Borstal	33	21	76	3	–	–				–	3	–	–	2	–
Otherwise dealt with	38	15	81	2	–	–	5	2	1	1	3	–	–	1	–

Register and Receptacles			Cannabis Cultivation			Larceny			Other drug Offences			Offences under other statutes			Total		
a	b	c	a	b	c	a	b	c	a	b	c	a	b	c	a	b	c
–	12	–	3	–	–	–	110	381	12	2	–	1	30	119	2734	680	2677
						–	2	6	2	–	–	–	–	6	339	49	189
															2	–	2
–	12	–	3	–	–	–	108	375	10	2	–	1	30	113	2393	631	2486
															12	4	17
															1	2	2
–	2	–	1	–	–	–	1	14				–	4	12	183	55	237
						–	–	1				–	–	1	6	1	3
						–	5	45	–	1	–	–	6	35	323	141	475
															–	–	1
–	10	–	2	–	–	–	21	114	8	–	–	–	3	24	1217	138	941
						–	2	3							1	8	4
															–	–	–
						–	8	34				–	2	–	42	27	131
						–	3	1							6	3	9
															1	–	–
						–	29	57	1	–	–	–	8	20	517	158	381
						–	15	35	–	1	–	–	–	6	36	42	117
						–	24	71	1	–	–	1	7	15	48	52	168

Table B Continued

	Unlawful Possession			Premises Offences			Unlawful Import			Unlawful Supply			Unlaw Procu
	a	b	c	a	b	c	a	b	c	a	b	c	a
Fines: (£)													
minimum imposed	1		1	10	4	–	3		25	5		50	–
maximum imposed	325		200	350		–	100		25	50		50	–
total imposed	40166	3472	22925	4610	29		419	75	25	230	140	50	–
Imprisonment:													
shortest sentence	1 d.		1 d.	2 m.	2 m.		6 m.		6 m.	6 m.	28 d.	–	9 m
longest sentence	7 y.		2 y.	3 y.	2 m.		4 y.	9 y.	6 m.	5 y.		–	9 m.

a – Cannabis
b – Drugs, other than Cannabis, controlled under the Dangerous Drugs Act 1965
c – Drugs controlled under the Drugs (Prevention of Misuse) Act 1964
d – Days   m – Months   y – Years
*Total no. of persons prosecuted under the Dangerous Drugs Act 1965 or the Drugs (Prevention of Misuse) Act 1964   a – 2639   b – 521   c – 2351

al g	Register and Receptacles			Cannabis Cultivation			Larceny			Other drug Offences		Offences under other statutes			Total		
	a	b	c	a	b	c	a	b	c	a	b	a	b	c	a	b	c
	–	7	–	10	–	–	–	5	2	10	–	–	10	4			
	–	25	–	25	–	–	–	50	100	100	–	–	75	50			
	–	124	–	35	–	–	–	605	2990	200	–		100	435	45660	50405	26425
							–	3 m.	2 m.	3 m.	–	–	3 m.	3 m.			
							–	5 y.	4½ y.	3 m.	–	–	18 m.	1 y.			

Table C   Analysis of Cannabis Prosecutions and Disposals Related to Age Groups and Weights of the Drug 1967

Up to 30 gm.

		Age Groups						
		15–20			21–25			
	Sex	Fine £50+	Imprison-ment	Other	Fine £50+	Imprison-ment	Other	Fin £50
No previous convictions	M	112	24	501	116	90	278	89
	F	11	1	91	11	4	61	3
Previous Offenders – Drugs offences only	M	1	1	13	2	7	8	1
	F	–	–	2	1	2	3	–
Previous Offender – Non-drug offences only	M	21	10	110	20	18	62	15
	F	–	–	7	3	–	2	2
Previous Offender – Drug and non-drug	M	3	2	28	5	12	23	3
	F	–	–	–	1	1	–	–
Total	M	137	37	652	143	127	371	108
	F	11	1	100	16	7	66	5

31 gm. up to 1 kg.

		15–20			21–25			
No previous convictions	M	2	1	27	7	23	14	7
	F	–	–	12	–	1	6	3
Previous Offender – Drugs offences only	M	–	–	–	–	–	–	–
	F	–	–	–	–	1	–	–
Previous Offender – Non-drug offences only	M	2	–	5	–	4	4	3
	F	–	–	1	–	–	3	–
Previous Offender – Drug and non-drug	M	1	–	1	–	1	2	1
	F	–	–	–	–	–	–	1
Total	M	5	1	33	7	28	20	13
	F	–	–	13	–	2	9	4

26–35		Over 35			No age			Total		
Imprisonment	Other	Fine £50+	Imprisonment	Other	Fine £50+	Imprisonment	Other	Fine £50+	Imprisonment	Other
66	135	42	44	79	10	5	43	369	229	1036
2	20	3	1	5	–	–	10	28	8	187
7	8	2	2	4	–	–	–	6	17	33
–	–	–	–	1	–	–	–	1	2	6
27	27	7	11	16	3	1	1	66	67	216
3	5	–	–	–	–	–	–	5	3	14
15	7	1	15	6	–	–	–	12	44	64
1	2	–	1	–	–	–	–	1	3	2
115	177	52	72	105	13	6	44	453	357	1349
6	27	3	2	6	–	–	10	35	16	209
22	9	9	24	10	1	1	–	26	71	60
2	6	–	1	2	–	1	–	3	5	26
4	1	1	–	–	–	–	–	1	4	1
–	–	–	–	–	–	–	–	–	1	–
4	4	2	2	3	–	–	–	9	10	16
–	3	–	–	–	–	–	–	–	–	7
7	–	3	3	–	–	–	–	5	11	3
–	1	–	2	–	–	–	–	1	2	1
37	14	15	29	13	1	1	–	41	96	80
2	10	–	3	2	–	1	–	4	8	34

Table C Continued

Over 1 kg.

| | | Age Groups | | | | | | | |
| | | 15–20 | | | 21–25 | | | | |
	Sex	Fine £50+	Imprison-ment	Other	Fine £50+	Imprison-ment	Other	Fine £50	
No previous convictions	M	–	–	–	–	3	1	–	
	F	–	–	–	–	1	–	–	
Previous Offender – Drugs offences only	M	–	–	–	–	–	–	–	
	F	–	–	–	–	–	–	–	
Previous Offender – Non-drug offences only	M	–	–	–	–	–	–	–	
	F	–	–	–	–	–	–	–	
Previous Offender – Drug and Non-drug	M	–	–	–	–	–	–	–	
	F	–	–	–	–	–	–	–	
Total	M	–	–	–	–	3	1	–	
	F	–	–	–	–	1	–	–	
Grand Total	M	142	38	685	150	158	392	121	
	F	11	1	113	16	10	75	9	

NOTE: These figures refer to the number of charges for cannabis offences and not to the number of persons concerned. Of these charges 339 were dismissed or withdrawn, and two were dealt with by Hospital or Guardianship Order, without proceeding to conviction. The table does not include three charges brought in respect of offences relating to the cannabis plant.

26–35		Over 35			No age			Total		
Imprisonment	Other	Fine £50+	Imprisonment	Other	Fine £50+	Imprisonment	Other	Fine £50+	Imprisonment	Other
15	1	1	10	–	–	2	2	1	30	4
1	–	–	–	–	–	–	–	–	2	–
–	1	–	3	–	–	–	–	–	3	1
–	–	–	–	2	–	–	–	–	–	2
3	1	–	1	–	–	–	–	–	4	1
1	–	–	–	–	–	–	–	–	1	–
–	–	–	–	–	–	–	–	–	–	–
–	–	–	–	–	–	–	–	–	–	–
18	3	1	14	–	–	2	2	1	37	6
2	–	–	–	2	–	–	–	–	3	2
70	194	68	115	118	14	9	46	495	490	1435
10	37	3	5	10	–	1	10	39	27	245

Acknowledgements and Sources

Acknowledgements and Sources

The editors wish to thank the following publishers, authors, and translators for their kind permission to quote from their works: Messrs Sidgwick & Jackson for A. L. Basham's 'The Wonder that Was India' from *The Wonder that Was India*, 1961; Pascal Brotteaux for 'The Ancient Greeks' from *Hachich, Herbe de Folie et de Rêve*, Editions Vega, 1934; Messrs Routledge & Kegan Paul Ltd for Mircea Eliade's 'Ancient Scythia and Iran' from *Shamanism: Archaic Techniques of Ecstasy*, 1964; Henry Miller's 'Utopian Speculations' from Norman O. Brown's *Life Against Death*, 1956; 'The Tale of Two Hashish Eaters' from *The Thousand Nights and One Night*, translated from the literal translation of Dr J. C. Mardrus and collated by E. Powys Mathers, 1937; 'Flying Saucers: A Modern Myth' from C. G. Jung's *Flying Saucers: A Modern Myth*, translated by R. F. C. Hull, 1959; *Ciba Symposia* for W. Reininger's 'Remnants from Prehistoric Times', 'Congo Cult' and 'Two Celebrated Hashish Eaters', Victor Robinson's 'Concerning Cannabis Indica', all of which appeared in vol. 8, nos. 5/6, 946; Sara Benetowa for 'Tracing One Word through Different Languages' from *Le Chanvre dans les Croyances et les Coutumes Populaires*, Warsaw Institute of Anthropological Sciences, 1936; Melvin Clay for 'Fragments from a Search'; Messrs MacMillan & Co. for 'The Assassins' from Philip K. Hitti's *History of the Arabs*, 1937; Taner Baybars for his version of 'The Hodja' from *Stories of the Hodja, fourteen century*; Penguin Books for 'The Herb Pantagruelion' from J. M. Cohen's translation of *The Histories of Gargantua and Pantagruel* by François Rabelais, 1955, and 'Yoga' from Ernest Wood's *Yoga*, 1959; Houghton Mifflin Co. for 'Diary Notes' from *The Diaries of George Washington*, 1925; Propyläen Verlag for 'Nietzsche's Letter to Peter Gast' from Friedrich Würzbach's *Nietzsche, Sein Leben in Selbstzeugnissen, Briefen und Berichten*, 1942; University of Nebraska Press for 'Black Elk Speaks of his Great Vision' from John Neihardt's *Black Elk Speaks*, 1932; Suhrkamp Verlag for 'Steppenwolf' from

Hermann Hesse's *Steppenwolf*, 1927; William Heinemann Ltd for 'Diego Rivera' from Errol Flynn's *My Wicked, Wicked Ways*, 1961; Mrs Laura Huxley for the late Aldous Huxley's 'Culture and the Individual'; Messrs Chatto & Windus for 'Island' from Aldous Huxley's *Island*, 1962; The Bodley Head for 'Light through Darkness' from their translation of Henri Michaux's *Connaissance par les Gouffres* by Haakon Chevalier, 1961; Messrs Calder & Boyars for 'Marijuana and Sex' from Alexander Trocchi's *Cain's Book*, 1961; Paul Bowles for 'Kif – Prologue and Compendium of Terms' and 'He of the Assembly' from *A Hundred Camels in the Courtyard*, City Lights, 1962; Ira Cohen for Mohammed Ben Abdullah Yussufi's 'The Three Alis'; Allen Ginsberg for 'Night at the Burning Ghat' from *Journals, Krittivas*, 1962; Simon Vinkenoog for 'High Season' from *Hoogseizoen*, De Bezige Bij, 1962; Oxford University Press for an extract from Gimlette & Thomson's *Dictionary of Malayan Medicine*, 1939; Messrs E. S. Livingstone Ltd for J. M. Watt's and M. G. Breyer-Brandwijk's *Medicinal and Poisonous Plants of Southern and Eastern Africa*, 1962; Ballière (Paris) for Pic & Bonnamour's 'Médicaments Végétaux' from *Bibliothèque de Thérapeutique*, 1932; Dr Boericke for *Materia Medica*, 1928; Roger Adams for 'Marihuana', Harvey Lecture Series, 1942; Louis S. Goldman & Alfred Gilman for *The Pharmacological Basis of Therapeutics*, 1955; Robert S. De Ropp for *Drugs and the Mind*, St Martin's Press, 1957; R. Polderman for *The Medical Use of Cannabis Sativa;* Pantheon Books Inc. for Esther Harding's 'The Psychological Significance of the Soma Ritual' from *Women's Mysteries Ancient and Modern*; University of Oklahoma Press for Stanley Vestal's 'Sitting Bull's Vision of Victory' from *Sitting Bull*, 1932; S. M. Groff for 'Marihuana and the "O" Effect'; William H. McGlothlin for 'Cannabis Intoxication and its Similarity to Peyote and LSD' from *Hallucinogenic Drugs: A Perspective with Special Reference to Peyote and Cannabis*, EFPC, 1964; R. D. Laing and A. Esterson for 'Two Letters', 1964; Dr Julian Reeves for *Recent Trends in Cannabis Research*; Information Canada for the extract from the *Interim Report of the Commission of Inquiry into the Non-Medical Use of Drugs* reproduced by permission of Information Canada; R. C. Zaehner for *Mysticism, Sacred and Profane*, 1957; Alan Watts for 'A Psychedelic Experience: Fact or Fantasy', 1964; Sir Julian Huxley for 'Psychometabolism' from *The Psychedelic Reader*, University Books, 1965; Porter Sargent Inc. for Oliver L. Reiser's

The Integration of Human Knowledge, 1958, and Mr Reiser for 'The Problem of Consciousness' which is taken from his forthcoming *The Universe: its Theory*; Royal Van Gorcum for 'Ecstasy' from Julius de Boer's *A System of Characterology,* 1965; William Burroughs for 'Cannabis and Opiates' from *Points of Distinction between Sedative and Consciousness-expanding Drugs, Evergreen Review,* December 1964; *The Harvard Review* for Timothy Leary's and Richard Alpert's 'The Politics of Consciousness Expansion', Summer 1963; Jonathan Cape Ltd for *The Process* by Brion Gysin; Carlos Castenada, *The Teachings of Don Juan*: originally published by the University of California Press; reprinted by permission of The Regents of the University of California; Messrs W. H. Allen Ltd for Lawrence Lipton's *The Holy Barbarians,* 1960; Michael Pickering for 'Memoirs of a Kif Smoker', June 1964; the *Colorado Daily News* for 'The Law in Colorado', 21 April, 1964; Henry Smith Williams for 'Abuse of American Law', 1938; Judge Murtagh for 'Two Statements'; *New York Daily News* for 'The Case of Timothy Leary', 11 March 1966; Akin Davies for 'Nigeria Whispers'; Neal Phillips for 'Notes from Tartaros'; Stephen Abrams for 'The Oxford Scene'; the *Sunday Times* for 'Marihuana and Alcohol' by Anthony Storr; extract from *Cannabis – Report by the Advisory Committee on Drug Dependence* reproduced by permission of Her Majesty's Stationery Office; *Marihuana: Is It Time for a Change in Our Laws? Newsweek* 7 September 1970, reprinted by permission of Newsweek Inc.; *The Gentle Moves to Legal Pot* by Peter Pringle, reproduced by permission of the author and the *Sunday Times*; *International Times* for letter and *Hell among the Turkish Delights; Case 4* reproduced from *The Release Report on Drug Offenders and the Law* by. Caroline Coon and Rufus Harris.

Other Sources: 'Sanskrit Sources' is taken from *The Materia Medica of the Hindus* by Uday Chand Dutt and George King, published by Thacker, Spink & Co., 1877; 'American Indians in 1626' from Jean Leander's *Traité du Tabac ou Panacée Universelle,* 1626; 'Concerning Hashish' from Charles Baudelaire's *Du Vin et du Hashish,* 1851; Gérard de Nerval's 'Supernaturalist' is quoted in André Breton's *Surrealist Manifesto*; 'Morning of Drunkenness' appeared as 'Matinée d'Ivresse' in Rimbaud's *Illuminations,* and 'Vowels' is translated from 'Voyelles', 1886; E. Whineray's 'The Herb Dangerous' appeared in *The Herb Dan-*

gerous: A Pharmaceutical Study of Cannabis Sativa, The Equinox, 1909; E. J. Waring's *Pharmacopoeia of India*, 1868, was published by The India Office, London; 'Varieties of Consciousness' is taken from William James's *Varities of Religious Experience*, Longmans, Green & Co., 1916.

More About Penguins

Penguinews, which appears every month, contains details of all the new books issued by Penguins as they are published. From time to time it is supplemented by *Penguins in Print*, which is a complete list of all available books published by Penguins. (There are well over three thousand of these.)

A specimen copy of *Penguinews* will be sent to you free on request, and you can become a subscriber for the price of the postage. For a year's issues (including the complete lists) please send 30p if you live in the United Kingdom, or 60p if you live elsewhere. Just write to Dept EP, Penguin Books Ltd, Harmondsworth, Middlesex, enclosing a cheque or postal order, and your name will be added to the mailing list.

Note: *Penguinews* and *Penguins in Print* are not available in the U.S.A. or Canada

Drugs

Medical, Psychological, and Social Facts

Peter Laurie

Second Edition

What are the known facts about the 'dangerous' drugs?
What actual harm, mental or physical, do they cause?
Which of them are addictive, and how many addicts are
there?

Peter Laurie has talked with doctors, policemen, addicts,
and others intimately involved with this problem. He has
tried some of the drugs for himself and closely studied the
medical literature (including little-known reports of American
research). The result of his inquiries into the
pharmacological uses and social effects of drugs today
appears in this book.

Originally published as a Penguin Special which went
through five printings, *Drugs* was the first objective study to
offer all the major medical, psychological and social facts
about the subject to a public which is too often fed with
alarmist and sensational reports. For this second edition in
Pelicans Peter Laurie has added fresh information and
statistics concerning English users of drugs and noted
changes in the law.

A Pelican Book

Also available
Scotland Yard
Beneath the City Streets

Writers at Work

The *Paris Review* Interviews

Selected by Kay Dick

For many years the *Paris Review* interviews have been justly
famous for giving deeper insight and understanding of the
creative process. In this selection from the interviews, fifteen
writers discuss what they think of their own, and other
people's work, their lives and the problems of writing in
the contemporary world.

Not for sale in the U.S.A. and Canada

On the Road

Jack Kerouac

And there was Dean in Denver. In San Francisco and New York. And Mexico. Riding the rails, hitching lifts, driving borrowed cars at a crazy hundred miles an hour. An unholy innocent abroad. Wild parties, girls, drink, drugs. Uncertainty, loneliness and dreams synthesized by bop. The beats roam America with irrepressible abandon. The narrator, Sal Paradise. His fabulous hero, Dean Moriarty. Problems, wives, problems, stars, longings, sadness and love . . .

'The beat generation', the post-war 'counter-culture' and the 'youth rebellion' begins with Jack Kerouac ('a strange, solitary, Catholic mystic') who was its chronicler – *On The Road* is its classic expression, its required text.

Not for sale in the U.S.A. and Canada

The Doors of Perception
and
Heaven and Hell

Aldous Huxley

When one of this century's finest minds underwent the mescalin experience . . .

Aldous Huxley was one of the first Western writers to experiment with consciousness-expanding drugs. In these two short essays he describes the mescalin-inspired visionary landscapes of the mind, which impressed themselves upon him with the force of revealed truth – visions of heavenly delights which could, in the wrong hands, be transformed into a schizophrenic hell.

Not for sale in the U.S.A.